Occupational and Environmental Neurology

Occupational and Environmental Neurology

Neil L. Rosenberg, M.D.

Associate Clinical Professor of Clinical Pharmacology and Medical
Toxicology, University of Colorado School of Medicine, Denver, Colorado;
Medical Director, Center for Occupational Neurology and
Neurotoxicology, Colorado Neurological Institute, Englewood, Colorado

With 12 contributing authors

Foreword by
Herbert H. Schaumburg, M.D.
Professor and Chairman, Unified Departments of Neurology,
Albert Einstein College of Medicine and Montefiore Medical Center,
Bronx, New York

Butterworth–Heinemann
Boston   Oxford   Melbourne   Singapore   Toronto   Munich   New Delhi   Tokyo

Every effort has been made to ensure that the drug dosage schedules within this text are accurate and conform to standards
accepted at time of publication. However, as treatment recommendations vary in the light of continuing research and clinical
experience, the reader is advised to verify drug dosage schedules
herein with information found on product information sheets.
This is especially true in cases of new or infrequently used drugs.

 Recognizing the importance of preserving what has been written, Butterworth-Heinemann prints its books on acid-free paper.

Library of Congress Cataloging-in-Publication Data

Rosenberg, Neil L.
    Occupational and environmental neurology / Neil L. Rosenberg;
  with 12 contributing authors; foreword by Herbert H. Schaumburg.
       p.   cm.
    Includes bibliographical references and index.
    ISBN 0-7506-9515-3 (alk. paper)
    1. Nervous system--Diseases.   2. Occupational diseases.
  3. Environmentally induced diseases.   4. Neurotoxicology.
  I. Title.
    [DNLM: 1. Nervous System Diseases. 2. Occupational Diseases.   WL
  140 R813o 1995]
  RC346.R66 1995
  616.8--dc20
  DNLM/DLC
  for Library of Congress   95-10373
                                              CIP

British Library Cataloguing-in-Publication Data

A catalogue record for this book is available from the British Library.

The publisher offers discounts on bulk orders of this book.
For information, please write:

Manager of Special Sales
Butterworth–Heinemann
313 Washington Street
Newton, MA 02158-1626

10 9 8 7 6 5 4 3 2 1

Printed in the United States of America

Contents

Contributing Authors

James W. Albers, M.D., Ph.D.
Professor of Neurology, University of Michigan Medical Center,
Ann Arbor, Michigan

Alan R. Berger, M.D.
Associate Professor of Neurology, Albert Einstein College of Medicine;
Director of Clinical Electromyography Laboratory and Attending
Neurologist, Montefiore Medical Center, Bronx, New York

Mark B. Bromberg, M.D., Ph.D.
Assistant Professor of Neurology, University of Michigan Medical Center,
Ann Arbor, Michigan

Julie H. Carter, R.N., M.N., A.N.P.
Assistant Professor of Neurology, School of Medicine and School of
Nursing, Oregon Health Sciences University; Academic Medical Staff,
Department of Neurology, University Hospital, Oregon Health Sciences
University, Portland, Oregon

Christopher M. Filley, M.D.
Associate Professor of Neurology and Psychiatry, University of Colorado
School of Medicine; Attending Physician, Department of Neurology,
University Hospital, Denver

Steven J. Gulevich, M.D.
Staff Neurologist and Associate Director of Center for Neurotoxicology,
Colorado Neurological Institute, Englewood, Colorado

John P. Hammerstad, M.D.
Professor of Neurology, School of Medicine, Oregon Health Sciences
University; Active Medical Staff, Department of Neurology, University
Hospital, Oregon Health Sciences University, Portland, Oregon

Steven Herskovitz, M.D.
Assistant Professor of Neurology, Albert Einstein College of Medicine;
Attending Neurologist, Montefiore Medical Center, Bronx, New York

James P. Kelly, M.A., M.D.
Assistant Professor of Rehabilitation Medicine and Neurology,
Northwestern University Medical School; Director, Brain Injury Program,
Rehabilitation Institute of Chicago, Chicago, Illinois

Richard J. Lederman, M.D., Ph.D.
Neurologist, Department of Neurology, Cleveland Clinic Foundation,
Cleveland, Ohio

Edward Lewin, M.D.
Professor of Neurology, University of Colorado Health Sciences Center;
Chief, Neurology Service, Veterans Administration Medical Center,
Denver, Colorado

Brent Lovejoy, D.O.
Staff Physician, Department of Occupational Medicine, Swedish Medical
Center, Englewood, Colorado

Neil L. Rosenberg, M.D.
Associate Clinical Professor of Clinical Pharmacology and Medical
Toxicology, University of Colorado School of Medicine, Denver; Medical
Director, Center for Occupational Neurology and Neurotoxicology,
Colorado Neurological Institute, Englewood, Colorado

Herbert H. Schaumburg, M.D.
Professor and Chairman, Unified Departments of Neurology, Albert
Einstein College of Medicine and Montefiore Medical Center, Bronx,
New York

Foreword

The field of occupational and environmental medicine is growing rapidly and evolving steadily. There are societies and professional associations devoted to this specialty, and several multiauthored textbooks have been published. Nevertheless, there are only a handful of academic departments or divisions in most North American medical schools and few formal courses devoted to this discipline.

Neurology's place in occupational medicine has either been negligible or, at best, fragmented. It is my experience that most neurologists lack sufficient exposure during their training to perform even a rudimentary occupational evaluation. Occupational physicians often must fend for themselves in sorting out whether neurologic dysfunction appearing in the worker represents a naturally occuring condition or is secondary to local exogenous factors. Rosenberg's *Occupational and Environmental Neurology* should help fill this gap in the occupational physician's clinical armamentarium.

This book has several advantages over the conventional "neurologic diseases" section of most texts in occupational medicine. First, the chapters are written by experienced academic clinical neurologists with experience in occupational issues. Second, it is unusually comprehensive, yet it adheres to issues relevant to occupational medicine (e.g., it doesn't have a section on brain tumors). Finally, 10 of the 13 chapters are authored or coauthored by Rosenberg, ensuring uniformity of style and minimal overlap. This text should become a standard in the field.

HERBERT H. SCHAUMBURG, M.D.

Preface

The field of occupational medicine has grown and developed over the past several decades, beginning with a focus on toxic exposures but gradually encompassing all issues relevant to the workplace. This has also had an effect on the practice of neurology in that many disorders of the workplace have their primary effect on the nervous system. The occupational medicine physician, with limited training in neurology, has had to rely on neurologic consultants who are often either ill-equipped or not interested in dealing with problems of the workplace, equating all such experiences with the distasteful task of having to deal with "worker's comp." Most neurologists, interested in practicing "real neurology," have not valued issues in occupational medicine as worthy of much time, until recent years.

This book has been written at the urging and with the encouragement of Herbert H. Schaumburg, M.D., Chair of the Department of Neurology at Albert Einstein College of Medicine, and leader in the field of neurotoxicology. Dr. Schaumburg has often stated that neurologists need to realize that occupational neurology is much more than dealing with classic, textbook descriptions of neurotoxic injuries. These types of problems are rarely, if ever, seen in this country or other industrialized nations. With that encouragement, much of the conceptualization for this book began in a course titled "Occupational Neurology and Neurotoxicology" at the annual meeting of the American Academy of Neurology. I have been surprised by how many neurologists have been dealing with occupational issues in their practices, by their great interest in the field, and by how many sought answers to their questions that were not addressed in other textbooks. This book expands on much of what is taught in that course, has been modified by the suggestions and questions of the participants, and I hope answers many of the questions that could only be superficially addressed in that course.

   This book also addresses many of the questions I receive from physicians working primarily in the occupational medicine arena, who are either uncomfortable in dealing with primary neurologic issues or who need to get more specific information from their neurology consultants. One of the goals of *Occupational and Environmental Neurology* is to address many of the neurologic questions that occupational medicine physicians and other occupational health professionals have and how to approach a neurologically injured worker in a logical fashion—and without panic. There is a considerable amount of anxiety in non-neurologic occupational health care providers in dealing with workers with primarily neurologic symptomatology—how to proceed (or if to proceed) with a neurologic work-up and what to do with results of tests that unexpectedly may be positive and need to be explained.

   I have intended both the style and content of this book to be readable. *Occupational and Environmental Neurology* is not intended to be encyclopedic in nature. It would be inappropriate if it attempted to be comprehensive, since so many other areas that impact occupational neurology, such as ergonomics, industrial hygiene, and epidemiology, among others, are covered in texts covering these fields in greater detail than could be given justice in this book. Each chapter is capable of standing alone, although there is still some unavoidable overlap. The overlap is important because it often represents critical areas of understanding.

   The first part of the book focuses on general aspects of occupational neurology, including clinical evaluation and performing a neurologic impairment rating. The remaining chapters cover many "typical" neurologic topics such as toxic neuropathies, encephalopathies, and movement disorders, but also many specific to certain occupations (e.g., performing artists), toxins (e.g., solvents), mechanisms of injury (e.g., cumulative trauma), and areas of specific discipline (e.g., neuroepidemiology). Many of the chapters address controversial areas of occupational neurology, and in some cases a strong position is taken by the author, rather than merely regurgitating what has been published in the literature. I thought that in certain situations, such as in dealing with the psycho-organic syndrome related to solvents or with cumulative trauma disorders, this approach was needed to bring up issues of concern, particularly to those readers who do not deal with these issues on a regular basis.

   I express my gratitude to many individuals, without whom this book would not have been possible. First, my thanks to all the contributors, who tolerated my many shortcomings as an editor, the delays in the realization of publication, and my incessant demands to keep revising and updating their chapters. Many thanks to everyone at Buttterworth-Heinemann, particularly Susan Pioli and Cindy Carlson, whose gentle urgings and suggestions helped tremendously in the final realization of the manuscript. I cannot thank enough Herbert Schaumburg, M.D., not only for his urging in my attempting this book but also for his support of my career and his friendship, which has been greater than that of any other individual. And finally, to my wife, Laura Watt, without whose support and toleration of my moodiness during the long course of the writing of this book, I would not have been up to the task.

NEIL L. ROSENBERG, M.D.

Occupational and Environmental Neurology

CHAPTER 1

Occupational Neurology: An Overview

Neil L. Rosenberg, M.D.

Occupational medicine is an evolving but clearly defined specialty of medicine concerning the health of workers and the prevention of workplace-associated disorders. Many excellent texts have been written over the years concerned with the medicine and science of occupational health.[1,2] However, the practice of occupational medicine and occupational health extends far beyond the science and includes the direct application of the knowledge of biology, medicine, industrial hygiene, epidemiology, engineering, education, economics, politics, and law. These and other disciplines combine to protect workers from diseases of the workplace; however, the pathology, physiology, chemistry, physics, and toxicology that help to form the scientific basis for occupational medicine are not unique to this specialty.

Neurology's place in occupational medicine has remained obscure. Most textbooks of occupational medicine fail to include a chapter on neurologic diseases, and those that do vary from discussing only neurotoxic disorders[3,4] to including general discussions of all major categories of neurological diseases.[5] This wide range of variability of depth and breadth of discussion of neurologic disorders in occupational medicine is confusing not only for neurologists, but for specialists in occupational medicine as well. Not a single neurology textbook has a chapter on occupational issues or disorders, which are instead discussed in chapters on specific diseases. Since most neurology textbooks are broken into chapters by either major disease category (e.g., infectious, tumors, cerebrovascular) or by symptom (e.g., pain, coma, dementia), issues of occupational neurology are dispersed throughout the text.

Despite the apparent lack of interest in defining a field of occupational neurology as a specialty area, a study of practice patterns by

TABLE 1.1
Occupation of Patients Seen in Neurologic Practices

Occupation	Percentage
Professional/technical	15.7
Office/clerical	12.5
Service worker	12.3
Skilled trade/craftsman	8.4
Managerial/administrative	6.3
Sales	5.7
Unskilled laborer	4.6
Manufacturing/processing	2.8
Vehicle operator	2.7
Agricultural worker	1.8
Marginally or unemployed, student, retired, homemaker	27.2

Colorado neurologists[6] emphasizes the importance of occupational issues to practicing neurologists. Of the private sector neurologists in this study, 22% identified occupational neurology as a clinical area that should receive more emphasis in neurology residency programs. In addition, 61% felt that back and neck disorders, neurologic problems of major importance as occupational issues, also needed to receive more emphasis in residency training. In other words, neurologists in practice deal with patients whose neurologic problem, or reason for referral for neurologic consultation, is primarily related to one or several occupational health concerns.

Neurologists see patients from all different forms of employment[7] and need to understand these various occupations, not only how the workplace may be causing the patient's problem but also how the patient's neurologic condition will impact job performance and/or that individual's ability to successfully return to work or function at his or her job. Table 1.1 shows the wide range of occupations of patients seen by neurologists in a study of outpatient neurologic practices.[7] Almost three-fourths of patients seen by neurologists in this study were gainfully employed, with one-fourth not considered part of the active workforce (those marginally employed or unemployed, retired, students, and homemakers).

Occupational neurology therefore not only encompasses those neurologic disorders caused by the workplace environment (Table 1.2) but also includes the impact of any idiopathic neurologic disorder on an individual's performance in his or her occupation.

In 1983, the National Institute for Occupational Safety and Health (NIOSH) developed a suggested list of the ten leading work-related diseases and injuries.[8] Of the ten (Table 1.3), four are commonly referred for neurologic consultation or come under the primary care of a neurologist;

TABLE 1.2
Major Categories of Occupationally Related Neurologic Disorders

Neurologic Disorder *(Chapters for Detailed Discussion)*	*Causative Factors/Agents*
Encephalopathy (2–5, 10)	Toxins, head trauma
Seizures (2, 6)	Toxins, trauma
Sleep disorders (6)	Shift work
Movement disorder (2–4, 7, 12)	Toxins, head trauma, cumulative trauma
Sensorineural hearing loss	Noise induced
Myelopathy (2–4, 10)	Toxins, spinal trauma
Peripheral neuropathy (2–4, 8, 9)	Toxins, cumulative trauma, focal trauma
Musculoskeletal injuries (7, 9, 11, 12)	Trauma, cumulative trauma
Psychological disorders (2–5)	Toxins, occupational stress, psychological mechanisms

TABLE 1.3
The Ten Leading Work-Related Disorders

1. Occupational lung diseases
2. Musculoskeletal injuries*
3. Nonpulmonary occupational concerns
4. Traumatic amputations, fractures, eye loss, lacerations, deaths
5. Cardiovascular diseases
6. Reproductive disorders
7. Neurotoxic disorders*
8. Noise-induced hearing loss*
9. Dermatologic conditions
10. Psychological disorders*

*Those disorders frequently evaluated by a neurologist.

these include musculoskeletal injuries, neurotoxic disorders, noise-induced hearing loss, and psychological disorders. Other common occupational neurologic disorders not included on this list, such as occupational carpal tunnel syndrome, are also very common; however, since there are no published epidemiologic data on their prevalence, it is difficult to know where to rank such disorders. NIOSH developed the list using these criteria: the disease's or injury's frequency of occurrence, its severity in the individual case, and its amenability to prevention. One of the three purposes of the list was to encourage deliberation and debate among professionals about the major problems in this field of public health; therefore, there is a clear need to define a field of occupational neurology to

TABLE 1.4
Reportable Occupational Neurologic Diseases (as of September 1, 1988)

Neurologic Disorder	*States*
Neurotoxic diseases	
Lead	CA, DE, KS, KY, LA, MA, MI, MN, NH, NY, OK, PA, RI, SC, TX, WV
Other heavy metals	IA, KS, ME, MI, NJ, WI
Pesticides	AR, CA, FL, IA, KS, ME, MI, MO, NJ, OR, TX, VA, WI
Other*	KS, ME, MI, NJ, WI
Carpal tunnel syndrome	IA
Noise-induced hearing loss	IA, MI
"Any occupational disease"	AK, KS, MD, MI, NH, NM, VA, WV, WI

*Other potential neurotoxins listed: carbon monoxide, benzene, cyanide, halogenated hydrocarbons, hydrogen sulfide, manganese, methanol, carbon tetrachloride, organic solvents, carbon disulfide, chlorinated hydrocarbons.

educate professionals dealing with these problems and to promote research in areas of diagnosis, treatment, and prevention of these disorders, as well as to assist in setting national priorities for efforts to prevent occupational neurologic disorders.

Surveillance

Surveillance is the systematic study of a wide variety of diseases, both infectious and noninfectious in nature.[9] It involves the systematic collection, analysis, and dissemination of information on groups or populations and is of great importance in identification of occupational disorders.[9–16]

One of the contributing factors to our lack of understanding of occupational neurologic disorders is the lack of disease surveillance in most states.[10] Case reporting by health care providers to public health authorities is one way of identifying sources of exposure toward which control measures can be directed.[11] A recently compiled list of reportable occupational diseases and occupational disease-related conditions as of September 1, 1988, reveals that 32 states have reportable occupational diseases (Table 1.4). Of these 28 (87.5%) list disorders associated with neurologic dysfunction. However, 18 states list lead or pesticide poisoning, or both, as the only example of occupational neurologic disorders, while most of the remaining states list "any occupational disease" as being reportable. Only one state (Iowa) lists carpal tunnel syndrome, and two states (Iowa and Michigan) specifically list noise-related hearing loss as reportable occupational diseases.[10]

Ten states are currently working with NIOSH in a program designed to establish reporting mechanisms for six occupational disorders. These disorders were selected by NIOSH because they appear to be particularly amenable to physician reporting. They include carpal tunnel syndrome, lead poisoning, noise-induced hearing loss, occupational asthma, pesticide poisoning, and silicosis. Four of these six conditions clearly fall in the area of occupational neurology, with neurologists commonly involved in the diagnosis and management of carpal tunnel syndrome, noise-induced hearing loss, and lead and pesticide poisoning. However, neurologists may be unaware of job-related issues when seeing such patients and a potential occupational-related disease may go unrecognized and unreported.[12]

Traditionally, surveillance of occupational disorders has relied mainly on data sources, such as patient self-report of symptoms or death certificates. Few rely on physician diagnosis, which, when it is relied on, often does not depend on the physician's recognition of the condition as being occupationally related.

Biological Monitoring

Biological monitoring of exposure to industrial chemicals is essentially surveillance of the internal exposure of the organism to a chemical agent(s) by sampling of a body tissue or compartment.

When surveillance is based on laboratory tests, such as occurs when monitoring for hematologic disorders where a complete blood count (CBC) can be done or for lead poisoning where serum lead concentrations are monitored, the problem becomes the ability to distinguish between statistical and clinical abnormality in interpretation of these tests. Choice of laboratory studies for surveillance purposes (i.e., biological monitoring) differs substantially from those chosen for clinical testing in that the former involves both the evaluation of ill patients and the regular screening of presumably healthy individuals. Results of these studies are unlikely to explain the etiology of the illness. Laboratory tests chosen for a surveillance program are in general those for which any abnormality is a matter of concern due to the type of occupation. These tests are not intended for diagnostic purposes, although they may be useful to supplement normal diagnostic testing. In an appropriately designed biological monitoring program, the aim is to prevent overt disease by picking up subtle changes in laboratory tests. Therefore, a slightly abnormal finding should prompt a review by a physician.

The greatest advantage of biological monitoring is that a biological parameter of exposure is more directly related to adverse health effects than is any environmental measurement. Another advantage is that environmental (nonoccupational) exposure can also be measured. The

TABLE 1.5
Neurotoxic Agents and Biological Monitoring Parameters

Neurotoxic Agent	Monitored Material	Tissue/Body Compartment
Organic Solvents		
N-Hexane	2,5-Hexanedione	Urine
	2,5-Hexanol	Urine
	N-Hexane	Blood, expired air
Methyl-N-butyl ketone	2,5-Hexanedione	Urine
Toluene	Hippuric acid	Urine
	Toluene	Blood, expired air
Trichloroethylene	Trichloroethanol	Urine, plasma
	Trichloracetic acid	Urine, plasma
	Trichloroethylene	Blood, expired air
Carbon disulfide	Iodine-azide test	Urine
	2-Thiothiazolidine-4-carboxylic acid	Urine
Metals		
Lead	Lead	Blood
	Zinc-protoporphyrin	Blood
	Coproporphyrin	Urine
	Delta-aminolevulinic acid	Urine
Inorganic arsenic	Inorganic arsenic	Urine
	Monomethylarsenic acid	
	Cacodylic acid	
Inorganic mercury	Mercury	Blood, urine
Methyl mercury	Mercury	Blood
Manganese	Manganese	Blood, urine
Gases		
Carbon monoxide	Carbon monoxide	Blood, expired air
	Carboxyhemoglobin	Blood
Pesticides		
Organophosphates	Cholinesterase	Blood, plasma, red blood cells
	Alkylphosphates	Urine

major disadvantage of biological monitoring in regard to neurotoxic illness is that laboratory tests are limited, because they do not exist for the body burden of most neurotoxins. Therefore, biological monitoring does not exist for the majority of neurotoxins in the workplace. Table 1.5 lists the most common neurotoxic compounds for which biological monitoring tests exist. Details of the difficulties of recognition of occupational neurotoxic disorders are discussed in the chapters on toxins in the workplace.

Summary

The field of occupational neurology encompasses areas of occupational and environmental medicine and general neurology. A working knowledge of these fields is essential for both occupational and preventive medicine physicians and neurologists to be able to diagnose and treat individuals with work-related or work-impacting neurologic disorders. Unlike specialists in occupational medicine, neurologists will only rarely work with industry, labor groups, or government; however, all neurologists deal with work-related problems. It is therefore important for neurologists to understand some of the basic issues related to occupational medicine, just as it is essential for full-time occupational medicine physicians to have an understanding of the evaluation of a worker with neurologic symptoms. As surveillance of occupational neurologic disorders increases, knowledge of these areas will become vital in the recognition and prevention of work-related neurologic disorders.

References

1. Raffle PAB, Lee WR, McCallum RI, Murray R (eds). Hunter's Diseases of Occupations. Boston: Little, Brown, 1987.
2. Zenz C (ed). Occupational Medicine: Principles and Practical Applications. Chicago: Year Book, 1988.
3. Baker EL Jr. Neurological Disorders. In WN Rom (ed), Environmental and Occupational Medicine. Boston: Little, Brown, 1983;313–327.
4. Baker EL Jr. Neurologic and Behavioral Disorders. In BS Levy, DH Wegman (eds), Occupational Health: Recognizing and Preventing Work-Related Disease. Boston: Little, Brown, 1988;399–413.
5. Swerdlow M, Schaumburg HH. Neurologic Diseases Important in Occupational Medicine. In MH Alderman, MJ Hanley (eds), Clinical Medicine for the Occupational Physician. New York: Marcel Dekker, 1982; 477–505.
6. Franklin GM, Ringel SP, Nelson LM, DeLapp C. Neurology practice patterns in Colorado. Neurology 1987;37:287–289.
7. Ringel SP, Franklin GM, DeLapp C, Boyko EJ. A cross-sectional comparative study of outpatient neurologic practices in Colorado. Neurology 1988;38:1308–1314.
8. Centers for Disease Control. Leading work-related diseases and injuries—United States. MMWR 1983;32:24–26.
9. Langmuir AD. William Farr: Founder of modern concepts of surveillance. Int J Epidemiol 1976;5:13–18.
10. Freund E, Seligman PJ, Chorba TL, Safford SK, Drachman JG, Hull HF. Mandatory reporting of occupational diseases by clinicians. JAMA 1989;262:3041–3044.
11. Baker EL, Melius JM, Millar JD. Surveillance of occupational illness and injury in the United States: Current perspectives and future directions. J Public Health Policy summer1988;198–221.

12. Seligman PL, Sieber WK Jr, Pedersen DH, Sundin DS, Frazier TM. Compliance with OSHA record-keeping requirements. Am J Public Health 1988;78:1218.
13. Muldoon JT, Wintermeyer LA, Eure JA, Fuortes L, Merchant JA, Van Lier SF, Richards TB. Occupational disease surveillance data sources, 1985. Am J Public Health 1987;77:1006–1008.
14. Halperin WE, Frazier TM. Surveillance for the effects of workplace exposure. Ann Rev Public Health 1985;6:419–432.
15. Rutstein DD, Mullan RJ, Frazier TM, Halperin WE, Melius JM, Sestito JP. Sentinel health events (occupational): a basis for physician recognition and public health surveillance. Am J Public Health 1983;73:1054–1062.
16. Frazier TM. Developing a national occupational health surveillance system in the United States. Scand J Work Environ Health 1981;7(Suppl 4):127–132.

CHAPTER 2

Recognition and Evaluation of Work-Related Neurologic Disorders

Neil L. Rosenberg, M.D.

Recognition of work-related neurologic disease is crucial in establishing the correct diagnosis and differentiating a naturally occurring disorder from a disorder caused by the work environment. Diagnosis of an occupational disorder is essential to be able to prevent recurrence of disease and determine if other workers are at similar risk.

Differentiation between work-related and occupational disorders is becoming an increasingly important distinction.[1] The World Health Organization (WHO) recently advocated distinguishing between these terms. By definition, work-related diseases may be partially caused by or exacerbated by workplace exposures, while an occupational disease is totally related to a workplace exposure. These distinctions are important when evaluating an individual with a possible work-related or occupational disease, because numerous elements, such as sociocultural, personality/psychological, and environmental factors, become issues in dealing with work-related disorders. A physician who fails to address these issues may wrongly diagnose a patient as having an occupational disease or fail to recognize a work-related disease.

Very few occupational neurologic disorders present with pathognomonic, clinical, or laboratory findings. This is particularly true with the occupational neurotoxic disorders, which tend to mimic metabolic, degenerative, nutritional, or demyelinating disorders. Therefore, recognition of a disorder as occupationally related is also important in discovering new relationships between work exposures and disease.

This chapter deals with recognizing occupational neurologic disorders in individuals by emphasizing a detailed occupational history that focuses

TABLE 2.1
Studies Used in the Evaluation of Occupational Neurologic Disorders

---

Focused occupational history
Neurologic examination
Neuropsychological studies
   Conventional test batteries
   Test batteries in neurotoxicology
      Conventional batteries
      Microcomputer batteries
Neurophysiologic studies
   Peripheral nervous system
      Electromyography (EMG)
      Nerve conduction studies (NCV)
      Quantitative sensory testing (QST)
   Central nervous system
      Evoked potentials (EP)
      Electroencephalography (EEG)
   Balance/vestibular system
      Posturography/Body sway
      Electronystagmography (ENG)
Neuroradiologic studies
   Structural/anatomic imaging
      Computed tomography (CT)
      Magnetic resonance imaging (MRI)
   Functional imaging
      Single photon emission computed tomography (SPECT)
      Positron Emission tomography (PET)

---

on workplace exposures and habits. Various aspects of the neurologic examination and additional studies that may be useful in evaluating individuals or groups of workers are discussed. Table 2.1 outlines the various studies that have been reported to be useful in the evaluation of a variety of work-related and occupational disorders, although they have primarily been used in the evaluation of occupational neurotoxic disorders. Because relatively few of these techniques have been validated in occupational settings, only the more important are discussed here.

Evaluation of the Patient

The same process used in the diagnosis of any condition should be used in the individual suspected of an occupationally related disorder: history of present illness, past medical history, review of systems, and family history. The specifics of the occupational history are discussed in detail in this section.

FOCUSED OCCUPATIONAL HISTORY

The key to the diagnosis of an occupational disorder is through a focused history. Occupational history taking is often an omitted or neglected portion of the medical and neurologic history.[2,3] The occupational history need not be detailed or time consuming.

When considering the workplace, one is concerned with various types of *exposures;* these may be chemical (e.g., solvents, pesticides, or metals), physical (e.g., radiation, noise, vibration), or psychological (e.g., stress). While exposure does not always lead to the development of disease or toxicity, certain questions need to be asked and certain basic principles of toxicology need to be understood to determine whether the workplace environment has caused or contributed to an individual's disease. The focus of the occupational history should be on those questions that will yield the most productive information. If the history fails to reveal an etiology in difficult cases that are still suspected of being work related, a workplace visit by the physician may be especially useful.

How to incorporate what is known about the basic mechanisms of neurotoxicity into a rational approach to the individual with possible occupational neurotoxic disease is less than perfect since these mechanisms are known for so few neurotoxins. In addition, the primary cellular and subcellular targets are also known for few industrial and environmental neurotoxins (Table 2.2). The basic principles of toxicology have been reviewed,[4,5] but below are listed some basic principles of toxicology that are of particular relevance to the understanding of neurotoxicology. When appropriate, relevant questions in the occupational history are listed that relate to that principle.

Proximity to Exposure and Improvement with
Removal of Toxin

Maximum symptoms generally occur with maximum exposure with little delay in the onset.

> What is the temporal relationship between your symptoms and the workplace?
>
> What happens to your symptoms before beginning work? During work? After leaving work? On weekends or holidays?

Although this principle has been one of the cornerstones in our understanding of clinical neurotoxicology, it may need redefining particularly in the area of neurodegenerative disorders, such as Parkinson's disease and Alzheimer's disease. Based on recent findings of individuals exposed to 1-methyl-4-phenyl-1,2,3,6-tetrahydropyridine (MPTP) and the search for environmental toxins as possible etiologic agents for these disorders, remote exposures (i.e., those that may have been symptomatic or even

TABLE 2.2
Classification of Neurotoxins Based on Basic Mechanisms and Cellular/
Subcellular Targets of Known Industrial and Environmental Toxins

I. Primary metabolic effects on neurons
    A. Neuronal membrane
        1. Membrane-channel blockers: tetraethylammonium, aminopyrides
        2. Membrane-channel openers: DDT, pyrethroid insecticides
    B. Neurotransmitters
        1. Cholinergic System
            a. Cholinergic agonist
            b. Anticholinesterases: organophosphate, carbamates
            c. Anticholinergic
            d. Presynaptic and postsynaptic cholinergic blockade
        2. Catecholaminergic system
            a. Cholinergic/adrenergic effects: organophosphates, carbamates
            b. Catecholaminergic
            c. Depletion of catecholamines: manganese
        3. Serotonergic pathways: ?
        4. GABAergic toxicity: ?
        5. Glutaminergic pathways: ?
    C. Structural integrity of the neuron
        1. Neuronal degeneration
            a. Central nervous system: thallium, organic mercury
            b. Peripheral nervous system: ?
            c. Special senses: methanol (vision)
        2. Axonal degeneration
            a. Central-peripheral distal axonopathy—*n*-Hexane, methyl butyl ketone (MBK), acrylamide, organophosphates, carbon disulfide, thallium
            b. Central distal axonopathy—clioquinol
II. Primary metabolic effects on myelin
    A. Metals: lead, triethyltin, thallium, copper
    B. Solvents: toluene (substance abuse only)
    C. Other: ammonia, hexachlorophene
III. Primary metabolic effects on blood vessels: lead, cadmium, indium, terbium,thallium, mercury, organotins, bismuth
IV. Primary metabolic effects on neuromuscular junction: organochlorine insecticides, pyrethrins, lead
V. Primary metabolic effects on muscle: dimethyl sulfoxide (DMSO), barium
VI. Secondary effects due to hypoxia/ischemia
    A. Anoxic anoxia
        1. Carbon monoxide (carboxyhemoglobinemia)
        2. Nitrites (methemoglobinemia)
    B. Ischemic anoxia: secondary to cardiac arrest
        1. Solvents
        2. Pesticides
        3. Metals
        4. Gases

TABLE 2.2 *(continued)*

   C. Cytotoxic anoxia
      1. Cyanide
      2. Azide
      3. Dinitrophenol
      4. Malononitrile
      5. Methionine sulfoximine

---

asymptomatic many years before the development of symptoms of a "neurodegenerative" disorder) may one day be linked to the much later development of progressive neurologic disorders. This concept also emphasizes the fear that the extremely low levels of industrial toxins in the environment, levels that are insufficient to produce neurologic symptoms, may actually predispose susceptible individuals to the later development of progressive neurodegenerative disorders (see Chapters 7 and 13).

Strong Dose-Response Relationship.

Dose-response is related both to level and duration of exposure. The higher the level of exposure, the more severe the symptoms. The greater the duration of exposure, the more likely the person is to have irreversible symptoms. In addition, with neurotoxins, there is very little variability in the effects on different individuals. Although extremes of age or health (especially severe liver disease) may be related to different effects from the same level of exposure, this does not generally occur in the occupational setting, where there is a narrower range of ages and most individuals are in good health.

Where do you work and how long have you worked there?

Do others at work have similar problems?

General Principles Related to Specific Exposures

Multiple Syndromes from a Single Toxin.   Depending on the level and duration of exposure (i.e., the dose-response relationship) widely different neurologic syndromes may develop. For example, acute high-level exposure to *n*-hexane produces a transient nonspecific encephalopathy, characterized by euphoria, disorientation, and a cerebellar ataxia. Chronic, lower-level exposure is associated with a peripheral neuropathy and a conspicuous lack of central nervous system (CNS) dysfunction. This principle emphasizes the need to not only know what an individual is exposed to, but also the general level of exposure.

Chemical Formula May Not Predict Toxicity.   Chemicals with similar structure may not have similar toxicity. Toluene (methylbenzene) produces a dramatic clinical syndrome, with chronic exposure characterized by dementia, anosmia, and cerebellar ataxia. Removing the methyl group from toluene produces a chemical with no clear chronic neurotoxicity, benzene, but it is thought to be carcinogenic.

Enhancement of Neurotoxicity by "Innocent Bystanders."   This principle, though important to recognize, will usually only add to confusion in the evaluation of exposed workers. Typically, workers are exposed to multiple chemicals or chemical mixtures (more common with organic solvents than with other chemicals). Although neurotoxicity may be known for an individual chemical, how it interacts with others in a mixture, and how that may contribute to or enhance neurotoxicity, is virtually never known. Mixtures of chemicals are generally believed to be more neurotoxic than individual chemicals, but evidence of this is lacking. There are few examples of enhancement of neurotoxicity by "innocent bystanders," but one should keep in mind the enhancement of *n*-hexane neurotoxicity by methyl ethyl ketone (see Chapter 4).

The preceding principles are important in understanding workplace exposures, and the questions relative to these principles that should be asked are as follows:

What type of product is produced or what kind of service is provided?

Describe specifically what you do at work.

With what materials, chemicals, or processes do you work? Do you work with liquids, vapors, aerosols, solids? Do you have skin contact with the materials?

Do you use protective equipment such as respirators, gloves, boots, separate work clothes?

Were you given instruction on the proper handling of the materials?

Were you given instruction on the proper cleaning and maintenance of equipment?

What are the general conditions of the workplace regarding ventilation and drainage?

Have you ever had symptoms severe enough that you needed assistance from coworkers or medical evaluation?

Limits of Clinical Laboratory Testing

In individuals with neurotoxic injuries, the clinical laboratory is generally not very useful. Clinical laboratory tests to assess industrial exposures are useful in acute exposures to assess the degree of exposure, but usually the history will identify the substance to which the individual was exposed. Acute exposures are usually completely reversible as far as neurotoxic injuries are concerned, and these individuals do not come to the attention of the neurologist.

Chronic low-level exposure, often associated with neurotoxicity, may occur at such low levels that clinical laboratory tests fail to establish a body burden for that particular chemical. Establishing a link between exposure and clinical dysfunction relies on a focused history of exposure and a neurologic examination, and not on the clinical laboratory.

Nonfocal Syndromes

This principle is one of the most useful when evaluating a patient with presumed neurotoxic injury. Neurotoxins generally affect the central and peripheral nervous systems in a *diffuse* or *bilaterally symmetric* fashion. Examples of diffuse injury include the distal axonopathy from acrylamide[6] or the diffuse CNS white matter changes due to chronic toluene abuse.[7] Bilaterally symmetric injuries are primarily related to those toxins that have specific cell targets, such as MPTP's effect on the dopaminergic neurons of the substantia nigra.[8]

Asymptomatic Neurotoxic Disease

Asymptomatic neurotoxic disease certainly occurs in nonoccupational settings and therefore would be expected to be found in the occupational setting as well.[9] Studies in workers in paint manufacturing facilities have been found to have subclinical neuropsychological deficits,[10] and further studies may reveal asymptomatic disease to be an extremely common phenomenon.

PHYSICAL AND NEUROLOGIC EXAMINATIONS

The physical examination should include a general examination, but with emphasis on the neurologic examination. The general examination should not be overlooked, since findings separate from the neurologic examination may lead to the appropriate diagnosis. For example, a bluish line on the gums (Burtonian lead line) may suggest lead poisoning in an individual whose principal complaints are gastrointestinal upset and wrist drop.

Completeness of the evaluation is also critical so that the diagnosis of an occupationally related disorder is not made when the correct diagnosis is actually a naturally occurring neurologic disease. For example, when an automotive spray painter develops dizziness, cognitive disturbance, and imbalance, the symptoms will commonly be attributed to chronic organic solvent intoxication. In some instances, certain aspects of the history and neurologic examination, and abnormalities on the spinal fluid and magnetic resonance imaging (MRI) examinations, may reveal a diagnosis of multiple sclerosis.

The history, physical and neurologic examinations, and additional laboratory and radiologic studies are particularly important in the recognition of occupational neurotoxic disease. Recognition of overt neurotoxic disease is not difficult if a worker develops a well-described clinical syndrome after exposure to a well-known industrial chemical, or if several workers at the same work site develop a similar clinical picture (e.g., peripheral neuropathy after chronic exposure to *n*-hexane). The more difficult and far more common situation is when a symptomatic individual is seen with either an unclear history of exposure or an apparently trivial exposure to a known or suspected neurotoxin. In this situation, careful evaluation for a naturally occurring disorder is essential so that a work-related or occupational disorder is not diagnosed incorrectly.

Neurologic Examination

The neurologic examination is the most systematized and quantitative part of the physical examination.[11] It is also one of the most neglected and seldom performed parts of the physical examination by non-neurologists. The examination generally comprises assessment of mental function (mental status exam), the function of the cranial nerves, muscle strength and tone, reflexes (muscle stretch and cutaneous), sensation, and station and gait. The data derived from the neurologic examination are important and are discussed here so that the non-neurologist evaluating a patient with a possible occupational neurologic disease can have a format to follow. The neurologic examination should be complete but does not have to take an inordinately long time. Table 2.3 represents an outline of a standard neurologic examination, which, when performed on a regular basis, can be completed in 15–20 minutes.

A complete and rigorously performed neurologic examination is important in defining the clinical neurologic syndrome. Once defined, a differential diagnosis can be entertained, and occupational versus nonoccupational causation can be determined. In regard to neurotoxic injuries, many neurotoxins produce relatively specific neurologic syndromes. Table 2.4 lists those common neurologic syndromes produced by various neurotoxins.

Quantification in Occupational Neurology

Quantitative assessment is essential in the evaluation of work-related neurologic problems. The primary reason for this importance is that work-related disabilities and a worker's ability to perform a work-related task will need to be determined by some quantitative measure. An attempt at quantification can be seen in the commonly used American Medical Association (AMA) guidelines to the evaluation of permanent impairment,[12] used as the standard for determining disability ratings. One of the major problems with these guidelines is that they use primarily nonquantitative (e.g., qualitative) measures. The neurologic examination,

TABLE 2.3
Outline of the Neurologic Examination

Mental status
    Orientation (person, place, time)
    Concentration (immediate recall, "serial sevens")
    Short-term memory (recall of three items at 15 minutes)
    Remote memory
    Affect (does the patient appear depressed?)
Cranial nerves
    I: olfaction (cloves, coffee, or other common odors)
    II: visual acuity, visual fields (to confrontation), fundoscopic examination
    III, IV, VI: Extraocular movements, pupillary responses
    V: facial sensation, strength of muscles of mastication
    VII: strength of facial muscles
    VIII: hearing to whispered word; tuning fork evaluation (e.g., Rinne's and
        Weber's tests with 256-hz tuning fork)
    IX, X: palatal movement
    XI: sternocleidomastoid and trapezius muscle strength
    XII: tongue strength; any atrophy of tongue; protrusion and lateral movement
Motor
    Tone and muscle bulk
    Manual strength testing graded using modified Medical Research Council (MRC)
        scale (0: no movement; 1: flicker of movement; 2: moves with gravity elimi-
        nated; 3: overcomes gravity; 4: some resistance, but not normal [4-, 4+ added
        when appropriate]; 5: normal).
Reflexes
    Muscle stretch reflexes of ankles, knees, brachioradialis, biceps, triceps; these
        reflexes are rated 0 to 4 (0: absent; 1: diminished; 2: normal; 3: hyperactive; 4:
        clonus). Of the cutaneous reflexes, the response to plantar stimulation is the
        most important.
Sensation
    Touch (light touch with finger or cotton wisp)
    Pain (pin prick)
    Temperature
    Position
    Vibration (128-hz tuning fork)
    Cortical sensation (i.e., double simultaneous stimulation, two-point
        discrimination, graphesthesia)
Cerebellar, station, and coordination
    Finger-to-nose and heel-to-shin testing
    Rapid alternating movements (i.e. finger tapping, opening-closing hand, prona-
        tion-supination, heel tapping)
    Romberg test (stability standing with eyes closed)
    Normal gait and tandem gait

TABLE 2.4
Major Neurologic Clinical Syndromes Produced by Various Neurotoxins*

Neurologic syndrome	Solvents	Metals	Pesticides	Gases
Seizures	Ethylene glycol Methanol Tin Carbon tetrachloride Aluminum Antimony Arsenic	Mercury Lead	Organochlorines Organophosphates	Carbon monoxide Hydrogen sulfide
Encephalopathy	All solvents	Aluminum Antimony Arsenic Bismuth Lead Manganese Mercury Silicon Tin Lithium	Organochlorines Carbamates Organophosphates	Hydrogen sulfide Carbon monoxide Methyl chloride Carbon disulfide Ethylene oxide Nitrous oxide
Cerebellar dysfunction	All solvents	Aluminum Bismuth Manganese Mercury Thallium Zinc Tin Lithium	Organophosphates Organochlorines	Carbon monoxide Methyl chloride

Disorder	Solvents	Metals	Pesticides	Gases
Peripheral neuropathy	n-Hexane MBK	Arsenic Gold Thallium Organotin Lithium Lead Mercury	Carbamates (?) Organophosphates Organochlorines	Nitrous oxide Carbon disulfide Carbon monoxide Ethylene oxide
Parkinsonism and other movement disorders	Methanol Toluene Trichloroethane Carbon tetrachloride	Lead Mercury Bismuth Manganese Thallium Bromides Zinc Aluminum Lithium	Organophosphates Organochlorines Carbamates	Carbon monoxide Carbon disulfide Hydrogen sulfide Methyl chloride
Cranial neuropathy	Methanol Ethylene glycol Trichlorethane n-Hexane MBK Benzene Toluene	Mercury Arsenic Thallium Gold Bromides Bismuth Lead	Organophosphates Organochlorides Carbamates	Nitrous oxide Carbon disulfide
	Carbon tetrachloride			

MBK = methyl butyl ketone.

*This table was developed from clinical reports (often anecdotal and not well documented) in the medical literature. Scientific evidence of an association between certain toxins and clinical disorders is often not present.

described previously, has the ability to be quantitative in many areas: Muscle strength is commonly graded using a standard or modified version of the Medical Research Council (MRC) rating scale,[13] and rating scales have been developed for evaluation of several common neurologic diseases such as multiple sclerosis[14] and Parkinson's disease.[15] In fact, in recent years efforts have begun to develop quantitative measures for all aspects of the neurologic examination.[16]

While these standard rating scales have been useful, they are insensitive and have poor interexaminer reproducibiity. Measures are needed that are sensitive and reproducible and can be applied in many different clinical situations. Sensitive quantitative methods are becoming even more important in occupational medicine with the 1990 passage of the Americans with Disabilities Act, which demands less subjective measures of an individual's ability to perform a job.

The three major areas of importance in quantifying neurologic performance related to occupational issues are those that deal with assessment of the peripheral nervous system (quantitative sensory testing and electromyography), cognitive function (neuropsychological and neurobehavioral testing techniques), and low back evaluations (discussed in Chapter 11).

COGNITIVE EVALUATION

Neurobehavioral testing is an accepted methodology for the assessment of the functional integrity of the CNS, and has been used extensively to evaluate the neurotoxic effects of occupational exposures.[17–21] The importance of neurobehavioral testing in occupational neurology can be seen by its discussion here and by how it relates to the neurobehavioral effects of organic solvents (see Chapter 4), other neurobehavioral disorders (see Chapter 5), and head trauma (see Chapter 10).

Neurobehavioral disorders and testing have been given a high priority by NIOSH.[22] Within its stated mission, NIOSH neurobehavioral research includes animal and human laboratory testing as well as the examination of workers in field studies.[23,24]

Between 1973 and 1983, NIOSH was involved in the evaluation of 11 industrywide studies to identify the possible neurobehavioral effects of various workplace exposures.[24] These have included studies to determine the possible neurobehavioral effects resulting from chronic exposure to inorganic mercury,[25] carbon monoxide,[26] lead,[27,28] methyl chloride,[29] carbon disulfide,[30,31] formaldehyde,[32] perchloroethylene,[33] velsicol pesticide,[34] and nonferrous smelter workers.[35] A wide variety of tests were used in these studies, making them difficult to compare.[23,24] NIOSH has not endorsed the use of a standard neurobehavioral test battery, although other investigators have advocated the use of standard batteries for occupational exposures.[36–39]

Neurobehavioral testing is generally administered by an examiner, but recently has also been adapted to the microcomputer.[40-46] Computerized tests have the advantages of standardization of test administration and easier manipulation of data but also have important disadvantages. Some important disadvantages are that only certain stimuli can be presented (primarily visual) and that only certain responses can be recorded (primarily motor). The major advantage for occupational neurotoxic studies is that they can be performed in large numbers of individuals in the field and in epidemiologic studies. Studies have also validated these computerized tests in certain occupational exposure settings.[43,44,46]

Neurobehavioral sequelae to chronic exposure to industrial chemicals is one of the most commonly evaluated clinical problems in occupational medicine. It is also one of the most controversial, particularly in regard to the "psycho-organic" syndrome allegedly related to chronic exposure to organic solvents (see Chapter 4). Most of the neuropsychological studies performed on workers have been in the setting of chronic exposure to organic solvents. One needs to interpret these studies critically, since invalid conclusions have been drawn from the results of many of these studies.

A skilled neuropsychologist is essential when evaluating occupationally exposed individuals. It is tempting to interpret abnormalities on neurobehavioral tests as being related to the worker's exposure, but often other, naturally occurring illnesses are to blame. In particular, one needs to pay careful attention to prior function (school performance history and evaluation of school records), alcohol and illicit substance abuse, prior head injuries, and psychological disorders (particularly affective disorders). Although with a focused history and attention to some basic principles of toxicology, it would seem that these issues would be adequately addressed, it is remarkable how often erroneous conclusions are reached because of the apparent need to attribute symptoms to an exogenous source, such as a toxin. No test(s), including neuropsychological tests, can replace the history, neurologic examination, and remembering some of the principles of toxicology described previously.

Screening test batteries, primarily used for evaluation of dementia in the elderly, such as enhanced cued recall[47] and brief mental status examinations,[48] which can be easily administered in a clinical setting, may also be sensitive enough to screen workers exposed to neurotoxins. Studies such as these have not been performed in exposed workers.

QUANTIFICATION OF SENSATION

The clinical assessment of sensation is the least reliable component of the neurologic examination and the most difficult to quantify. Clinical neurologists will continue to test sensation at the bedside with the usual hand-held instruments that have been used since the neurologic examination became systematized. However, for some purposes, better instruments and testing procedures are available and should be used.

Such instruments use sensitive and precisely defined quantifiable stimuli and use methods of testing and scoring to assess sensation accurately and objectively. In addition, automation of this testing has allowed optimum efficiency and the elimination of both testing and observer variability, thus obtaining responses that are quantifiable as well as reproducible. Collectively, this group of procedures is referred to as quantitative sensory testing (QST). QST is not a new procedure, and its origins can be traced to the roots of experimental psychology and human factors testing. It has become an integral part of the clinical evaluation of the auditory and visual systems.

Historically, assessment of the somatosensory system has been less quantitative due primarily to lack of available devices for the accurate control of stimulus characteristics and intensities. Workers in several laboratories have developed a variety of somatosensory QST methods and instruments that have been useful for the assessment of peripheral nerve function.[49–52] In the past decade, as a result of the development of these methods, a large number of portable, relatively inexpensive devices have been introduced for the QST of a variety of sensory modalities, in particular vibration and thermal thresholds. These instruments use sensitive and precisely defined quantifiable stimuli and the best available methods of testing and scoring to assess sensation accurately and objectively.

Standard electrophysiologic studies of the peripheral nervous system, nerve conduction velocity studies (NCV), are limited in their ability to test different sensory modalities. NCV studies use methods that involve stimulation of large-diameter myelinated fiber and recording of the evoked muscle action potential or sensory nerve action potential in the same fibers. Therefore, many fiber populations cannot be tested. In particular, the small myelinated and unmyelinated fibers are not evaluated on standard NCV studies.

There are several purposes of performing QST. These include obtaining positive evidence of peripheral nerve dysfunction when other tests are negative, particularly in those pathologic conditions that predominantly affect small-fiber function, specifically the distal axonopathies produced by toxic or metabolic conditions. Potential uses in the occupational setting where quantitative measurement of sensory thresholds can provide useful information are listed in Table 2.5.

A wide variety of tests are available to test all aspects of sensation (Table 2.6). However, because of time and cost constraints, one needs to consider what tests should be done based on the particular clinical situation as well as the cost of the equipment. One must also be cognizant of the fact that, since sensory pathways also can result from dysfunction in the central nervous system, lesions of the brain and spinal cord may also produce abnormalities on QST.[49,53]

TABLE 2.5
Potential Occupational Uses for QST

I. Positive evidence of peripheral nerve dysfunction with normal NCVs
    A. Suspected toxic neuropathy
    B. Cumulative trauma syndrome with suspected carpal tunnel syndrome
II. Monitoring of individuals in "at risk" groups
    A. Workers exposed to neurotoxic chemicals
    B. Workers "at risk" for development of carpal tunnel syndrome
    C. Individuals at increased risk for development of an occupational neuropathy (e.g., those with naturally occurring disorders that can affect peripheral nerves, such as diabetes, uremia, and AIDS, and those receiving neurotoxic drugs)
III. Monitoring response to treatment
    A. Individual patients with toxic neuropathy or carpal tunnel syndrome
    B. Large numbers of patients in clinical trials

TABLE 2.6
Methods of Quantifying Specific Sensory Modalities

Sensory modality	*Method of quantification*
Large fiber	
A—Beta mechanoreceptors	Vibration perception threshold
	Sensory nerve action potential current perception threshold (high-frequency stimulation)
	Tactile threshold
Small fiber	
A—Delta cold receptors	Cold threshold
B—Delta fast pain sensors	Pinch-pain threshold
C—Warm receptors	Warm threshold
C—Nociceptors	Pinch-pain threshold
	Current perception threshold (low-frequency stimulation)

Types of Sensation Quantified

Many types of sensory modalities and virtually all fiber types can be quantified (see Table 2.6). In addition to sensation, motor and autonomic function can also be quantified by a variety of techniques. However, this review focuses only on the following sensory modalities: tactile, thermal, vibration, and current perception threshold testing.

Tactile. Tests for quantifying tactile sensation, mediated by rapidly adapting intracutaneous mechanoreceptors and large diameter nerve fibers, were first introduced by von Frey. The clinical tool, referred to as "Frey hairs" or "Frey filaments," usually consists of a series of 10 or 12 nylon filaments mounted in plastic handles with different bending pressures.[54–56] Although a variety of methodologies have been employed using this technique, all test tactile threshold—i.e., "What is the filament of lowest bending pressure that can be perceived?" The advantages of this method are that it can be performed quickly and cheaply and that it can be applied anywhere on the body. The disadvantages of this method are that mixed sensory modalities are stimulated and that the rate of application is undefined.

Tactile thresholds can also be obtained by using mechanical stimulators.[57,58] These devices provide precise and adequate stimuli of the low-threshold cutaneous mechanoreceptors and are probably the best controlled and most sensitive measures of tactile threshold. The disadvantages of these mechanical stimulators are that they are expensive and time consuming.

Thermal. Small-diameter nerve fibers principally process pain and temperature. The clinical assessment of small-fiber function is so imprecise that only the complete absence of sensation can be determined. In addition, as noted previously, standard NCV studies are heavily weighted toward the assessment of large-fiber function. Pathologic changes of small-diameter nerve fibers are related to the painful, dysesthetic (or hyperesthetic) condition that occurs with many peripheral neuropathies and may be the presenting symptom of specific metabolic neuropathies such as diabetes. Tests of thermal discrimination measure small fiber function using precise psychophysical procedures[59,60]. The two most commonly used testing procedures are the Marstock method and the "two-alternative forced choice" procedure. Both use a thermoelectric (Peltier) module.

The Marstock method was so named because of collaboration between investigators at institutions located in Marburg, Germany, and Stockholm, Sweden.[59] The stimulator is applied to the skin of the patient and both warm/cold thresholds and cold pain/heat pain thresholds are determined.

Our laboratory uses a thermal device for quantitative assessment of thermal thresholds. This device consists of two identical 25-cm squared, nickel-coated copper plates that are connected to separate power units and perfused with water in series. The plates can be contacted by either hand or foot. Temperature can be adjusted by gradients as small as 0.1°C and span 50.0°C range. The temperature of each plate and the difference in temperature between the plates are continuously displayed on digital monitors with resolution of 0.1°C.

Testing using the "two-alternative forced choice" procedure is done by having the patient determine which of the two plates is colder. Initially, a wide temperature difference is set; it is then successively reduced until the individual can no longer detect a difference in temperature between the stages. The actual temperature difference can be read directly from the digital readout of the differential thermometer.

Vibration.   In clinical testing, pallesthesia is the ability to perceive the presence of vibrations when an oscillating tuning fork (usually 128 Hz) is placed over certain bony prominences and from the skin, such as the pads of the fingertips. Both the intensity and duration of the stimulus perceived at the various sites are noted. It is emphasized, however, that both intensity and duration depend on the force at which the tuning fork is struck and the interval between the time it is struck and the time it is applied. For clinical testing, the vibrating tuning fork is placed on a bony prominence (e.g., great toe or lateral or medial malleolus) until the patient no longer feels vibration. The examiner compares the patient's ability to feel when the fork has almost stopped vibrating with his or her own. The drawbacks of this type of clinical testing are well known to clinicians and have been augmented by the determination of vibration threshold using electromagnetic devices.

Vibration perception thresholds (VPTs) are a proven method for detection of large-fiber dysfunction.[61–63] A large number of commercially available devices assess vibratory sensation, including Vibratron II (Physitemp Instruments, Inc., Clifton, NJ), Optacon (Telesensory Systems, Inc., Mountain View, CA), Vibrameter (Somedic Ab, Sweden), and Bio-Thesiometer (Bio-Medical Instruments Co., Newbury, OH), among others.

Our laboratory uses an electromechanical device for quantitative assessment of VPT. It is a simple, inexpensive, portable device that measures VPT in the hands and feet. The vibrating surface area is 12 mm in diameter, constructed of hard rubber, and vibrates at a frequency of 120 Hz. There is a vibration intensity control unit and two vibrating post units. The control unit contains the power supply, switches, and digital readout meter. The vibrating post units are separately attached to the control unit with adjoining cables. Each vibrating rod protrudes through a metal case and can be contacted by either the hands or feet. Vibration is achieved by driving the electromagnetic unit of one post and using the "two alternative forced choice procedure" described previously. The subject is required to determine which of the two posts is actually vibrating. A dual position switch connected in series with the vibrating units controls which post vibrates, while a "dummy" switch is used to imitate the sounds of switching. The amplitude (intensity) of vibration is proportional to the square of the applied voltage and is continuously displayed on the digital readout meter to the nearest 0.1 vibration units. The range of amplitude available to test with this device is 0–20 vibration units.

Both normal populations at different ages and patients with peripheral neuropathy have been studied with these devices[64,65] and are discussed in more detail below.

Current Perception Threshold.   The study of cutaneous senses by their response to electrical stimulation has been in use for over 80 years.[66] In 1952, Sigel[67,68] published results of stimulation of the forearm with square-wave electrical currents to assess cutaneous sensory thresholds. If square-wave stimulation is used, separate variation of the frequency and duration of the stimulus can be achieved, while the rate of current increase during each pulse remains constant. Square-wave stimulation is thus a method of analyzing the frequency-intensity functions obtained with sinusoidal currents.

Thus, frequency, amplitude, duration, and waveform of the current pulse are parameters that govern the electrical excitation of nervous tissue.[66,69–76]Intensity and perception of electrical stimulation correlate best with the current applied,[67,68,75] and the reproducible application of current requires standardization of skin impedance.[71,72] Because skin impedance, the frequency-dependent resistance of the skin, is difficult to standardize, until recently it has been difficult to quantify sensory threshold to an applied current.[77–80]

A recently developed device for current perception threshold (CPT) determination can generate a variable frequency sinusoidal waveform stimulus at 5,250, and 2,000 Hz at digitally calibrated levels of 0–10 mA. The current is delivered to the skin surface by a pair of 1-cm diameter electrodes coated with standard conductive gel and then taped to the body site being tested. The controls are hidden from the view of the patient. The unit is then turned on and the electrical stimulus is gradually increased until the patient reports feeling the stimulus. The intensity level is then decremented/reincremented until the same threshold measurement is obtained on at least three consecutive trials using the "two alternative forced choice" procedure described previously.

CPT has been shown to correlate with standard nerve conduction tests and has the additional advantages of being painless, quick, and easy to perform.[80] An additional potential benefit of this device is its ability to stimulate at three different frequencies, possibly stimulating three different nerve fiber populations.[81]

A recent study in diabetic patients demonstrated a significant relationship between high-frequency (2,000 Hz) stimulation and tests of large-fiber function (nerve conduction tests and vibration perception thresholds) and between low-frequency (5 Hz) stimulation and a measure of small-fiber function (thermal thresholds).[82] Thus, CPT measurement at different frequencies may provide useful information about different nerve fiber types and increase our understanding of the physiology of different types of peripheral neuropathies by using one stimulus modality rather than several to gain the same information. However, before endorsing the widespread clinical use of such a device, additional studies are necessary, especially those correlating with sensory testing where there are known receptors in the nervous system, such as thermal and vibration.

Quantification of Sensation in Specific Conditions

The basic physiology of the various sensory modalities described forms a solid foundation for the development and use of mechanical devices for QST.

The main clinical application of QST has been in the evaluation of peripheral nerve disorders. Despite their solid foundation in basic neurophysiology and their clinical utility, QST methods are still not widely used in clinical practice. In the following section, those peripheral nerve disorders that have been most closely studied using quantitative methods are discussed.

Occupational Exposures and Injuries. Occupational injuries and exposures for which quantitative sensory testing would be of value in assessment are neurotoxic exposures and cumulative trauma syndrome, specifically carpal tunnel syndrome.

Neurotoxic exposures Toxic exposure in the workplace may occur with exposure to numerous chemicals and metals. Toxic neuropathies are often first suspected by distal symmetric sensory dysfunction, and because of this, QST has been recommended in the evaluation of workers exposed to neurotoxic agents.[83–85] In spite of these recommendations, few studies have been performed using QST to evaluate workers exposed to neurotoxic agents.[86,87]

Vibration perception thresholds were tested in 257 individuals working at two different chemical plants that manufacture acrylamide monomer, a known peripheral nerve toxin.[86] This study demonstrated the utility of this testing under field conditions, with consistent data being obtained on repeated testing of individuals. An age-related decrease in vibration thresholds was found, and a subclinical neuropathy was detected in two individuals, one neuropathy related to acrylamide.

Another recent study has evaluated vibration and thermal thresholds in 93 construction trade painters and 105 nonpainter control subjects.[87] A number of statistical analyses were performed and comparison to standard neurophysiologic studies was not done. In general, both vibration and thermal thresholds were higher in painters than controls, suggesting that exposure to the organic solvents present in paint may be associated with sensory system dysfunction.

Cumulative trauma syndrome/carpal tunnel syndrome QST has proved useful in the evaluation of focal traumatic neuropathies[88] and carpal tunnel syndrome.[89–95]

Eleven patients with painful traumatic focal nerve injuries were studied with both thermal and mechanical sensory stimuli.[88] All patients had raised thresholds for temperature, touch, or both. Thermal pain thresholds (Marstock method) were variably raised or lowered (indicating hyperesthesia). This study demonstrates the utility of QST for assessing hyperesthetic conditions that cannot be quantified by other methodologies.

Carpal tunnel syndrome (CTS) is the most common nerve compression syndrome, initially presenting with sensory impairment and only later developing motor dysfunction. Early in the course of CTS, the clinical examination often fails to demonstrate sensory dysfunction and past reported results with a variety of QST modalities reveal several discrepancies.[89–92]

A detailed study assessing a variety of QST methods in 22 patients with CTS (33 hands) revealed that at least one test was abnormal in 27 of 33 CTS hands (82%). QST methods used in this study included vibration perception thresholds, tactile pulses, von Frey hairs, two-point discrimination, graphesthesia, and thermal thresholds.[92] The results of this study suggest that, although QST methods are useful in the evaluation of CTS, no one method will suffice. In addition, increase in sensitivity of QST can be expected for any test if it is combined with provocation, such as wrist flexion.[93,96]

One study used an occupationally relevant functional tactile inspection task to evaluate CTS.[95] In this study, a ridge detection threshold task was administered to patients with CTS and compared to reference controls without CTS. Sixteen hands with CTS and 30 normal hands were assessed for detection of ridge height changes, ridge gradient, and direction of shearing against the skin in ridge detection thresholds. Normals had ridge detection thresholds that were two and one-half times lower than hands with CTS (0.08 mm versus 0.20 mm), with no effect being seen with age. These studies suggest that workers with CTS may not detect an edge or surface defect in a tactile inspection task unless it was more than twice as high as edges detected by workers without CTS.

Peripheral Neuropathy: Multiple Etiologies.   Using an automated method of determining thermal thresholds, Jamal and coworkers[97] found abnormalities in 99% of individuals with peripheral neuropathies of diverse etiologies. Of this same group, 89% also showed one or more abnormalities on conventional electromyographic studies. Of interest was the fact that 39 of 40 patients with completely normal sensory nerve studies using conventional techniques had abnormalities of one or more thermal thresholds. This study demonstrated that abnormalities of thermal thresholds are present and often antedate the appearance of abnormalities on conventional electrophysiologic studies in the majority of patients with peripheral neuropathy irrespective of etiology.

In a similar study, patients with signs and symptoms of small-fiber peripheral neuropathy were studied with the same technique of detection of thermal thresholds.[98] All patients had abnormalities of thermal thresholds, despite all having normal conventional electrophysiologic studies and vibration thresholds. This study demonstrates the importance of using techniques that test more than one nerve fiber population to detect abnormalities.

Diabetes Mellitus.   Diabetic neuropathy has been the most widely studied of the peripheral neuropathies by QST methods.[99–105] Thermal,[99–104] vibration,[99,102] and current perception[105] thresholds have all been utilized in the evaluation of diabetic neuropathy and were found to be superior to conventional electrophysiologic studies in the detection of abnormalities.

A conference on diabetic neuropathy, jointly sponsored by the American Diabetes Association and the American Academy of Neurology, was held in

1988.[106] During this conference, presentations were made in a number of areas regarding diabetic neuropathy, including sensory testing. The panel recommended that QST be included in the evaluation of diabetic polyneuropathy for several reasons: (1) They are sensitive, reproducible, and noninvasive; (2) they can test a broad range of sensory modalities, thus evaluating the integrity of a range of primary cutaneous sensory nerve fibers that are not easily accessible to conventional electrophysiologic studies; and (3) they can document and measure a parameter that no other test can measure, hyperalgesia.

In conclusion, a wide range of QST measures have been made in diabetic neuropathy and are accepted methodologies in the evaluation of this disorder. These simple, noninvasive measures are also suitable for long-term studies of its natural history and response to treatment. When evaluating an individual for possible occupational neuropathy, whether diffuse (e.g., toxic neuropathy) or focal (e.g., CTS due to cumulative trauma), one also needs to be constantly aware of the possible coexistence of diabetic neuropathy, the most common cause of peripheral neuropathy.

Uremia. In nondiabetic dialysis patients, peripheral nerve integrity has been one parameter of insufficient dialysis.[107] The health of the peripheral nerve is one of the important quantitative longitudinal measures of dialytic adequacy in the nondiabetic patient, and QST measures have been used to assess uremic neuropathy.[80,108–110] Current perception thresholds,[80,108] vibration thresholds,[109] and thermal thresholds[110] have all been shown to be sensitive indicators of peripheral nerve function in these patients and correlate well with conventional nerve conduction tests.

SUMMARY OF QST

QST methods are sensitive measures of peripheral nervous system integrity and are useful adjuncts to the evaluation of disorders of sensation of occupational and nonoccupational origin. They have proved to be valuable in the evaluation of toxic neuropathies and carpal tunnel syndrome, the most common occupational disorders of the peripheral nerve. QST can augment information gained from the clinical evaluation and conventional electrophysiologic studies and are sensitive enough in certain conditions to detect subclinical peripheral nerve dysfunction, such as in occupational toxic neuropathy or carpal tunnel syndrome. Because they are extremely well tolerated, as well as sensitive, repeat evaluations can be performed with a high rate of patient compliance. They should also be considered in conditions in which peripheral nerve involvement is suspected but not documented by conventional nerve conduction velocity studies. In cases of suspected occupational peripheral nerve dysfunction, one must interpret test results with caution. Because of the sensitivity of QST, the clinician must be certain that no other cause of peripheral nerve dysfunction, such as diabetes, is causing the abnormalities.

OTHER NEUROPHYSIOLOGIC STUDIES

Several types of neurophysiologic tests are valuable in evaluating a wide variety of neurologic conditions but are rarely helpful in diagnosing neurologic injuries related to occupational exposures. The primary reasons for this is that these tests are either normal or are only mildly, nonspecifically abnormal.

Electromyography/Nerve Conduction Studies

Electromyography (EMG) and nerve conduction studies (NCV) are discussed in the evaluation of toxic neuropathies (see Chapter 8) and occupational carpal tunnel syndrome (see Chapter 9). In a suspected toxic neuropathy, typically a distal axonopathy, EMG/NCV studies may be normal in early cases or may reveal evidence of mild axonal changes. If these studies reveal demyelinating changes, the polyneuropathy is unlikely to be related to occupational toxic exposure.

NCVs are a widely used quantitative tool for the evaluation of peripheral nerve function.[111] Standard motor and sensory NCVs determine the maximal velocity of the fastest conducting fibers within a nerve. NCVs are extremely sensitive to demyelination changes but, as noted above, are a relatively poor and insensitive method for quantification of changes in axonopathies. Even if only a small number of fibers continue to conduct at normal velocities, NCVs can remain within normal limits. Measurement of amplitude of responses, though a more sensitive measure in axonopathies than NCVs, have wide variation of the response when recorded with standard methods using surface electrodes. The primary value of NCVs in the diagnosis of toxic neuropathies is in confirming the presence of a polyneuropathy and ruling out other causes of peripheral nerve dysfunction. Mononeuropathies and nerve entrapments, especially carpal tunnel syndrome, can also be documented.

The value of NCVs can be enhanced by using different special techniques. Collision techniques can be used to measure the conduction of slower-conducting fibers; measurement of long latency responses (F waves and H responses) may assess proximal segments of the nerve that are not accessible to direct stimulation; and paired stimuli or trains can be used to assess refractory periods and fatigue.

Evoked Potentials

Evoked potentials (EVPs) have rarely been used to evaluate occupational or other neurotoxic exposures and their value in detecting and characterizing these disorders is limited.

EVPs have been made possible by both recent advances in electrophysiologic procedures and microcomputer technology. They are in widespread use in clinical neurology as an index of the integrity of the sensory CNS pathways. When properly administered and interpreted,

EVPs can be used to assess a sensory pathway from receptor to cortex. The most widely used in the evaluation of neurotoxic disease and in the evaluation of other neurologic disorders are the visual evoked potential (VEP), auditory evoked potential (AEP), and somatosensory evoked potential (SEP).

EVPs have been used extensively to aid in the diagnosis of neurotoxic disease, but those studies related to occupational exposures have revealed limited abnormalities and must be interpreted with caution.[112] Marked AEP abnormalities have been seen related to toluene exposure,[113,114] but these studies were in toluene abusers, exposed to much higher levels than those in the occupational setting. Abnormalities on SEPs have been seen in association with the CNS manifestations of toxic distal axonopathies.[112]

Electroencephalography

With the advent of recent technological advances in the area of neuroimaging, electroencephalography (EEG), a method that has been used extensively in clinical neurology for decades, is now used less frequently as a neurodiagnostic method and more appropriately in the evaluation of epilepsy. EEG has been supplanted by computed tomographic (CT) scanning and MRI (see below) for the diagnosis of structural disorders of the CNS, though it is still widely used in the evaluation of epilepsy, encephalitides, and toxic and metabolic encephalopathies.

Conventionally performed EEG has been used in the evaluation of occupational neurotoxic exposures of many kinds.[115,116] However, the abnormalities seen are not specific for diagnosing neurotoxic disease, and its value in detecting and characterizing neurotoxicity is extremely limited.

Newer techniques, such as automated frequency and power analysis, available because of the use of microcomputers, permit a more quantitative assessment of the EEG. These techniques may be useful in studying groups of individuals exposed to various industrial chemicals, but have not yet been performed in the occupational setting.[117]

Neuroimaging Studies

Neuroimaging methods either evaluate anatomic or structural changes of the CNS (CT and MRI), or evaluate functional (e.g. metabolic, neurochemical, blood flow) characteristics of the CNS (positron emission tomography [PET] and single-photon emission CT [SPECT]). None of these expensive, labor-intensive techniques has been widely used in the evaluation of occupational or nonoccupational neurotoxic exposures, and their primary role is in diagnosis or evaluation of naturally occurring neurologic diseases. Neuroimaging studies are either normal or have not yet been studied in most neurotoxic disorders.

Structural Neuroimaging

Computed tomographic scanning   With the advent of CT scanning in the mid 1970s, visualization of the nervous system and other tissues was capable in detail that had previously not been available. In particular, visualization of the brain and spinal cord can now be identified in sub-millimeter detail and can be performed with such speed (with exposure times of 1–2 seconds) that studies can be performed even in individuals who are not fully cooperative. Ability to detect size and location of abnormalities based on anatomic changes is superior to that of prior methods; however, lack of specificity of these changes as well as the lack of metabolic information makes CT almost useless in the evaluation of neurotoxic injuries.

CT is valuable in ruling out other naturally occurring disorders of the nervous system. The use of CT in the evaluation of neurobehavioral disorders, traumatic head injuries, and occupational low back injuries is discussed elsewhere in the text.

CT scanning of the brain has revealed nonspecific changes, such as cerebral atrophy, in individuals chronically exposed to organic solvents in the workplace,[118] but other studies in similar populations have been negative.[119] The primary value of CT in the evaluation of dementias in the workplace setting has been to rule out other causes of dementia.[120] For a more detailed discussion of the use of CT in solvent-induced encephalopathies, see Chapter 4.

Magnetic resonance imaging   Combined with the discovery of nuclear magnetic resonance (1940s), CT technology (1970s), and improved signal detection in the 1980s, MRI was developed.[121] Major advantages of MRI over CT in imaging of the brain have been the ability to visualize abnormalities in the white matter[122] and a variety of traumatic, inflammatory, degenerative, and metabolic disorders.[123]

Neurotoxic disorders, as noted above, tend to mimic clinically these types of disorders; however, MRI has not been widely applied in the evaluation of neurotoxic disorders. It has been used in the evaluation of chronic toluene exposure, but only in the setting of inhalant abuse.[124–127] These studies have revealed that chronic high-level toluene, such as the kind seen in inhalant abuse, produces diffuse white matter changes[124–127] (Figure 2.1A). Studies using a 1.5 Tesla MRI scanner have revealed that in addition to the white matter changes, low signal intensity in the thalamus on T2-weighted images is also seen[128] (Figure 2.1B). Such abnormalities have not been seen in individuals exposed to the lower levels of toluene that occur in the occupational setting, but MRI has not been widely studied in exposed workers.

Several points are worthy of emphasis regarding this apparently unique finding in chronic toluene abuse and its relationship to lower-level exposures in industry. First, MRI may still become a useful tool

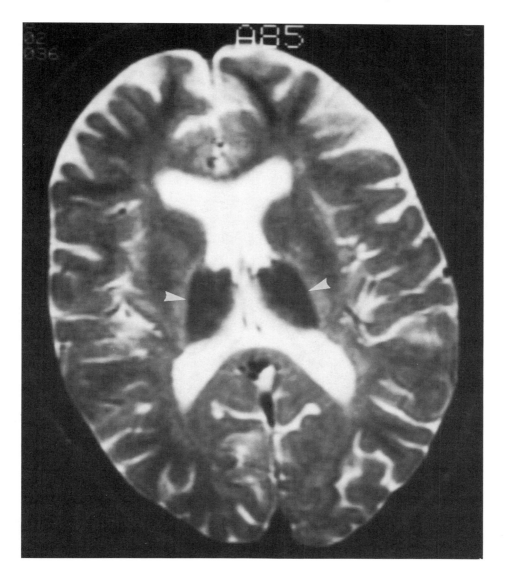

FIGURE 2.1A   T2-weighted image using a 1.5 Tesla magnetic resonance scanner in a chronic toluene inhalant abuser shows the low signal intensity in the thalamus bilaterally (arrows), in addition to the diffuse white matter changes.

for the study of neurotoxic exposures as it becomes applied more widely in the evaluation of neurotoxic disorders. Second, the extremely high-level exposures seen in the abuse setting emphasize the dose-response principle: The MRI changes seen in abuse but not occupation-

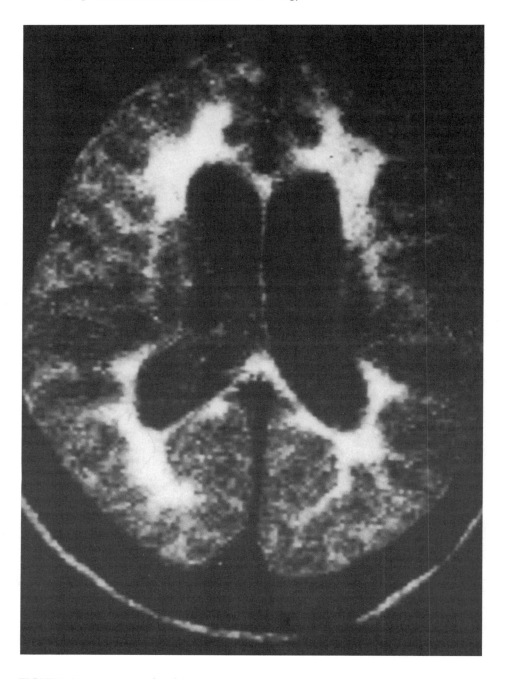

FIGURE 2.1B   T2-weighted image using a 0.35 Tesla magnetic resonance scanner in a chronic toluene inhalant abuser shows high signal intensity diffusely throughout the cerebral white matter.

al settings suggest that occupational-level exposures are insufficient to cause these changes. Third, the diffuse (or bilaterally symmetric) changes are in keeping with the principle that neurotoxins produce nonfocal disorders.

Finally, with the rapid advances occurring with MRI technology, we may soon see increasing use of MRI in the evaluation of neurotoxic injuries. This may be especially true as magnetic resonance spectroscopy (MRS) enters the clinical arena.[129] MRS may also increase the sensitivity so that nervous system abnormalities may even be detected after occupational-level exposures.

Functional Neuroimaging

Positron emission tomography   Many disorders affecting the nervous system, including neurotoxic disorders, fail to reveal anatomic changes of sufficient degree to produce abnormalities that can be visualized with CT or MRI, or reveal only nonspecific abnormalities. When this occurs, the ability to noninvasively measure metabolic activity, blood flow, or neurotransmitter receptors would be a tremendous advantage in the evaluation of these disorders. PET has been developed over the past two decades to look at these areas and is developing increasing applications in clinical neurology.[130]

During a PET scan, a tracer molecule tagged with a positron-emitting radioisotope is injected into the body. Positron decay results in an annihilation reaction that is the basis of PET imaging. When annihilation occurs, two photons of equal energy are given off in opposite directions. The PET scanner then produces images of the distribution of these photons in a single plane, thereby accurately localizing the tracer's biodistribution. PET has already been found to be valuable in the study and evaluation of several neurologic disorders, including epilepsy, stroke, and other types of cerebral ischemia; brain tumors; schizophrenia; Parkinson's disease and other movement disorders; and the dementias.[131,132] Many isotopes are available; however, the most commonly used in the evaluation of neurologic disorders are ^{15}O-labeled water (cerebral blood flow), [^{18}F]-fluorodeoxyglucose (glucose metabolism in the brain), and [^{18}F]- fluorodopa (for dopamine receptor mapping).

PET would appear to be an ideal tool to study the effects of neurotoxins on cerebral function, since most produce nonspecific or no anatomic changes visualized by CT or MRI. Unfortunately, PET has only been used to evaluate a few isolated cases of neurotoxic exposures. These have been in individuals in whom parkinsonism develops after exposure to MPTP (see Chapter 7 for details)[133] and cyanide.[134]

PET has been studied preliminarily in traumatic brain injuries[135–137] and may be used more in the future in the evaluation of both occupational (see Chapter 10) and nonoccupational head injuries.

As use of PET increases and becomes more accessible, studies on the use of PET in neurotoxic disorders and head trauma will increase and may someday become a valuable tool in the evaluation of these disorders.

Single photon emission computed tomography   SPECT is often referred to as "the poor man's PET" for obvious but inappropriate reasons. PET is complicated and expensive and requires on-site access to a cyclotron, which is generally beyond the capabilities of most medical centers. SPECT allows the study of regional cerebral metabolism and neurotransmitter receptor imaging with relatively good spatial resolution using equipment available in most nuclear medicine departments. While most studies of neurologic disorders have measured only regional cerebral blood flow, as newer radiopharmaceuticals become available, SPECT may be applied to the evaluation of a wider range of disorders and may rival PET in some areas.

Like PET, SPECT has primarily been used in the evaluation of Alzheimer's disease and other dementias[138–142] but has also been used in the evaluation of a variety of neuropsychiatric disorders,[143–145] epilepsy,[146,147] and traumatic brain injury.[148]

SPECT has not been utilized in the evaluation of neurotoxic disorders, although other methods of evaluating regional cerebral blood flow (by xenon[133] inhalation) have been studied in occupational organic solvent exposure.[149,150]

Because of the availability of SPECT and the development of new radioisotopes, studies of occupational neurotoxic and traumatic brain injuries will probably occur in the near future. Currently, although SPECT's utility has not been widely validated, there are some clinical situations related to occupational injuries in which use of SPECT may add useful clinical information (Plate 1).

Conclusions

A large number of neurodiagnostic tests are available in the clinical setting that allow the clinician to obtain a large amount of anatomic and physiologic information on an individual. In the evaluation of both naturally occurring and especially occupationally related neurologic disorders, a great deal of frustration can be avoided by the clinician and patient if the clinician spends more time obtaining a focused occupational history and performing a careful neurologic examination. This should avoid the random ordering of expensive tests, which will most likely only add confusion to an already complicated clinical situation if an abnormality on one of these tests needs to be explained.

References

1. World Health Organization. Identification and control of work-related diseases. Technical Report No. 174. Geneva: WHO, 1985.
2. Lee WR, McCallum RI. The Occupational History. In PAB Raffle, WR Lee, RI McCallum, R Murray (eds), Hunter's Diseases of Occupation. Boston: Little, Brown, 1987:229–236.
3. Imbus HR. Clinical Aspects of Occupational Medicine. In C Zenz (ed), Occupational Medicine. Chicago: Year Book, 1988:107–119.
4. Klaassen CD. Principles of Toxicology. In CD Klaassen, MO Amdur, J Doull (eds), Cassarett and Doull's Toxicology. The Basic Science of Poisons (3rd ed). New York: Macmillan, 1986:11–32.
5. Ballantyne B, Sullivan JB. Basic Principles of Toxicology. In JB Sullivan Jr, GR Krieger (eds), Hazardous Materials Toxicology. Baltimore: Williams & Wilkins, 1992:9–23.
6. Spencer PS, Schaumburg HH. Review of acrylamide neurotoxicity. II: Experimental animal neurotoxicity and pathologic mechanisms. Can J Neurol Sci 1974;1:152–169.
7. Rosenberg NL, Kleinschmidt-DeMasters BK, Davis KA, Dreisbach JN, Hormes JT, Filley CM. Toluene abuse causes diffuse central nervous system white matter changes. Ann Neurol 1988;23: 611–614.
8. Burns RS, Chiueh CC, Markey SP, Ebert MH, Jacobowitz DM, Kopin IJ. A primate model of parkinsonism: selective destruction of dopaminergic neurons in the pars compacta of the substantia nigra by n-methyl-4-phenyl-1,2,3,6 tetrahydropyridine. Proc Natl Acad Sci 1983;80:4546–4550.
9. Schaumburg HH, Spencer PS. Recognizing neurotoxic disease. Neurology 1987;37:276–278.
10. Bolla KI, Schwartz BS, Agnew J, Ford PD, Bleecker ML. Subclinical neuropsychiatric effects of chronic low-level solvent exposure in US paint manufacturers. J Occup Med 1990;32: 671–677.
11. DeJong RN (ed). The Neurologic Examination (4th ed). Hagerstown, MD: Harper & Row, 1979.
12. Engelberg, AL (ed). Guides to the Evaluation of Permanent Impairment (3rd ed). Chicago: American Medical Association, 1988.
13. Medical Research Council of United Kingdom. Aids to Examination of the Peripheral Nervous System. London: Pendragon House of North America, 1976.
14. Kurtzke JF. Disability rating scales in multiple sclerosis. Ann NY Acad Sci 1984;436:347–360.
15. Fahn S, Elton RL, and Members of the UPDRS Development Committee. Unified Parkinson Disease Rating Scale. In S Fahn, CD Marsden, M Goldstein et al. (eds), Recent Developments in Parkinson's Disease II. New York: Macmillan 1987;153–163.
16. Munsat TL (ed). Quantification of Neurologic Deficit. Newton, MA: Butterworth-Heinemann, 1989.
17. Hartman DE. Neuropsychological Toxicology: Identification and Assessment of Human Neurotoxic Syndromes. New York: Pergamon, 1988.
18. Hanninen H. Psychological test methods: sensitivity to longterm chemical exposure at work. Neurobehav Toxicol 1979;1:157–161.

19. White RF, Proctor SP. Research and clinical criteria for development of neu-robehavioral test batteries. J Occup Med 1992;34:140–148.
20. Tilson HA. Behavioral indices of neurotoxicity. Toxicologic Pathol 1990;18:96–104.
21. Hawkins KA. Occupational neurotoxicology: some neuropsychological issues and challenges. J Clin Exp Neuropsychol 1990;12:664–680.
22. National Institute for Occupational Safety and Health (NIOSH). Neurobehavioral research section publications: 1972 to present. Washington, DC: 1988.
23. Anger WK. Neurobehavioral testing of chemicals: impact on recommended standards. Neurobehav Toxicol Teratol 1984;6:147–153.
24. Anger WK. Neurobehavioral tests used in NIOSH-supported worksite studies, 1973–1983. Neurobehav Toxicol Teratol 1985;7:359–368.
25. Chaffin DB, Miller JM. Behavioral and Neurologic Evaluation of Workers Exposed to Inorganic Mercury. In C Xintaras, BL Johnson, I deGroot (eds), Behavioral Toxicology: Early Detection of Occupational Hazards. US Department of Health and Human Services (NIOSH) Publication No. 74-126. Washington, DC: US Government Printing Office, 1974.
26. Johnson BL, Cohen HH, Struble R, Setzer JV, Anger WK, Gutnik BD, McDonough T, Hauser P. Field Evaluation of Carbon Monoxide Exposed Toll Collectors. In C Xintaras, BL Johnson, I deGroot (eds), Behavioral Toxicology: Early Detection of Occupational Hazards. US Department of Health and Human Services (NIOSH) Publication No. 74-126. Washington, DC: US Government Printing Office, 1974.
27. Morgan BB, Repko JD. Evaluation of Behavioral Function in Workers Exposed to Lead. In C Xintaras, BL Johnson, I deGroot (eds), Behavioral Toxicology: Early Detection of Occupational Hazards. US Department of Health and Human Services (NIOSH) Publication No. 74-126. Washington, DC: US Government Printing Office, 1974.
28. Repko JD, Corum CR, Jones PD, Garcia LS Jr. The Effects of Inorganic Lead on Behavior and Neurologic Function. US Department of Health and Human Services (NIOSH) Publication No. 78-128. Washington, DC: US Government Printing Office, 1978.
29. Repko JD, Jones PD, Garcia LS, Schneider EJ, Roseman E, Corum CR. Behavioral and Neurologic Effects of Methyl Chloride. US Department of Health and Human Services (NIOSH) Publication No. 77-125. Washington, DC: US Government Printing Office, 1976.
30. Tuttle TC, Wood GD, Grether CB. Behavioral and Neurologic Evaluation of Workers Exposed to Carbon Disulfide. US Department of Health and Human Services (NIOSH) Publication No. 77-128. Washington, DC: US Government Printing Office, 1976.
31. Putz-Anderson V, Albright BE, Lee ST, Johnson BL, Chrislip DW, Taylor BJ, Brightwell WS, Dickerson N, Culver M, Zentmeyer D, Smith P. A behavioral examination of workers exposed to carbon disulfide. Neurotoxicology 1983;4:67–78.
32. Wayne LG, Bryan RJ, Ziedman K. Irritant Effects of Industrial Chemicals: Formaldehyde. US Department of Health and Human Services (NIOSH) Publication No. 777-117. Washington, DC: US Government Printing Office, 1976.

33. Tuttle TC, Wood GD, Grether CB, Johnson BL, Xintaras C. A Behavioral and Neurologic Evaluation of Dry Cleaners Exposed to Perchloroethylene. US Department of Health and Human Services (NIOSH) Publication No. 77-214. Washington, DC: US Government Printing Office, 1977.

34. Xintaras C, Burg JR, Tanaka S, Lee ST, Johnson BL, Cottrill CA, Bender J. NIOSH Health Survey of Velsicol Pesticide Workers. US Department of Health and Human Services (NIOSH) Publication No. 78-136. Washington, DC: US Government Printing Office, 1978.

35. Johnson BL, Burg JR, Xintaras C, Handke JL. A neurobehavioral examination of workers from a primary nonferrous smelter. Neurotoxicology 1980;1:561–581.

36. Ryan CM, Morrow LA, Bromet EJ, Parkinson DK. Assessment of neuropsychological dysfunction in the workplace: normative data from the Pittsburgh Occupational Exposures Test Battery. J Clin Exp Neuropsychol 1987;9:665–679.

37. Baker EL Jr, Feldman RG, White RF, Harley JP, Dinse GE, Berkey CS. Monitoring neurotoxins in industry: development of a neurobehavioral test battery. J Occup Med 1983;25:125–130.

38. Hanninen H, Lindstrom K. Behavioral Test Battery for Toxicopsychological Studies: Used at the Institute of Occupational Health in Helsinki. Helsinki: Institute of Occupational Health, 1979.

39. Valciukas JA, Lilis R. Psychometric techniques in environmental research. Environ Res 1980; 21: 275–297.

40. Letz R. Occupational screening for neurotoxicity computerized techniques. Toxicol 1988;49:417–424.

41. Letz R, Baker EL. Computer-administered neurobehavioral testing in occupational health. Semin Occup Med 1:197–203, 1986.

42. Baker EL, Letz R. Neurobehavioral testing in monitoring hazardous workplace exposures. J Occup Med 1986;28:987–990.

43. Baker EL, Letz R, Fidler A. A computer-administered neurobehavioral evaluation system for occupational and environmental epidemiology. Rationale, methodology and validation studies. J Occup Med 1985;27:206–212.

44. Baker EL, Letz RE, Fidler AT, Shalat S, Plantamura D, Lyndon M. A computer-based neurobehavioral evaluation system for occupational and environmental epidemiology: methodology and validation studies. Neurobehav Toxicol 1985; 7:369–377.

45. Letz R. Quantitative neurobehavioral testing in humans for assessing potential effects of occupational exposure. J Am Coll Toxicol 1989;8:303–309.

46. Agnew J, Schwartz BS, Bolla KI, Ford DP, Bleecker ML. Comparison of computerized and examiner-administered neurobehavioral testing techniques. J Occup Med 1991;33:1156–1162.

47. Grober E, Buschke H, Crystal H, Bang S, Dresner R. Screening for dementia by memory testing. Neurology 1988;38:900–903.

48. Schmitt FA, Ranseen JD, DeKosky ST. Cognitive mental status examinations. Clin Geriatric Med 1989;5:545–564.

49. Lindblom V, Tegner R. Quantification of Sensibility Inmononeuropathy, Polyneuropathy and Central Lesions. In TL Munsat (ed). Quantification of Neurologic Deficit. Boston: Butterworth-Heinemann, 1989;171–185.

50. Dyck PJ, O'Brien PC. Approaches to Quantitative Cutaneous Sensory Assessment. In TL Munsat (ed), Quantification of Neurologic Deficit. Newton, MA: Butterworth-Heineman, 1989:187–195.
51. O'Brien PC, Dyck PJ, Kosanke JL. A Computer Evaluation of Quantitative Algorithms for Measuring Detection Thresholds of Cutaneous Sensation. In TL Munsat (ed), Quantification of Neurologic Deficit. Boston: Butterworth-Heinemann, 1989;197–206.
52. LeQuesne PM, Fowler CJ, Parkhouse N. Quantitative Tests to Determine Peripheral Nerve Fiber Integrity. In TL Munsat (ed), Quantification of Neurologic Deficit. Boston: Butterworth-Heineman, 1989;207–220.
53. Adams RW, Burke D. Deficits of thermal sensation in patients with unilateral cerebral lesions. Electroenceph Clin Neurophysiol 1989;73:443–452.
54. Johansson RS, Vallbo AB, Westling G. Thresholds of mechanosensitive afferents in the human hand as measured with Von Frey hairs. Brain Res 1980;184:343–351.
55. Sekuler R, Nash D, Armstrong R. Sensitive objective procedure for evaluating response to light touch. Neurology 1973;23:1282–1291.
56. Levin S, Pearsall G, Ruderman RJ. Von Frey's method of measuring pressure sensibility in the hand: an engineering analysis of the Weinstein-Semmes pressure aesthesiometer. J Hand Surg 1978;3:211–216.
57. Lindblom V. Touch perception threshold in human glabrous skin in terms of displacement amplitude on stimulation with single mechanical pulses. Brain Res 1974;82:205–210.
58. Dyck PJ, Zimmerman IR, O'Brien PC, Ness A, Caskey PE, Karnes J, Bushek W. Introduction of automated systems to evaluate touch-pressure, vibration and thermal cutaneous sensation in man. 1978;Ann Neurol 4: 502–510.
59. Fruhstorfer H, Lindblom V, Schmidt WG. Method for quantitative estimation of thermal estimation of thermal thresholds in patients. J Neurol Neurosurg Psychiatry 1976;39:1071–1075.
60. Jamal GA, Hansen S, Weir AI, Ballantyne JP. An improved automated method for the measurement of thermal thresholds. 1. Normal subjects. J Neurol Neurosurg Psychiatry 1985;48:354–360.
61. Steiness IB. Vibratory perception in normal subjects. A biothesiometric study. Acta Med Scand 1957;158:315–325.
62. Goldberg JM, Lindblom V. Standardized method of determining vibratory perception thresholds for diagnosis and screening in neurologic investigation. J Neurol Neurosurg Psychiatry 1979;42:793–803.
63. Haloren P. Quantitative vibration perception thresholds in healthy subjects of working age. Eur J Appl Physiol 1986;54: 647–655.
64. Arezzo JC, Schaumburg HH, Laudadio C. The vibratron: a simple device for quantitative evaluation of tactile/vibratory sense. Neurology 1985;35(Suppl 1):169.
65. Bleecker ML. Quantifying sensory loss in peripheral neuropathies. Neurobehav Toxicol Teratol 1985;7:305–308.
66. Hahn JF. Cutaneous vibratory thresholds for square-wave electrical pulses. Science 1958;127:879–880.
67. Sigel H. Cutaneous sensory threshold stimulation with high frequency square-wave current. I. Relationship of electrode dimensions to sensory threshold. J Invest Dermatol 1952;18:441–445.

68. Sigel H. Cutaneous sensory threshold stimulation with high frequency square-wave current. II. Relationship of body site and of skin disease to the sensory threshold. J Invest Dermatol 1952;18:447–451.
69. Conomy JP, Barnes KL. Quantitative assessment of cutaneous sensory function in subjects with neurologic disease. J Neurol Sci 1976;30:221–235.
70. Bütikofer R, Lawrence PD. Electrocutaneous nerve stimulation. I. Model and experiment. IEEE Trans Biomed Eng BME 1978;25:526–531.
71. Joss G. Unusual phenomenon in electrical properties of mammalian skin. Nature 1964;201:418–419.
72. Davis DR, Kennard DW. Influence of electric current on skin. Nature 1962;193:1186–1187.
73. Mueller EE, Loeffel R, Mead S. Skin impedance in relation to pain threshold testing by electrical means. J Appl Physiol 1953;5:746–752.
74. Notermans SLH. Measurement of pain threshold determined by electrical stimulation and its clinical application. Part I. Method and factors possibly influencing the pain threshold. Neurology 1966;16:1071–1086.
75. Tursky B, Watson PD. Controlled physical and subjective intensities of electric shock. Psychophysiology 1964;1:151–162.
76. Sjölund BH, Eriksson MBE. Influence of naloxone on analgesia produced by peripheral conditioning stimulation. Brain Res 1979;173:295–301.
77. Katims JJ, Naviasky EH, Ng LKY, Rendell M, Bleecker ML. New screening device for assessment of peripheral neuropathy. J Occup Med 1986;28:1219–1221.
78. Katims JJ, Naviasky EH, Rendell M, Ng LKY, Bleecker ML. Constant current sine wave transcutaneous nerve stimulation for the evaluation of peripheral neuropathy. Arch Phys Med Rehab 1987;68:210–213.
79. Katims JJ, Long DM, Ng LKY. Transcutaneous nerve stimulation: Frequency and waveform specificity in humans. Appl Neurophysiol 1986;49:86–91.
80. Weseley SA, Sadler B, Katims JJ. Current perception: preferred test for evaluation of peripheral nerve integrity. ASAIO Trans 1988;34:188–193.
81. Katims JJ, Long DM, Ng LKY. Transcutaneous nerve stimulation (TNS): frequency and waveform specificity in humans. Appl Neurophysiol 1986;49:86–91.
82. Masson EA, Boulton AJM. The "neurometer": validation and comparison with conventional tests for diabetic neuropathy. Diabetic Med 1991;8:S63–66.
83. Arezzo JC, Schaumburg HH. The use of the Optacon® as a screening device: a new technique for detecting sensory loss in individuals exposed to neurotoxins. J Occup Med 1980;22:461–464.
84. Moody L, Arezzo JC, Otto D. Evaluation of workers for early peripheral neuropathy: the role of existing diagnostic tools. Semin Occup Med 1986;1:153–162.
85. Bove F, Litwak MS, Arezzo JC, Baker EL Jr. Quantitative sensory testing in occupational medicine. Semin Occup Med 1986;1:185–189.
86. Arezzo JC, Schaumburg HH, Petersen CA. Rapid screening for peripheral neuropathy: a field study with the Optacon. Neurology 1983;33:626–629.
87. Bove FJ, Letz R, Baker EL Jr. Sensory thresholds among construction trade painters: a cross-sectional study using new methods for measuring temperature and vibration sensitivity. J Occup Med 1989;31:320–325.
88. Lindblom V, Verrillo RT. Sensory functions in chronic neuralgia. J Neurol Neurosurg Psychiatry 1979;42:422–435.

89. Werner JL, Omer GE Jr. Evaluating cutaneous passive sensation of the hand. Am J Occup 1970;24:347–356.
90. Dellon AL. The moving two-point discrimination test: clinical evaluation of the quickly adapting fiber/receptor system. J Hand Surg 1978;3:474–481.
91. Dellon AL. Clinical use of vibratory stimuli to evaluate peripheral nerve injury and compression neuropathy. Plast Reconstr Surg 1980;65:466–476, 1980.
92. Szabo RM, Gelberman RH, Dimick MP. Sensibility testing in patients with carpal tunnel syndrome. J Bone Joint Surg 1984;66A:60–64.
93. Borg K, Lindblom V. Diagnostic value of quantitative sensory testing (QST) in carpal tunnel syndrome. Acta Neurol Scand 1988;78:537–541.
94. Jetzer TC. Use of vibration testing in the early evaluation of workers with carpal tunnel syndrome. J Occup Med 1991;33:117–120.
95. Radwin RG, Wertsch JJ, Jeng O-J, Casanova J. Ridge detection tactile deficits associated with carpal tunnel syndrome. J Occup Med 33:730–736, 1991.
96. Borg K, Lindblom V. Increase of vibration threshold during wrist flexion in patients with carpal tunnel syndrome. Pain 1986;26:211–219.
97. Jamal GA, Weir AI, Hansen S, Ballantyne JP. An improved automated method for the movement of thermal thresholds. 2. Patients with peripheral neuropathy. J Neurol Neurosurg Psychiatry 1985;48:361–366.
98. Jamal GA, Hansen S, Weir AI, Ballantyne JP. The neurophysiologic investigation of small fiber neuropathies. Muscle Nerve 1987;10:537–545.
99. Guy RJC, Clark CA, Malcolm PN, Watkins PJ. Evaluation of thermal and vibration sensation in diabetic neuropathy. Diabetologia 1985;28:131–137.
100. Bertelsmann FW, Heimans JJ, Weber EJM, van der Veen EA. Thermal discrimination thresholds in normal subjects and in patients with diabetic neuropathy. J Neurol Neurosurg Psychiatry 1985;48:686–690.
101. Arezzo JC, Schaumburg HH, Laudadio C. Thermal sensitivity tester: device for quantitative assessment of thermal sense in diabetic neuropathy. Diabetes 1986;35:590–592.
102. Dyck PJ, Bushek W, Spring EM, Karnes JL, Litchy WJ, O'Brien PC, Service FJ. Vibrations and cooling detection thresholds compared with other tests in diagnosing and staging diabetic neuropathy. Diabetes Care 1987;10:432–440.
103. Sosenko JM, Kato M, Soto RA, Gadia MT, Ayyar DR. Specific assessments of warm and cool sensitivities in adult diabetic patients. Diabetes Care 1988;11: 481–483.
104. Levy D, Abraham R, Reid G. A comparison of two methods for measuring thermal thresholds in diabetic neuropathy. J Neurol Neurosurg Psychiatry 1989;52:1072–1077.
105. Rendell MS, Katims JJ, Richter R, Rowland F. A comparison of nerve conduction velocities and current perception thresholds as correlates of clinical severity of diabetic sensory neuropathy. J Neurol Neurosurg Psychiatry 1989;52:502–511.
106. Report and recommendations of the San Antonio conference on diabetic neuropathy. Diabetes 1988;37:1000–1004.
107. Lindsay R, Henderson L. Adequacy of dialysis. Kidney Int 1988;33:592–599.
108. Weseley SA, Katims JJ, Liebowitz B. Neuropathy of uremia: assessment by nerve conduction times versus current perception thresholds. Kidney Int 1988;31:241.

109. Tegner R, Lindholm B. Vibratory perception threshold compared with nerve conduction velocity in the evaluation of uremic neuropathy. Acta Neurol Scand 1985;71:284–289.
110. Lindblom V, Tegner R. Thermal sensitivity in uremic neuropathy. Acta Neurol Scand 1985;71:290–294.
111. Kimura J. Electrodiagnosis in diseases of nerve and muscle: principles and practice. Philadelphia: FA Davis, 1983.
112. Arezzo JA, Simson R, Brennan NE. Evoked potentials in the assessment of neurotoxicity in humans. Neurobehav Toxicol Teratol 1985;7:299–304.
113. Metrick SA, Brenner RP. Abnormal brainstem auditory evoked potentials in chronic paint sniffers. Ann Neurol 1982;12:553–556.
114. Rosenberg NL, Spitz MC, Filley CM, Davis KA, Schaumburg HH. Central nervous system effects of chronic toluene abuse—clinical, brainstem evoked response and magnetic resonance imaging studies. Neurotoxicol Teratol 1988;10:489–495.
115. Seppalainen AM. Neurotoxic effects of industrial solvents. Electroenceph Clin Neurophysiol 1973;34:702–703.
116. Seppalainen AM. Neurophysiological findings among worker exposed to organic solvents. Acta Neurol Scand 1982;66(Suppl 92):109–116.
117. Eccles CU. EEG correlates of neurotoxicity. Neurotoxicol Teratol 1988;10:423–428.
118. Jensen PB, Nielsen P, Nielsen NO, Olivarius B deF, Hansen JH. Chronic toxic encephalopathy following occupational exposure to organic solvents. The course after cessation of exposure illustrated by a neurophysiological follow-up investigation. Ugeskr Laeg 1984;146:1387–1390.
119. Orbaek P, Lindgren M, Olivecrona H, Haeger-Aronsen B. Computed tomography and psychometric test performances in patients with solvent induced chronic toxic encephalopathy and healthy controls. Br J Ind Med 1987;44:175–179.
120. Bradshaw JR, Thomson JLG, Campbell MJ. Computed tomography in the investigation of dementia. Br Med J 1983;286:277–280.
121. Edelman RR, Kleefield J, Wentz KU, Atkinson DJ. Basic Principles of Magnetic Resonance Imaging. In RR Edelman, JR Hesselink (eds), Clinical Magnetic Resonance Imaging. Philadelphia: Saunders, 1990:3–38.
122. Hesselink JR, Hicks RJ. Brain: Periventricular White Matter Abnormalities. In RR Edelman, JR Hesselink (eds), Clinical Magnetic Resonance Imaging. Philadelphia: Saunders, 1990:545–562.
123. Hicks RJ, Hesselink JR, Wismer GL, Davis KR Brain: Trauma, Inflammation, and Degenerative and Metabolic Disorders. In RR Edelman, JR Hesselink (eds), Clinical Magnetic Resonance Imaging. Philadelphia: Saunders, 1990:563–597.
124. Rosenberg NL, Kleinschmidt-DeMasters BK, Davis KA, Dreisbach JN, Hormes JT, Filley CM. Toluene abuse causes diffuse central nervous system white matter changes. Ann Neurol 1988;23:611–614.
125. Rosenberg NL, Spitz MC, Filley CM, Davis KA, Schaumburg HH. Central nervous system effects of chronic toluene abuse—clinical, brainstem evoked response and magnetic resonance imaging studies. Neurotoxicol Teratol 1988;10:489–495.
126. Filley CM, Franklin GM, Heaton RK, Rosenberg NL. White matter dementia: clinical disorders and implications. Neuropsychiatry Neuropsychol Behav Neurology 1989;1:239–254.

127. Filley CM, Heaton RK, Rosenberg NL. White matter dementia in chronic toluene abuse. Neurology 1990;40(3):532–534.
128. Rosenberg NL, Dreisbach J, Seibert C, Latchaw R, Brown M. 1.5 Tesla MRI findings in toluene patients. Neurology 1991;41(Suppl 1):237.
129. Atkinson DJ, Martin JF, Brown MA, Koutcher JA, Burt CT, Ballon D. Clinical Spectroscopy. In RR Edelman, JR Hesselink (eds), Clinical Magnetic Resonance Imaging. Philadelphia: Saunders, 1990:269-312.
130. Hubner KF, Collmann J, Buonocore E, Kabalka GW (eds). Clinical Positron Emission Tomography. St. Louis: Mosby-Year Book, 1992.
131. Council on Scientific Affairs: Positron emission tomography—a new approach to brain chemistry. JAMA 1988;260:2704-2910.
132. Fulham MJ. Clinical Applications of PET in Neurology. In KF Hubner, J Collmann, E Buonocore, GW Kabalka (eds), Clinical Positron Emission Tomography. St. Louis: Mosby-Year Book, 1992:42–49.
133. Calne DB, Langston JW, Martin WRW, Stoessel AJ, Ruth TJ, Adam MJ, Pate B, Schulzer M. Positron emission tomography after MPTP: Observations relating to the cause of Parkinson's disease. Nature 1985;317:246–248.
134. Rosenberg NL, Myers JA, Martin WRW. Cyanide-induced parkinsonism: clinical, MRI, and fluorodopa PET studies. Neurology 1989;39:142–144.
135. Alavi A. Functional and anatomical studies of head injury. J Neuropsych 1989;1:S45–50.
136. Alavi A, Fazekas T, Alves W et al. Positron emission tomography in the evaluation of head injury. J Cereb Blood Flow Metab 1987;7:S646.
137. Rao N, Turski PA Polcyn RE et al. [18]F positron emission computed tomography in closed-head injury. Arch Phys Med Rehab 1984;5:780–785.
138. Jagust WJ, Budinger TF, Reed BR. The diagnosis of dementia with single photon emission computed tomography. Arch Neurol 1987;44:258–262.
139. Celsis P, Agniel A, Puel M, Rascol A, Marc-Vergnes J-P. Focal cerebral hypoperfusion and selective cognitive deficit in dementia of the Alzheimer type. J Neurol Neurosurg Psychiatry 1987;50:1602–1612.
140. Neary D, Snowden JS, Shields RA, Burjan AW, Northen B, Macdermott N, Prescott MC, Testa HJ. Single photon emission tomography using ^{99m}Tc-HM-PAO in the investigation of dementia. J Neurol Neurosurg Psychiatry 1987;50:1101–1109.
141. Johnson KA, Mueller ST, Walshe TM, English RJ, Holman BL. Cerbral perfusion imaging in Alzheimer's disease: use of single photon emission computed tomography and iofetamine hydrochloride I 123. Arch Neurol 1987;44:165–168.
142. Johnson KA, Holman L, Mueller SP, Rosen J, English R, Nagel JS, Growdon JH. Single photon emission computed tomography in Alzheimer's disease: abnormal iofetamine I 123 uptake reflects dementia severity. Arch Neurol 1988;45:392–396.
143. Paulman RG, Devous MD Sr, Gregory RR, Herman JH, Jennings L, Bonte FJ, Nasrallah HA, Raese JD. Hypofrontality and cognitive impairment in schizophrenia: dynamic single-photon tomography and neuropsychological assessment of schizophrenic brain function. Biol Psychiatry 1990;27:377–399.
144. Smith FW, Besson JAO, Gemmell HG, Sharp PF. The use of technetium-99m-HM-PAO in the assessment of patients with dementia and other neuropsychiatric conditions. J Cereb Blood Flow Metab 1988;8:S116–S122.

145. Trzepacz PT, Hertweck M, Starratt C, Zimmerman L, Adatepe MH. The relationship of SPECT scans to behavioral dysfunction in neuropsychiatric patients. Psychsomatics 1992;33:61–71.

146. Ryding E, Rosen I, Elmqvist D, Ingvar DH. SPECT measurements with ^{99m}Tc-HM-PAO in focal epilepsy. J Cereb Blood Flow Metab 1988;8:S95–S100.

147. Duncan R, Patterson J, Hadley DM, Macpherson P, Brodie MJ, Bone I, McGeorge AP, Wyper DJ. CT, MR and SPECT imaging in temporal lobe epilepsy. J Neurol Neurosurg Psychiatry 1990;53:11–15.

148. Gray BG, Ichise M, Chung D-G, Kirsh JC, Franks W. Technetium-99m-HMPAO SPECT in the evaluation of patients with a remote history of traumatic brain injury: a comparison with x-ray computed tomography. J Nuclear Med 1992;33:52–58.

149. Hagstadius S, Risberg J. Regional Cerebral Blood Flow in Subjects Occupationally Exposed to Organic Solvents. In R Gilioli, MG Cassitto, V Foa V (eds), Neurobehavioral Methods in Occupational Health. Oxford, England: Pergamon, 1983:211–217.

150. Arlien-Soborg P, Henriksen L, Gade A, Glydensted C, Paulson, OB. Cerebral blood flow in chronic toxic encephalopathy in house painters exposed to organic solvents. Acta Neurol Scand 1982;66:34–41.

CHAPTER 3

Determination of Causality and the Impairment Rating Process

Neil L. Rosenberg, M.D.

Determinations of work-relatedness (causality) and impairment are processes that are not enthusiastically undertaken by most physicians. Determining causality is often difficult but very important in the workers' compensation arena. The treating physician often is asked to determine causality based on a worker's word against someone else. With this in mind, however, an approach that uses the scientific method will be discussed, which will allow the physician to differentiate between a possible relationship between the workplace and disease and a probable cause.

The determination of impairment related to a work-related injury is a commonly performed process, which varies greatly from state to state depending on the requirements of the worker's compensation system. Many states have adopted laws requiring the use of the American Medical Association's (AMA's) *Guides to the Evaluation of Permanent Impairment*[1] in the physician's evaluation of a patient for the purpose of determining impairment rating. Many have criticized the *Guides'* use for this purpose because of the lack of scientific basis for how impairment percentages are derived; the *Guides* nevertheless represent an attempt to quantify impairment by using clinical parameters. It is also certain that in the near future more states will adopt use of the *Guides* as part of attempts to achieve greater degrees of standardization among physicians performing impairment ratings, which should help reduce the often adversarial situation that exists in many state systems of worker's compensation.

This chapter uses the fourth edition of the *Guides* as a critical part of determining impairment rating in individuals with occupational neurologic injuries. Although the focus is on determining neurologic impairment, general aspects of use of the *Guides* and impairment evaluations are discussed.

Causation

Analysis of cause-and-effect relationships is often the weakest link in cases involving workplace exposures and injuries. Understanding of basic principles of causation analysis, particularly in cases of toxic exposures, is critical for the physician to have a methodology that is scientifically rigorous and defensible. Defensibility is required in situations of the workplace since the legal system is usually used for workers to obtain compensation for alleged injuries, whether through worker's compensation or through tort systems.[2] The following descriptions of terminology and concepts relate generally to issues of causality:

1. Cause: an agent, circumstance, or event capable of producing a new effect or aggravating an already existing effect.
2. Effect: a diagnosis, status, function, or condition that can result from or be aggravated by a cause.
3. Medical probability: from a medical standpoint, something that is more likely (greater than 50%) than not to be true.
4. Medical possibility: from a medical standpoint, a notion that is less likely (less than 50%) than not to be true.
5. Aggravation: a stimulus that can worsen the existing state of affairs of a susceptible condition.
   a. Temporary: occurs when the existing status of an ongoing problem is temporarily worsened compared to what the status would have been predicted to have been had the exposure or event not occurred; in these situations, the individual is expected to eventually recover to the status that was predicted by the natural history of the problem.
   b. Permanent: occurs when the existing status of an ongoing problem is permanently worsened compared to what the status would have been predicted to have been had the exposure or event not occurred; in these situations, the individual is *not* expected to recover to the status that was predicted by the natural history of the problem.

When attempting to assess causation in most cases in the workplace setting, the circumstances will be very similar to those in the nonoccupational setting. Identification of medically probable cause-and-effect relationships will usually be a logical process. In many situations related to the occupational setting, however, a case will present in which the diagnosis is straightforward but the identification of probable cause is more difficult. This is particularly true when several possible causes are identified, making the job of separating work-related and non–work-related factors even more difficult. Much of this can be minimized as long as an accurate history is obtained, complete examination is performed, and key principles

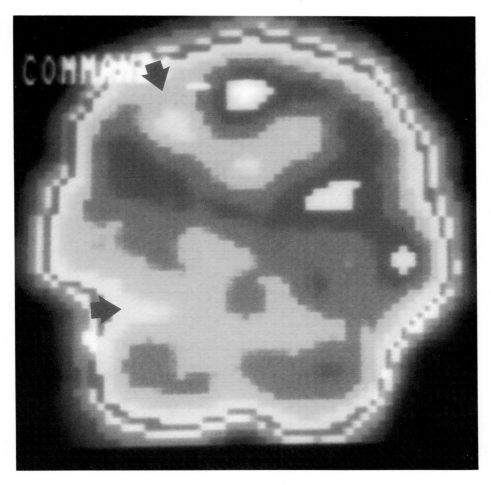

PLATE 1A Single-photon emission computed tomography (SPECT) scan (after intravenous injection of technetium-99m-HM-PAO) of the brain in an individual in whom complex partial epilepsy developed after an acute occupational exposure to hydrochloric acid gas emitted from a chemical reaction involved in a photographic equipment cleaning process. SPECT reveals decreased activity in the right temporal and frontal regions (arrow) correlating to an EEG abnormality. MRI and CT scans were normal.

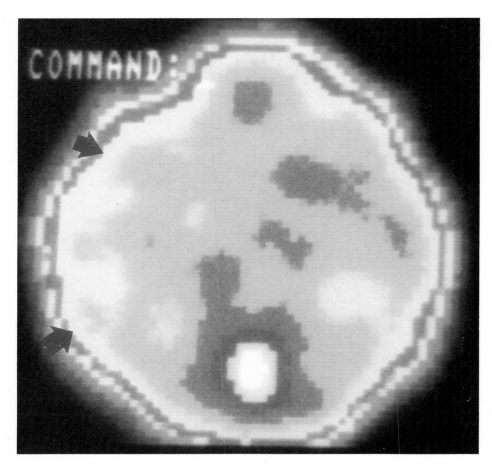

PLATE 1B   SPECT scan (after intravenous injection of technetium-99m-HM-PAO) of the brain in a 27-year-old woman in whom persistent mild cognitive impairment developed after a moderate carbon monoxide exposure (mild transient encephalopathy but no loss of consciousness) at work from a faulty furnace. CT and MRI scans were normal, but an EEG revealed some mild intermittent slowing over the right hemisphere, correlating with decreased activity over the right frontal, temporal, and parietal lobes on this SPECT scan.

are followed (see Chapter 2). There will still be certain situations, particularly those related to possible neurotoxic injuries, where additional approaches to assessing causation are needed.

The Scientific Methodology for Causation Analysis in Neurotoxic Exposures

Neurotoxic disorders represent some of the more common problems that require evaluation related to workplace exposures.[3] Because of this, alleged neurotoxic disorders create problems for physicians arising from worker's compensation or tort litigation, in proving that an injury did (or did not) arise from workplace exposure to a potentially neurotoxic substance. The evaluating physician should adhere to a formalized process of cause and effect analysis. This will allow the physician to be consistent in his or her methodology of assessing causation and applying those methods to the facts in any case.

Before presenting a method of assessing causation, several definitions of terms are offered:

1. Exposure: the opportunity for contact with a chemical. Exposure is assessed by measuring through analytical techniques the presence of a chemical in the environment (air, water, soil, clothing).
2. Dose: the amount of a chemical that is absorbed by the body. Dose is assessed by measuring the amount of a chemical present in body fluids and tissues. It is possible to have been exposed to a chemical but not to have received a dose.
3. Dose-response: a fundamental principle of toxicology discussed in more detail in Chapter 2. Dose-response is often described mathematically and is the extent of the response to an agent that will be directly related to the dose. All effects are related to the dose. If a sufficient dose occurs to produce an effect, then the extent of the response will be proportionate to the dose. This principle was first stated by Paracelsus in the sixteenth century: "All substances are poisons: There is none that is not a poison. The right dose differentiates a poison and a remedy."[4] All chemicals are toxic to some tissues in some species at some dose. Conversely, there is some dose at which no toxicity is apparent.
4. Threshold: the amount (dose) of a substance below which no effect will occur.
5. Effect: a change from a baseline state that is produced in response to a chemical. An effect may not be a toxic effect. Note: The definition for effect as it is used here is different from that used previously for causality.

6.   Toxic effect: an effect that, if sustained at a sufficient degree of intensity, may become an adverse health consequence. A chemically caused toxic effect on the nervous system should be completely reversible if exposure is terminated before pathologic alteration of the nervous system (neurotoxic effect).

7.   Adverse health effect: a condition that can impair one's ability to carry out normal activities of daily living or potentially shorten life.

8.   Neurotoxic effect: a toxic effect that is sustained for a sufficient period of time at a sufficient intensity to produce pathologic alteration to the peripheral or central nervous systems. A neurotoxic effect has the potential for not being completely reversible.

ASSOCIATION AND CAUSATION

Identification of toxic hazards is often inferred through epidemiologic studies. Epidemiologic studies have led both to overestimating and underestimating risk, based on different interpretations of the data.[5] In most situations in which epidemiologic studies have found an increased association between a toxic exposure and a disease (see Chapter 13), the association is weak and not sufficient to reliably assume that the exposure caused the disease. Unfortunately, the uncertainties in epidemiologic studies are frequently large enough to be significant in the legal arena, where the standards for scientific causation are not stringently adhered to.[6] The apparent correlations or associations produced in epidemiologic studies do not by themselves establish the existence of a cause and effect relationship between a chemical exposure and a particular health condition for a given individual.

ASSESSING CAUSATION

When evaluating for human toxicity to a chemical, two criteria must be established: First, an individual must be exposed to a chemical agent that is capable of producing the particular toxic effect. Second, the chemical must produce the particular toxic effect at the specific dose level the individual received. As simple as these concepts appear, often cases come into question in which an individual has either not been known to be exposed to an agent capable of causing toxic effects in humans at any dose, or it is not known if the person was exposed to any chemical in the workplace at all.

Causation analysis is a formalized process with principles and methods that have been refined with the advancements of scientific knowledge.[7] Any physician asked to assess cause-and-effect relationships for exposure to a chemical and some clinical situation must follow a general methodology that is scientifically rigorous and defensible. Causation analysis is not simply a matter for personal experience or opinion in the absence of such a defined scientific methodology. Thus, one needs to consider such factors as the qualitative toxicology of the chemical in question, the individual's opportunity for exposure, the degree and duration of exposure, the dose of the chemical received, the clinical condition of the individual (including a differential diagnosis), and the biologic plausibility of the association.

Henle-Koch-Evans (HKE) Postulates

Most physicians are familiar with the first efforts to develop a formalized process for causation analysis. First proposed over a century ago by Robert Koch, bacteriologist and Nobel Prize winner, Koch's postulates were developed for establishing the causes of infectious diseases. Some of these postulates were first attributed to Koch's teacher, Henle. These were later restated by Evans[8,9] and then referred to as Henle-Koch-Evans (HKE) postulates.[10] These criteria are listed in Table 3.1.

Most physicians and scientists would agree that if evidence is available that fulfills HKE postulates, causation would not be in doubt. However, it is not very common that these criteria, most easily satisfied for infectious diseases, are satisfied for the toxic effects of chemicals.

The Hill Criteria

In 1965, Sir Bradford Hill[11] further developed this same scientific method for the characterization of chemical hazards in the occupational setting. These criteria are listed in Table 3.2. Most scientists apply Hill's criteria particularly when assessing causation from epidemiologic studies, but these are also used in some form as the basis of the scientific method for establishing medical causation in general. Others have also contributed to the development of similar criteria in other settings.[12,13]

SPECULATION IN THE APPROACH TO CAUSATION ANALYSIS

The current set of criteria that have been proposed as the scientific basis for establishing causation include the strength of the association, its consistency, specificity, time course, dose-response, biological plausibility, experimental association, analogy, confounders, and the coherence of evidence. This widely accepted scientific method to establish a causal link between a chemical and disease requires review of the data, including a critical analysis of the toxicologic literature to determine whether these criteria are met.

In cases in which worker's compensation or tort litigation is involved, a physician or other expert must consider a number of factors in order to express an opinion regarding causation of a particular exposure to a medical diagnosis. However, in the legal arena, where a jury decides in favor of the side that has established its claim by the "preponderance of evidence," causation is not necessarily determined by the scientific method. Rather, the determination in the legal setting is based on being

TABLE 3.1
Henle-Koch-Evans Postulates

1. The disease is significantly more prevalent in those exposed to the hypothe-sized cause than in unexposed control subjects.
2. Exposure is more frequent among those with the disease than in controls without the disease.
3. Prospective studies show a significantly higher incidence of disease in those exposed than in those unexposed.
4. Disease should follow exposure after an incubation period that tracks a log-normal curve.
5. Host responses should follow exposure along a logical biological gradient from mild to severe.
6. Exposure should produce a measurable response with high probability (e.g., antibodies, cancer cells) or increase the magnitude of the response if already present before exposure occurred. This pattern should occur infrequently or never in unexposed persons.
7. Reproduction of the disease in experimental animals or human subjects (vol-unteers) or by controlled regulation of natural exposure should occur more frequently in those exposed than in those not exposed.
8. Elimination or modification of the suspected agent should decrease the inci-dence of disease.
9. Prevention or modification of the host's response on exposure should decrease or eliminate the disease.
10. All of the relationships and findings should be biologically plausible and make scientific sense.

TABLE 3.2
Hill's Criteria of Causation in Occupational Settings

1. Strength of association
2. Consistency of association
3. Specificity of association
4. Temporality
5. Biologic gradient (referring to dose-response relationship)
6. Plausibility (biological plausibility)
7. Coherence (should not conflict with known facts of natural history and biolo-gy of disease)
8. Experiment (i.e., does preventive action prevent the disease?)
9. Analogy (i.e., is a similar situation known to occur from a different exposure?)

medically probable (more likely than not), and is a judgmental decision the jury must make on the basis of often conflicting evidence presented by medical experts on both sides in a case. It is hoped, and is probably true in most incidences, that a case is decided in a way that is consistent with mainstream scientific opinion. However, in cases in which witnesses present radically different views, differentiating what is considered accepted scientific opinion versus what represents interpretations of an extreme minority of scientists can be extremely confusing to a lay jury.

The opinion of the scientific community is that "experts" who do not follow the established scientific approach to causation analysis engage in nothing more than speculation.[2,5,6] It has been suggested that certain criteria need to be applied in the assessment of expert witnesses in order to improve the quality of testimony, particularly in toxic tort situations.[14,15]

Most of the problems involved in "experts" assigning causation of a disorder to an exposure is reasoning by the use of *post hoc, ergo propter hoc* (after the fact, therefore, because of the fact). This circular "logic" is illustrated in the following situation: A person is possibly exposed to an agent and then symptoms or some type of medical condition develops. It is argued that the symptoms or medical condition "prove" that sufficient exposure occurred to cause the injury. Then, it is argued that since there is proof of sufficient exposure, the exposure to the alleged agent is the likely cause of the symptoms or medical condition. In essence, the symptoms become the basis for explaining themselves. Such "logic" should not be acceptable to the scientific and medical communities and should be guarded against. The scientific standards for causation analysis should be followed as outlined previously. When all data needed to make such a scientific analysis are not available, they either need to be obtained (by obtaining additional records or by doing additional studies) or one must admit the limits of the analysis. Scientific speculation should be avoided at all costs.

Basic Principles of the Impairment Rating Process

Once causation of an illness or injury is determined to be related to an occupational factor, determination of impairment is usually undertaken. The impairment rating process for work-related injuries is usually determined by the division of worker's compensation of a state's department of labor. In a growing number of instances, determination of impairment involves the use of the *AMA Guides to the Evaluation of Permanent Impairment*.[1] Determination of neurologic impairment, the focus of this section, is relatively easy to perform, if one obtains the appropriate clinical information.

HISTORY OF THE AMERICAN MEDICAL ASSOCIATION GUIDES

The creation of the *Guides* dates to 1956, when the Board of Trustees of the American Medical Association created a committee to address issues of medical impairment. As a result of the meetings of this committee, 13 publications appeared in the *Journal of the American Medical Association (JAMA)* between 1958 and 1970 related to issues of medical impairment. In 1971, the first edition of the *Guides* was published as a compilation of these 13 articles.

An advisory panel was established in 1981 that included 12 panels of experts, each of which was to address a major organ system. Subsequent editions of the *Guides* appeared in 1984 (2nd edition), 1988 (3rd edition), 1990 (3rd edition, revised), and most recently 1993 (4th edition). Each subsequent edition has included significant changes from prior editions. The increasing rate of change is only partly due to increasing knowledge, with much change related to expanded use of the *Guides*.

The use of the *Guides* has expanded to the point that 40 of 53 jurisdictions (38 of 50 states, Puerto Rico, and the Virgin Islands) reported that use of the *Guides* is either mandated or recommended by law in worker's compensation cases, or that the *Guides* is frequently used in the evaluation of such cases. States and other jurisdictions that do not frequently use or mandate use of the *Guides* include Alabama, California, the District of Columbia, Illinois, Michigan, Minnesota, Missouri, New Jersey, New York, North Carolina, Pennsylvania, West Virginia, and Wisconsin. At the time of this 1991 survey of chief executives of the 50 state worker's compensation agencies and those of Puerto Rico, the Virgin Islands, and Washington, DC, mandatory use of the *Guides* was in litigation in the state of Texas.[16] It is essential that one is familiar with the laws of the state(s) in which one is practicing. For example, in the state of Colorado, a law has been passed (Senate Bill 218) that states: "All physical impairment ratings shall be based on the revised 3rd edition of the American Medical Association *Guides to the Evaluation of Permanent Impairment* in effect as of July 1, 1991." This is being done in spite of the recommendations of the American Medical Association that only the most recent edition of the *Guides* be used, to ensure that the most recent material is used in the assessment process.

PURPOSE OF THE GUIDES

The primary purpose for the use of the *Guides* in states that have adopted it for the purpose of determining impairment is to provide a referential framework within which physicians may evaluate and report impairments. This purpose is achieved by providing objective data, when available (and estimated, when not available), on accepted methods of evaluating organ function. It is acknowledged by the contributors to the *Guides*, however, that it is not possible to provide answers about every kind and degree of impairment because of limitations in knowledge of some areas, the wide variety of disease, and ongoing changes in medicine.

STANDARDIZATION

The *Guides* provides a set of standards and method of analysis for the acquisition, communication, and use of medical information about the impairments of any organ system.

MEDICAL DOCUMENTATION

Medical documentation may include not only the medical evaluation performed by the assessing physician but also any prior evaluations present in the medical record of the patient. These include consultation reports, progress notes, outpatient laboratory and other diagnostic tests, and the entire record of any hospital admissions.

When assigning medical impairment, one cannot apply a rating if there is no documentation in the medical record to support subjective symptoms. In other words, application of an impairment rating depends on objective findings.

ACTIVITIES OF DAILY LIVING

In the process of developing the *Guides,* the authors believed that determination of impairment should be based on activities of daily living and not work. The activities specified in the *Guides* include the following:

1.   Self-care and personal hygiene, including dressing, bathing, toileting, shaving, eating
2.   Communication, including speech, writing, or signing (when applicable)
3.   Normal living postures: standing, sitting, and lying
4.   Ambulation
5.   Travel by automobile, train, plane, public transportation
6.   Nonspecific hand activities such as grasping
7.   Sexual function
8.   Sleep
9.   Social and recreational activities

DEFINITIONS FOR THE RATING PROCESS

1.   Impairment: the loss of, the loss of use of, or the derangement of any body part, system, or function.
2.   Permanent impairment: impairment that has become static or well stabilized with or without medical treatment, or that is not likely to remit despite medical treatment of the impairing condition.
3.   Disability: the loss or absence of the capacity of an individual to meet personal, social, or occupational demands or to meet statutory or regulatory requirements.
4.   Permanent disability: when the disability becomes static or well stabilized and is not likely to change in spite of continuing medical or rehabilitation measures.
5.   Handicap: a barrier or obstacle to functional activity. An impairment results in a handicap "if there are barriers to accomplishment of tasks or life activities that can be overcome only by compensating in some

way for the effects of the impairment." Therefore, if the individual compensates successfully, there is no disability.

6. Employability: the ability of an individual to commute to and from work and to perform the job for which the employer is willing to pay wages. To be able to answer questions of employability, the physician needs to know several things:
   a. What are the job tasks that need to be performed?
   b. What are the work expectations of the employer?
   c. Does the patient have the capacity to perform the required job?

WHOLE PERSON VERSUS SCHEDULED RATINGS

The AMA *Guides* recommends that all impairment ratings should be combined (e.g., combining neurologic and musculoskeletal impairments) to express the impairment of the whole person, since all physical and mental impairments affect the whole person. Some states may require reporting impairment in terms of the whole person or by using scheduled (e.g., extremity) ratings, or both.

PROCESS OF IMPAIRMENT EVALUATION

1. Medical evaluation: includes the narrative history with special focus to onset and course of illness, physical examination, other testing (e.g., clinical laboratory, radiologic, electrophysiologic), assessment of current clinical status and diagnosis, and plans for future treatment.
2. Review of prior medical evaluations: This includes a review of any previous examination findings, treatment, and response to treatment. Review of records before the alleged workplace injury is essential in order to deal with possible impairments/medical conditions that impact the patient's current impairment. There may be a need to apportion impairment between work-related and non–work-related injuries.
3. Analysis of findings: Once the medical evaluation and review of prior medical records is completed, an analysis should include the following items:
   a. Impact of the impairment on activities of daily living
   b. Determination of maximum medical improvement (when the underlying condition has stabilized and no further medical intervention will improve the condition)
   c. Determination of prognosis
   d. Determination of restrictions
4. Comparison of results to criteria in AMA *Guides:* Listing of specific clinical findings for each impairment and how these findings relate to criteria set forth in the *Guides.*
5. Rating of impairment: This refers to the mechanical process of taking

the clinical information noted above and applying it to the appropriate system chapter in the *Guides* in order to determine a percentage of impairment. This is discussed in detail for the nervous system in the following section.

The Neurologic Impairment Rating Process

Provided that one has followed the basic concepts above related to use of the AMA *Guides* and causation analysis, the actual mechanics of the evaluation of neurologic impairment are quite easy. The criteria for the evaluation and rating of permanent impairment of the nervous system are based on findings on the neurologic examination (see Chapter 2) and applying those findings to one or more of 22 tables found in the chapter in the AMA *Guides* related to the nervous system. The following examples illustrate this process.

TOXIC NEUROPATHY

The opportunities to assess impairment in a case of occupational toxic peripheral neuropathy are extremely uncommon for two major reasons: First, toxic neuropathies that occur in the workplace are rare, and second, if they do occur, most will resolve over time (except in the most severe cases), with no impairment or disability being sustained.

Case Example

A 57-year-old man was determined to have a peripheral neuropathy due to occupational exposure to mercury. He had worked for 35 years in a chlorine-alkali plant and was exposed to inorganic mercury vapor on a daily basis. Neither he nor any coworkers had ever been treated for acute mercury intoxication, and all workers in the facility had monthly urine screens for mercury over the last 15 years. In no instances were levels found to be elevated in the patient during that time.

Over the past 4 years, the patient had complained of initially intermittent numbness and paresthesias in his hands and feet. More recently, these symptoms had become constant and he was now also complaining of dysesthesias in the same distribution. His neurologic examination was normal except for a stocking-glove loss of temperature sense, touch, and pain perception to the wrists in the upper extremities and to the midcalf in the lower extremities. Vibration sense was mildly diminished at the toes, but all other sensory modalities were intact. Achilles reflexes were judged to be slightly diminished bilaterally, but all other reflexes and the remainder of the neurologic examination was normal.

As to activities of daily living, the patient was able to rise to a standing position and to walk, but had trouble with walking stairs and long distances because of increasing pain in his feet and legs. He was able to use his upper

TABLE 3.3
Station and Gait Impairment Criteria

Impairment Description	Percent Impairment of the Whole Person
Patient can rise to a standing position and can walk but has difficulty with elevations, grades, stairs, deep chairs, and walking long distances	1–9
Patient can rise to a standing position and can walk some distance with difficulty and without assistance but is limited to level surfaces	10–19
Patient can rise to a standing position and can maintain it with difficulty but cannot walk without assistance	20–39
Patient cannot stand without the help of others, mechanical support, and a prosthesis	40–60

Source: American Medical Association. The Nervous System. In Guides to the Evaluation of Permanent Impairment (4th ed). Chicago: American Medical Association, 1993;148.

extremities for self-care and daily activities but had difficulty holding objects because of "weakness" and pain.

Determining Impairment

The Guides does not have a method for the determination of impairment of a peripheral polyneuropathy. Although individual nerves can be rated and the results combined, it is not possible to do this for every peripheral nerve that is affected in a polyneuropathy (since all will be affected to a similar degree). It is reasonable in this situation to determine impairment by rating the patient just as one would rate an individual with spinal cord injury based on functional impairments. In this case, one would have to determine impairment for the categories of station and gait (Table 3.3) and two impaired upper extremities (Table 3.4).

Using Table 3.3, one sees that this patient would have between a 1 and 9% impairment of the whole person based on the mildest impairment description, which states, "Patient can rise to a standing position and can walk but has difficulty with elevations, grades, stairs, deep chairs, and walking long distances." Notice that it does not qualify the *type* of difficulty (i.e., spasticity, motor weakness, etc.). Although any percentage between 1 and 9 is acceptable, we will choose 5% as the impairment in this case.

Next, using Table 3.4, one can see that the upper-extremity impairment for this patient will be between 1 and 19% impairment of the whole person based on the mildest impairment description, which states, "Patient can use both upper extremities for self-care, grasping, and holding, but has difficulty with digital dexterity." Though one may be tempted to

TABLE 3.4
Criteria for Two Impaired Upper Extremities

Impairment Description	*Percent Impairment of the Whole Person*
Patient can use both upper extremities for self-care, grasping, and holding but has difficulty with digital dexterity	1–19
Patient can use both upper extremities for self-care, can grasp and hold objects with difficulty, but has no digital dexterity	20–39
Patient can use both upper extremities but has difficulty with self-care activities	40–79
Patient cannot use upper extremities	80+

Source: American Medical Association. The Nervous System. In Guides to the Evaluation of Permanent Impairment (4th ed). Chicago: American Medical Association, 1993;148.

rate this area of the patient's dysfunction as moderate because he can "grasp and hold objects with difficulty," it is clearly out of line to rate his upper-extremity dysfunction between 20 and 39% whole person, because motor strength is normal and the difficulty in holding objects is a subjective complaint (without any corresponding objective findings) and is probably influenced by pain, fatigue, or other factors. Because motor weakness is not seen, one can choose not to assign any impairment in this category, or to assign a low percent impairment. For the purposes of this example, we will assign a 3% impairment.

Total Impairment

The total impairment is obtained by using the combined values chart (see chapter appendix): Combining 5 and 3%, one comes up with a total impairment of 8% of the whole person. Whenever determining impairment at a spinal cord level, one should always combine the values.

TOXIC ENCEPHALOPATHY

Toxic encephalopathy is one of the most common of all suspected neurotoxic injuries that occur in the workplace. It results both from high-level acute exposures, which can be associated with cardiorespiratory arrest and hypoxic brain injury, or from lower-level chronic exposure, which can result in direct toxic injury to the brain.

Case Example

A 42-year-old petroleum refinery worker suffered a "knock-down" (loss of consciousness) from exposure to hydrogen sulfide. He was found by a co-worker, slightly cyanotic, with depressed respiration, but after a few minutes he was awake and conversant. He was evaluated and released from the emergency room of a local hospital, but he continued to have persistent cognitive complaints. Complaints consisted of memory disturbance (particularly short-term memory difficulty), generalized fatigue, headaches, decreased libido, depression, and sleep disturbance. He had reduced daytime alertness, falling asleep for brief periods three to four times per day, but is able to carry out all of his daily activities.

Neurologic examination revealed mild impairment of short-term recall, but the the remainder of the mental status and neurologic examination was normal.

Determination of Impairment

This patient has impairment resulting from central nervous system injury that includes mental status (i.e., short-term memory disturbance; Table 3.5), emotional or behavioral disturbances (i.e., depression; Table 3.6), and sleep and arousal disorder (Table 3.7). The greatest impairment was determined to be in the area of mental status. His impairment was considered to be mild, described as "impairment exists, but ability remains to perform satisfactorily most activities of daily living." This category of mental status impairment has a range of 1–14% of the whole person. Based on mental status testing and further neuropsychological evaluation, this patient was determined to have an impairment of 10% of the whole person. When determining impairment related to cerebral function, one should never combine values, even when the patient has more than one type of cerebral dysfunction. The most severely affected of the five areas of cerebral dysfunction (disturbances of consciousness and awareness, aphasia or communication disturbances, mental status and integrative functioning abnormalities, emotional or behavioral disturbances, special types of preoccupation or obsession) should be used to represent the cerebral impairment.

CARPAL TUNNEL SYNDROME

Occupational carpal tunnel syndrome (OCTS) is a common diagnosis believed to be related to repetitive trauma (see Chapter 9). OCTS evaluations for determination of disability are becoming increasingly important for worker's compensation systems throughout the United States.

Case Example

A 36-year-old key punch operator began to develop pain in the right hand as well as numbness and paresthesias in a median nerve distribution. These symptoms began within 2 weeks after she started to use new equipment at work. Evaluation of her work station revealed that her wrist supports were placing her hands in a position of extension with the new equipment, rather than the previous neutral position. Despite rotating jobs for 2 weeks

TABLE 3.5
Mental Status Impairments

Impairment Description	Percent Impairment of the Whole Person
Impairment exists, but ability remains to perform satisfactorily most activities of daily living	1–14
Impairment requires direction and supervision of daily living activities	15–29
Impairment requires directed care under continued supervision and confinement in home or other facility	30–49
Individual is unable without supervision to care for self and be safe in any situation	50–70

Source: American Medical Association. The Nervous System. In Guides to the Evaluation of Permanent Impairment (4th ed). Chicago: American Medical Association, 1993;142.

TABLE 3.6
Emotional or Behavioral Impairments

Impairment Description	Percent Impairment of the Whole Person
Mild limitation of daily social and interpersonal functioning	0–14
Moderate limitation of some but not all social and interpersonal daily living functions	15–29
Severe limitation impeding useful action in almost all social and interpersonal daily functions	30–49
Severe limitation of all daily functions requiring total dependence on another person	50–70

Source: American Medical Association. The Nervous System. In Guides to the Evaluation of Permanent Impairment (4th ed). Chicago: American Medical Association, 1993;142.

and later taking time off work, her symptoms did not improve. Electrodiagnostic studies revealed a right carpal tunnel syndrome. The patient underwent surgical decompression of the right median nerve but was unable to successfully return to work after six months.

At the time of neurologic evaluation, her symptoms were numbness and paresthesias in a right median nerve distribution and pain in the right hand that only allowed her to work 10–15 minutes at a time. Neurologic examination revealed slight decreases to pin, temperature, and light touch in a right median nerve distribution. Grip and thumb abduction strength were mildly decreased, perhaps secondary to pain. Phalen's sign was present on the right and a Tinel's sign was present over the right median nerve at the wrist. No other abnormalities were seen on examination.

TABLE 3.7
Impairment Criteria for Sleep and Arousal Disorders

Impairment Description	Percent Impairment of the Whole Person
Reduced daytime alertness with sleep pattern such that patient can carry out most daily activities	1–9
Reduced daytime alertness requiring some supervision in carrying out daytime activities	10–19
Reduced daytime alertness that significantly limits daily activities and requires supervision by caretakers	20–39
Severe reduction of daytime alertness that causes the patient to be unable to care for self in any situation or manner	40–60

Source: American Medical Association. The Nervous System. In Guides to the Evaluation of Permanent Impairment (4th ed). Chicago: American Medical Association, 1993;143.

Determination of Impairment

1. Determination of pain or sensory deficit. First one needs to identify the nerve involved. In this case, the clinical picture is that of carpal tunnel syndrome, a mononeuropathy of the median nerve at the wrist. Using Table 3.8, the location of the injury to the median nerve is below the midforearm. The maximum percentage of upper-extremity impairment due to sensory deficit or pain at this area is 38%. Next, one should grade the severity of the sensory deficit or pain according to the classification scheme in Table 3.9. This patient would be grade 3: "decreased sensibility with or without abnormal sensation or pain, which interferes with but does not prevent activity." The range of deficit is 26–60%. For this patient, we will choose 40% impairment. Next one should multiply the severity of the sensory deficit (40%) by the maximum impairment value (38%), to obtain a value of 15% impairment related to pain or sensation.

2. Determine impairment due to loss of power and motor deficits. Returning to Table 3.8, one identifies that the maximum motor deficit of the median nerve below the midforearm is 10%. Next, one should grade the severity of the motor deficit of the individual muscle or group of muscles according to the classification scheme in Table 3.10. This patient would be grade 4: "active movement against gravity with some resistance." The range of deficit is 1–25%. For this patient, we choose 10% impairment. Next, the severity of the motor deficit (10%) should be multipled by the maximum impairment value (10%) to obtain a value of 1% impairment related to loss of power and motor deficits.

3. Combine sensory and motor deficits. Next, to determine the upper extremity impairment for the median nerve, one combines the sensory

TABLE 3.8
Maximum Upper-Extremity Impairments Due to Unilateral
Sensory or Motor Deficits or Combined Deficits of the Median Nerve

Nerve	*Maximum % Upper-Extremity Impairment*		
	Due to Sensory Deficit or Pain	*Due to Motor Deficit*	*Due to Combined Motor and Sensory Deficits*
Median (above midforearm)	38	44	65
Median (anterior interosseous branch)	0	15	15
Median (below midforearm)	38	10	44
Radial palmar digital—thumb	7	0	7
Ulnar palmar digital—thumb	11	0	11
Radial palmar digital—index finger	5	0	5
Ulnar palmar digital—index finger	4	0	4
Radial palmar digital—middle finger	5	0	5
Ulnar palmar digital—middle finger	4	0	4
Radial palmar digital—ring finger	2	0	2

Source: American Medical Association. The Nervous System. In Guides to the Evaluation of Permanent Impairment (4th ed). Chicago: American Medical Association, 1993;54.

TABLE 3.9
Determining Impairment of the Upper Extremity Due to
Pain or Sensory Deficit Resulting From Peripheral Nerve Disorders

Grade	Description of Sensory Deficit or Pain	Percent Sensory Deficit
1	No loss of sensibility, abnormal sensation, or pain	0
2	Decreased sensibility with or without abnormal sensation or pain, which is forgotten during activity	1–25
3	Decreased sensibility with or without abnormal sensation or pain, which interferes with activity	26–60
4	Decreased sensibility with or without abnormal sensation or pain, which may prevent activity, and/or minor causalgia	61–80
5	Decreased sensibility with abnormal sensations and severe pain, which prevents activity, and/or major causalgia	81–100

Source: American Medical Association. The Nervous System. In Guides to the Evaluation of Permanent Impairment (4th ed). Chicago: American Medical Association, 1993;48.

TABLE 3.10
Determining Impairment of the Upper Extremity Due
to Loss of Power and Motor Deficits Resulting From
Peripheral Nerve Disorders Based on Individual Muscle Rating

Grade	Description of Muscle Function	% Motor Deficit
5	Active movement against gravity with full resistance	0
4	Active movement against gravity with some resistance	1–25
3	Active movement against gravity only, without resistance	26–50
2	Active movement with gravity eliminated	51–75
1	Slight contraction and no movement	76–99
0	No contraction	100

Source: American Medical Association. The Nervous System. In Guides to the Evaluation of
Permanent Impairment (4th ed). Chicago: American Medical Association, 1993;49.

(15%) and motor (1%) values using the combined values chart (see
chapter appendix) to obtain a value of 16%.
4.   Convert to whole-person impairment. Using Table 3.11, an upper-extremity impairment of 16% converts to a whole-person impairment of 10%.

When multiple peripheral nerves are affected, the respective impairments of each nerve are combined using the combined values chart to
obtain the total upper extremity impairment due to peripheral nerve disorders. If multiple extremities are involved, one should first determine the
extremity impairment for each individual extremity, convert to a whole-
person rating, then combine the extremity values using the combined values chart (see chapter appendix).

Conclusions

Determination of causation is of critical importance when dealing with a
potential occupational injury and is not always an easy task. If one follows
the scientific approach to causation analysis outlined in this chapter, the
task will at least be performed in a uniform and consistent fashion and will
avoid many of the pitfalls that commonly occur in the assessment of causation in occupational cases. Once causation is found to be related to the
workplace, determination of impairment usually will need to be performed,
using the AMA *Guides to the Evaluation of Permanent Impairment*. The
latter process is much easier to perform than causation analysis but equally
important in the management of work-related injuries.

TABLE 3.11
Relationship of Impairment of the
Upper Extremity to Impairment of the Whole Person

Upper Extremity/ Whole Person	Upper Extremity/ Whole Person	Upper Extremity/ Whole Person
0/0	35/21	70/42
1/1	36/22	71/43
2/1	37/22	72/43
3/2	38/23	73/44
4/2	39/23	74/44
5/3	40/24	75/45
6/4	41/25	76/46
7/4	42/25	77/46
8/5	43/26	78/47
9/5	44/26	79/47
10/6	45/27	80/48
11/7	46/28	81/49
12/7	47/28	82/49
13/8	48/29	83/50
14/8	49/29	84/50
15/9	50/30	85/51
16/10	51/31	86/52
17/10	52/31	87/52
18/11	53/32	88/53
19/11	54/32	89/52
20/12	55/33	90/54
21/13	56/34	91/55
22/13	57/34	92/55
23/14	58/35	93/56
24/14	59/35	94/56
25/15	60/36	95/57
26/16	61/37	96/58
27/16	62/37	97/58
28/17	63/38	98/59
29/17	64/38	99/59
30/18	65/39	100/60
31/19	66/40	
32/19	67/40	
33/20	68/41	
34/20	69/41	

Source: American Medical Association. The Nervous System. In Guides to the Evaluation of Permanent Impairment (4th ed). Chicago: American Medical Association, 1993;20.

References

1. American Medical Association. Guides to the Evaluation of Permanent Impairment (4th ed). Chicago: American Medical Association, 1993.
2. Muscat JE, Huncharek MS. Causation and disease: biomedical science in toxic tort litigation. J Occup Med 1989;31:997–1002.
3. Centers for Disease Control. Leading work-related diseases and injuries— United States. MMWR 1983;32:24–26.
4. Doull J, Bruce MC. Origin and Scope of Toxicology. In MO Amdur, J Doull, CD Klaassen (eds). In Casarett and Doull's Toxicology: The Basic Science of Poisons (4th ed). New York: Pergammon, 1991.
5. Foster KR, Bernstein DE, Huber PW. A Scientific Perspective. In KR Foster, DE Bernstein, PW Huber (eds), Phantom Risk: Scientific Inference and the Law. Cambridge, MA: MIT Press, 1993.
6. Black B. Evolving legal standards for the admissibility of scientific evidence. Science 1988;239:1508–1512.
7. Evans AS. Causation and Disease: A Chronological Journey. New York: Plenum, 1993.
8. Evans AS. Causation and disease: the Henle-Koch postulates revisted. Yale J Biol Med 1976;49:175–195.
9. Evans AS. Limitations of Koch's postulates. Lancet 1977;2:1277.
10. Black B, Lilienfeld DE. Epidemiological proof in toxic tort litigation. Fordham Law Rev 1984;52:723–785.
11. Hill AB. The environment and disease: association or causation? Proc Royal Soc Med 1965;58:295–300.
12. Doll R. Occupational cancer: problems in interpreting human evidence. Ann Occup Hyg 1984;28:291–305.
13. Hackney JD, Linn WS. Koch's postulates updated: a potentially useful application to laboratory research and policy analysis in environmental toxicology. Am Rev Resp Dis 1979;119:849–852.
14. Brent RL. The irresponsible expert witness: a failure of biomedical graduate education and professional accountability. Pediatrics 1982;70:754–762.
15. Brent RL. Improving the quality of expert witness testimony. Pediatrics 1988; 82:511–513.
16. Impairment Evaluation. In American Medical Association, Guides to the Evaluation of Permanent Impairment (4th ed). Chicago: American Medical Association, 1993.

Appendix to Chapter 3

The values are derived from the formula A + B (1–A)=*combined* value of A and B, where A and B are the decimal equivalents of the impairment ratings. In the chart all values are expressed as percents. To *combine* any two impairment values, locate the larger of the values on the side of the chart and read along that row until you come to the column indicated by the smaller value at the bottom of the chart. At the intersection of the row and the column is the combined value.

For example, to combine 35% and 20% read down the side of the chart until you come to the larger value, 35%. Then read across the 35% row until you come to the column indicated by 20% at the bottom of the chart. At the intersection of the row and column is the number 48. Therefore, 35% *combined* with 20% is 48%. Due to the construction of this chart, the larger impairment value must be identified at the side of the chart.

If three or more impairment values are to be combined, select any two and find their combined value as above. Then use that value and the third value to locate the combined value of all. This process can be repeated indefinitely, the final value in each instance being the combination of all the previous values. In each step of this process the larger impairment value must be identified at the side of the chart.

Note: If impairments from two or more organ systems are to be *combined* to express a whole-person impairment, each must first be expressed as a whole-person impairment percent.

	1	2	3	4	5	6	7	8	9	10	11	12	13	14	15	16	17	18	19	20	21	22	23	24	25	26	27	28	29	30	31	32	33	34	35	36	37	38	39	40	41	42	43	44	45	46	47	48	49	50
1	2																																																	
2	3	4																																																
3	4	5	6																																															
4	5	6	7	8																																														
5	6	7	8	9	10																																													
6	7	8	9	10	11	12																																												
7	8	9	10	11	12	13	14																																											
8	9	10	11	12	13	14	14	15																																										
9	10	11	12	13	14	15	15	16	17																																									
10	11	12	13	14	15	15	16	17	18	19																																								
11	12	13	14	15	15	16	17	18	19	20	21																																						
12	13	14	15	16	16	17	18	19	20	21	22	23																																					
13	14	15	16	16	17	18	19	20	21	22	23	23	24																																				
14	15	16	17	17	18	19	20	21	22	23	23	24	25	26																																			
15	16	17	18	18	19	20	21	22	23	24	24	25	26	27	28																																		
16	17	18	19	19	20	21	22	23	24	24	25	26	27	28	29	29																																	
17	18	19	19	20	21	22	23	24	24	25	26	27	28	29	29	30	31																																
18	19	20	20	21	22	23	24	25	25	26	27	28	29	29	30	31	32	33																															
19	20	21	21	22	23	24	25	25	26	27	28	29	30	30	31	32	33	34	34																														
20	21	22	22	23	24	25	26	26	27	28	29	30	30	31	32	33	34	34	35	36																													
21	22	23	23	24	25	26	27	27	28	29	30	30	31	32	33	34	34	35	36	37	38																												
22	23	24	24	25	26	27	27	28	29	30	31	31	32	33	34	34	35	36	37	38	38	39																												
23	24	25	25	26	27	28	28	29	30	31	31	32	33	34	35	35	36	37	38	38	39	40	41																											
24	25	26	26	27	28	29	29	30	31	32	32	33	34	35	35	36	37	38	39	40	41	41	42																											
25	26	27	27	28	29	30	30	31	32	33	33	34	35	36	36	37	38	39	39	40	41	42	42	43	44																									
26	27	28	28	29	30	30	31	32	33	33	34	35	36	37	38	38	39	39	40	41	42	42	43	44	45	45																								
27	28	28	29	30	30	31	32	33	34	34	35	36	36	37	38	39	39	40	41	42	42	43	44	45	45	46	47																							
28	29	29	30	31	32	32	33	34	34	35	36	36	37	38	38	39	40	40	41	42	42	43	44	45	45	46	47	47	48																					
29	30	30	31	32	33	33	34	35	35	36	37	38	38	39	40	40	41	42	42	43	44	45	45	46	47	47	48	49	50																					
30	31	31	32	33	34	34	35	36	36	37	38	38	39	40	41	41	42	43	43	44	45	45	46	47	48	48	49	50	50	51	52																				
31	32	32	33	34	34	35	36	37	37	38	39	39	40	41	41	42	43	44	44	45	46	46	47	48	48	49	50	50	51	52	52	53	54																		
32	33	33	34	35	35	36	37	37	38	39	39	40	41	42	42	43	44	44	45	46	46	47	48	48	49	50	50	51	52	52	53	54	54	55																	
33	34	34	35	36	36	37	38	38	39	40	40	41	42	42	43	44	45	45	46	47	47	48	49	49	50	51	51	52	53	53	54	54	55	56																	
34	35	35	36	37	37	38	39	39	40	41	41	42	43	43	44	45	45	46	47	47	48	49	49	50	51	51	52	52	53	54	54	55	56	56																	
35	36	36	37	38	38	39	40	40	41	42	42	43	43	44	45	45	46	47	47	48	49	49	50	51	51	52	53	53	54	55	55	56	56	57	58																
36	37	37	38	39	39	40	41	42	42	43	44	44	45	46	46	47	48	48	49	50	50	51	51	52	53	53	54	55	55	56	56	57	57	58	58	59															
37	38	38	39	40	40	41	41	42	43	43	44	45	45	46	46	47	48	48	49	50	50	51	51	52	53	53	54	55	55	56	57	57	58	58	59	60	60														
38	39	39	40	40	41	42	42	43	44	44	45	45	46	47	47	48	49	49	50	50	51	52	52	53	54	54	55	55	56	57	57	58	58	59	59	60	61	62													
39	40	40	41	41	42	43	43	44	45	45	46	46	47	48	48	49	49	50	51	51	52	52	53	54	54	55	55	56	57	57	58	59	59	60	60	61	62	62	63												
40	41	41	42	42	43	44	44	45	45	46	47	47	48	48	49	50	50	51	51	52	53	53	54	54	55	56	56	57	57	58	59	59	60	60	61	62	62	63	63	64											
41	42	42	43	43	44	45	45	46	46	47	47	48	49	49	50	50	51	52	52	53	53	54	55	55	56	56	57	57	58	59	59	60	60	61	61	62	63	63	64	64	65										
42	43	43	44	44	45	45	46	47	47	48	48	49	50	50	51	51	52	52	53	54	54	55	55	56	57	57	58	58	59	60	60	61	61	62	62	63	63	64	65	65	66	66									
43	44	44	45	45	46	46	47	48	48	49	49	50	50	51	51	52	52	53	54	54	55	55	56	57	57	58	58	59	59	60	61	61	62	62	63	64	64	65	65	66	66	67	68								
44	45	45	46	46	47	47	48	48	49	50	50	51	51	52	52	53	54	54	55	55	56	56	57	57	58	59	59	60	60	61	62	62	63	64	64	65	65	66	66	67	68	68	69								
45	46	46	47	47	48	48	49	49	50	50	51	52	52	53	53	54	54	55	55	56	57	57	58	58	59	59	60	60	61	62	62	63	63	64	64	65	65	66	66	67	68	68	69	69	70						
46	47	47	48	48	49	49	50	50	51	51	52	52	53	53	54	54	55	55	56	56	57	57	58	58	59	60	60	61	61	62	63	63	64	64	65	66	66	67	67	68	68	69	69	70	70	71					
47	48	48	49	49	50	50	51	51	52	52	53	53	54	54	55	55	56	57	57	58	58	59	59	60	60	61	61	62	62	63	63	64	64	65	66	66	67	67	68	68	69	69	70	70	71	71	72				
48	49	49	50	50	51	51	52	52	53	53	54	54	55	55	56	56	57	57	58	58	59	60	60	61	61	62	62	63	63	64	64	65	65	66	67	67	68	68	69	69	70	70	71	71	72	72	73				
49	50	50	51	51	52	52	53	53	54	54	55	55	56	56	57	57	58	58	59	59	60	60	61	61	62	62	63	63	64	64	65	65	66	66	67	67	68	68	69	69	70	70	71	71	72	72	73	73	74		
50	51	51	52	52	53	53	54	54	55	55	56	56	57	57	58	58	59	59	60	60	61	61	62	62	63	63	64	64	65	65	66	66	67	67	68	68	69	69	70	70	71	71	72	72	73	73	74	74	75	75

	1	2	3	4	5	6	7	8	9	10	11	12	13	14	15	16	17	18	19	20	21	22	23	24	25	26	27	28	29	30	31	32	33	34	35	36	37	38	39	40	41	42	43	44	45	46	47	48	49	50
51	51	52	52	53	53	54	54	55	55	56	56	57	57	58	58	59	59	60	60	61	61	62	62	63	63	64	64	65	65	66	66	67	67	68	68	69	69	70	70	71	71	72	72	73	73	74	74	75	75	76
52	52	53	53	54	54	55	55	56	56	57	57	58	58	59	59	60	60	61	61	62	62	63	63	64	64	64	65	65	66	66	67	67	68	68	69	69	70	70	71	71	72	72	73	73	74	74	75	75	76	76
53	53	54	54	55	55	56	56	57	57	58	58	59	59	60	60	61	61	61	62	62	63	63	64	64	65	65	66	66	67	67	68	68	69	69	69	70	70	71	71	72	72	73	73	74	74	75	75	76	76	77
54	54	55	55	56	56	57	57	58	58	59	59	59	60	60	61	61	62	62	63	63	64	64	65	65	66	66	66	67	67	68	68	69	69	70	70	71	71	71	72	72	73	73	74	74	75	75	76	76	77	77
55	55	56	56	57	57	58	58	59	59	60	60	60	61	61	62	62	63	63	64	64	64	65	65	66	66	67	67	68	68	69	69	69	70	70	71	71	72	72	73	73	73	74	74	75	75	76	76	77	77	78
56	56	57	57	58	58	59	59	60	60	60	61	61	62	62	63	63	63	64	64	65	65	66	66	67	67	67	68	68	69	69	70	70	71	71	71	72	72	73	73	74	74	74	75	75	76	76	77	77	78	78
57	57	58	58	59	59	60	60	60	61	61	62	62	63	63	63	64	64	65	65	66	66	66	67	67	68	68	69	69	69	70	70	71	71	72	72	72	73	73	74	74	75	75	75	76	76	77	77	78	78	79
58	58	59	59	60	60	61	61	61	62	62	63	63	63	64	64	65	65	66	66	66	67	67	68	68	68	69	69	70	70	71	71	71	72	72	73	73	74	74	74	75	75	76	76	76	77	77	78	78	79	79
59	59	60	60	61	61	61	62	62	63	63	64	64	64	65	65	66	66	66	67	67	68	68	68	69	69	70	70	70	71	71	72	72	73	73	73	74	74	75	75	75	76	76	77	77	77	78	78	79	79	80
60	60	61	61	62	62	62	63	63	64	64	64	65	65	66	66	66	67	67	68	68	68	69	69	70	70	70	71	71	72	72	72	73	73	74	74	74	75	75	76	76	76	77	77	78	78	78	79	79	80	80
61	61	62	62	63	63	63	64	64	65	65	65	66	66	66	67	67	68	68	68	69	69	70	70	70	71	71	72	72	72	73	73	73	74	74	75	75	75	76	76	77	77	77	78	78	79	79	79	80	80	81
62	62	63	63	64	64	64	65	65	65	66	66	67	67	67	68	68	68	69	69	70	70	70	71	71	72	72	72	73	73	73	74	74	75	75	75	76	76	76	77	77	78	78	78	79	79	79	80	80	81	81
63	63	64	64	64	65	65	66	66	66	67	67	67	68	68	69	69	69	70	70	70	71	71	72	72	72	73	73	73	74	74	74	75	75	76	76	76	77	77	77	78	78	79	79	79	80	80	80	81	81	82
64	64	65	65	65	66	66	67	67	67	68	68	68	69	69	69	70	70	70	71	71	72	72	72	73	73	73	74	74	74	75	75	76	76	76	77	77	77	78	78	78	79	79	79	80	80	81	81	81	82	82
65	65	66	66	66	67	67	67	68	68	69	69	69	70	70	70	71	71	71	72	72	72	73	73	73	74	74	74	75	75	76	76	76	77	77	77	78	78	78	79	79	79	80	80	80	81	81	81	82	82	83
66	66	67	67	67	68	68	68	69	69	69	70	70	70	71	71	71	72	72	72	73	73	73	74	74	75	75	75	76	76	76	77	77	77	78	78	78	79	79	79	80	80	80	81	81	81	82	82	82	83	83
67	67	68	68	68	69	69	69	70	70	70	71	71	71	72	72	72	73	73	73	74	74	74	75	75	75	76	76	76	77	77	77	78	78	78	79	79	79	80	80	80	81	81	81	82	82	82	83	83	83	84
68	68	69	69	69	70	70	70	71	71	71	72	72	72	72	73	73	73	74	74	74	75	75	75	76	76	76	77	77	77	78	78	78	79	79	79	80	80	80	80	81	81	81	82	82	82	83	83	83	84	84
69	69	70	70	70	71	71	71	71	72	72	72	73	73	73	74	74	74	75	75	75	76	76	76	76	77	77	77	78	78	78	79	79	79	80	80	80	80	81	81	81	82	82	82	83	83	83	84	84	84	85
70	70	71	71	71	72	72	72	72	73	73	73	74	74	74	75	75	75	75	76	76	76	77	77	77	78	78	78	78	79	79	79	80	80	80	81	81	81	81	82	82	82	83	83	83	84	84	84	84	85	85
71	71	72	72	72	72	73	73	73	74	74	74	74	75	75	75	76	76	76	77	77	77	77	78	78	78	79	79	79	79	80	80	80	81	81	81	81	82	82	82	83	83	83	83	84	84	84	85	85	85	86
72	72	73	73	73	73	74	74	74	75	75	75	75	76	76	76	76	77	77	77	78	78	78	78	79	79	79	80	80	80	80	81	81	81	82	82	82	82	83	83	83	83	84	84	84	85	85	85	85	86	86
73	73	74	74	74	74	75	75	75	75	76	76	76	77	77	77	77	78	78	78	78	79	79	79	79	80	80	80	81	81	81	81	82	82	82	82	83	83	83	84	84	84	84	85	85	85	85	86	86	86	87
74	74	75	75	75	75	76	76	76	76	77	77	77	77	78	78	78	78	79	79	79	79	80	80	80	81	81	81	81	82	82	82	82	83	83	83	83	84	84	84	84	85	85	85	85	86	86	86	86	87	87
75	75	76	76	76	76	77	77	77	77	78	78	78	78	79	79	79	79	80	80	80	80	81	81	81	81	82	82	82	82	83	83	83	83	84	84	84	84	85	85	85	85	86	86	86	86	87	87	87	87	88
76	76	76	77	77	77	77	78	78	78	78	79	79	79	79	80	80	80	80	81	81	81	81	82	82	82	82	82	83	83	83	83	84	84	84	84	85	85	85	85	86	86	86	86	87	87	87	87	88	88	88
77	77	77	78	78	78	78	79	79	79	79	80	80	80	80	80	81	81	81	81	82	82	82	82	83	83	83	83	83	84	84	84	84	85	85	85	85	86	86	86	86	86	87	87	87	87	88	88	88	88	89
78	78	78	79	79	79	79	80	80	80	80	80	81	81	81	81	82	82	82	82	82	83	83	83	83	84	84	84	84	84	85	85	85	85	85	86	86	86	86	87	87	87	87	87	88	88	88	88	89	89	89
79	79	79	80	80	80	80	80	81	81	81	81	82	82	82	82	82	83	83	83	83	83	84	84	84	84	84	85	85	85	85	86	86	86	86	86	87	87	87	87	87	88	88	88	88	88	89	89	89	89	90
80	80	80	81	81	81	81	81	82	82	82	82	82	83	83	83	83	83	84	84	84	84	84	85	85	85	85	85	86	86	86	86	86	87	87	87	87	87	88	88	88	88	88	89	89	89	89	89	90	90	90
81	81	81	82	82	82	82	82	83	83	83	83	83	83	84	84	84	84	84	85	85	85	85	85	86	86	86	86	86	87	87	87	87	87	87	88	88	88	88	88	89	89	89	89	89	90	90	90	90	90	91
82	82	82	83	83	83	83	83	83	84	84	84	84	84	85	85	85	85	85	85	86	86	86	86	86	87	87	87	87	87	87	88	88	88	88	88	88	89	89	89	89	89	90	90	90	90	90	90	91	91	91
83	83	83	84	84	84	84	84	84	85	85	85	85	85	85	86	86	86	86	86	86	87	87	87	87	87	87	88	88	88	88	88	88	89	89	89	89	89	89	90	90	90	90	90	90	91	91	91	91	91	92
84	84	84	84	85	85	85	85	85	85	86	86	86	86	86	86	87	87	87	87	87	87	88	88	88	88	88	88	88	89	89	89	89	89	89	90	90	90	90	90	90	91	91	91	91	91	91	92	92	92	92
85	85	85	85	86	86	86	86	86	86	87	87	87	87	87	87	87	88	88	88	88	88	88	88	89	89	89	89	89	89	90	90	90	90	90	90	90	91	91	91	91	91	91	91	92	92	92	92	92	92	93
86	86	86	86	87	87	87	87	87	87	87	88	88	88	88	88	88	88	89	89	89	89	89	89	89	90	90	90	90	90	90	90	90	91	91	91	91	91	91	91	92	92	92	92	92	92	92	93	93	93	93
87	87	87	87	88	88	88	88	88	88	88	88	89	89	89	89	89	89	89	89	90	90	90	90	90	90	90	91	91	91	91	91	91	91	91	92	92	92	92	92	92	92	92	93	93	93	93	93	93	93	94
88	88	88	88	88	89	89	89	89	89	89	89	89	90	90	90	90	90	90	90	90	91	91	91	91	91	91	91	91	91	92	92	92	92	92	92	92	92	93	93	93	93	93	93	93	93	94	94	94	94	94
89	89	89	89	89	90	90	90	90	90	90	90	90	90	91	91	91	91	91	91	91	91	91	92	92	92	92	92	92	92	92	92	93	93	93	93	93	93	93	93	93	94	94	94	94	94	94	94	94	94	95
90	90	90	90	90	91	91	91	91	91	91	91	91	91	91	92	92	92	92	92	92	92	92	92	92	93	93	93	93	93	93	93	93	93	93	94	94	94	94	94	94	94	94	94	94	95	95	95	95	95	95
91	91	91	91	91	91	92	92	92	92	92	92	92	92	92	92	92	93	93	93	93	93	93	93	93	93	93	93	94	94	94	94	94	94	94	94	94	94	94	95	95	95	95	95	95	95	95	95	95	95	96
92	92	92	92	92	92	92	93	93	93	93	93	93	93	93	93	93	93	93	94	94	94	94	94	94	94	94	94	94	94	94	94	95	95	95	95	95	95	95	95	95	95	95	95	96	96	96	96	96	96	96
93	93	93	93	93	93	93	93	94	94	94	94	94	94	94	94	94	94	94	94	94	94	95	95	95	95	95	95	95	95	95	95	95	95	95	95	96	96	96	96	96	96	96	96	96	96	96	96	96	96	97
94	94	94	94	94	94	94	94	94	95	95	95	95	95	95	95	95	95	95	95	95	95	95	95	95	96	96	96	96	96	96	96	96	96	96	96	96	96	96	96	96	96	97	97	97	97	97	97	97	97	97
95	95	95	95	95	95	95	95	95	95	96	96	96	96	96	96	96	96	96	96	96	96	96	96	96	96	96	96	96	96	96	97	97	97	97	97	97	97	97	97	97	97	97	97	97	97	97	97	97	97	98
96	96	96	96	96	96	96	96	96	96	96	96	96	97	97	97	97	97	97	97	97	97	97	97	97	97	97	97	97	97	97	97	97	97	97	97	97	97	98	98	98	98	98	98	98	98	98	98	98	98	98
97	97	97	97	97	97	97	97	97	97	97	97	97	97	97	97	97	98	98	98	98	98	98	98	98	98	98	98	98	98	98	98	98	98	98	98	98	98	98	98	98	98	98	98	98	98	98	98	98	98	99
98	98	98	98	98	98	98	98	98	98	98	98	98	98	98	98	98	98	98	98	98	98	98	98	98	99	99	99	99	99	99	99	99	99	99	99	99	99	99	99	99	99	99	99	99	99	99	99	99	99	99
99	99	99	99	99	99	99	99	99	99	99	99	99	99	99	99	99	99	99	99	99	99	99	99	99	99	99	99	99	99	99	99	99	99	99	99	99	99	99	99	99	99	99	99	99	99	99	99	99	99	100
	1	**2**	**3**	**4**	**5**	**6**	**7**	**8**	**9**	**10**	**11**	**12**	**13**	**14**	**15**	**16**	**17**	**18**	**19**	**20**	**21**	**22**	**23**	**24**	**25**	**26**	**27**	**28**	**29**	**30**	**31**	**32**	**33**	**34**	**35**	**36**	**37**	**38**	**39**	**40**	**41**	**42**	**43**	**44**	**45**	**46**	**47**	**48**	**49**	**50**

Combined Values Chart (continued)

R\C	51	52	53	54	55	56	57	58	59	60	61	62	63	64	65	66	67	68	69	70	71	72	73	74	75	76	77	78	79	80	81	82	83	84	85	86	87	88	89	90	91	92	93	94	95	96	97	98	99
99																																																	100
98																																																100	100
97																																															100	100	100
96																																														100	100	100	100
95																																													100	100	100	100	100
94																																												100	100	100	100	100	100
93																																											100	100	100	100	100	100	100
92																																										99	99	100	100	100	100	100	100
91																																									99	99	99	99	100	100	100	100	100
90																																								99	99	99	99	99	100	100	100	100	100
89																																							99	99	99	99	99	99	99	100	100	100	100
88																																						99	99	99	99	99	99	99	99	100	100	100	100
87																																					98	98	99	99	99	99	99	99	99	99	100	100	100
86																																				98	98	98	98	99	99	99	99	99	99	99	100	100	100
85																																			98	98	98	98	98	99	99	99	99	99	99	99	100	100	100
84																																		97	98	98	98	98	98	98	99	99	99	99	99	99	100	100	100
83																																	97	97	97	98	98	98	98	98	98	99	99	99	99	99	99	100	100
82																																97	97	97	97	97	98	98	98	98	98	99	99	99	99	99	99	100	100
81																															96	97	97	97	97	97	98	98	98	98	98	98	99	99	99	99	99	100	100
80																														96	96	96	97	97	97	97	97	98	98	98	98	98	99	99	99	99	99	100	100
79																													96	96	96	96	96	97	97	97	97	97	98	98	98	98	99	99	99	99	99	100	100
78																												95	95	96	96	96	96	96	97	97	97	97	98	98	98	98	98	99	99	99	99	100	100
77																											95	95	95	95	96	96	96	96	97	97	97	97	97	98	98	98	98	99	99	99	99	100	100
76																										94	94	95	95	95	95	96	96	96	96	97	97	97	97	98	98	98	98	99	99	99	99	100	100
75																									94	94	94	95	95	95	95	96	96	96	96	97	97	97	97	98	98	98	98	99	99	99	99	100	100
74																								93	94	94	94	94	95	95	95	95	96	96	96	96	97	97	97	97	98	98	98	98	99	99	99	99	100
73																							93	93	93	94	94	94	94	95	95	95	95	96	96	96	96	97	97	97	98	98	98	98	99	99	99	99	100
72																						92	92	93	93	93	94	94	94	94	95	95	95	96	96	96	96	97	97	97	97	98	98	98	99	99	99	99	100
71																					92	92	92	92	93	93	93	94	94	94	94	95	95	95	96	96	96	97	97	97	97	98	98	98	99	99	99	99	100
70																				91	91	92	92	92	93	93	93	93	94	94	94	95	95	95	96	96	96	96	97	97	97	98	98	98	99	99	99	99	100
69																			90	91	91	91	92	92	92	93	93	93	93	94	94	94	95	95	95	96	96	96	97	97	97	98	98	98	98	99	99	99	100
68																		90	90	90	91	91	91	92	92	92	93	93	93	94	94	94	95	95	95	96	96	96	96	97	97	97	98	98	98	99	99	99	100
67																	89	89	90	90	90	91	91	91	92	92	92	93	93	93	94	94	94	95	95	95	96	96	96	97	97	97	98	98	98	99	99	99	100
66																88	89	89	89	90	90	90	91	91	92	92	92	93	93	93	94	94	94	95	95	95	96	96	96	97	97	97	98	98	98	99	99	99	100
65															88	88	88	89	89	90	90	90	91	91	91	92	92	92	93	93	93	94	94	94	95	95	95	96	96	97	97	97	98	98	98	99	99	99	100
64														87	87	88	88	88	89	89	90	90	90	91	91	91	92	92	92	93	93	94	94	94	95	95	95	96	96	96	97	97	97	98	98	99	99	99	100
63													86	87	87	87	88	88	89	89	89	90	90	90	91	91	91	92	92	93	93	93	94	94	94	95	95	96	96	96	97	97	97	98	98	99	99	99	100
62												86	86	86	87	87	87	88	88	89	89	89	90	90	91	91	91	92	92	92	93	93	94	94	94	95	95	95	96	96	97	97	97	98	98	98	99	99	100
61											85	85	86	86	86	87	87	88	88	88	89	89	89	90	90	91	91	91	92	92	93	93	93	94	94	95	95	95	96	96	96	97	97	98	98	98	99	99	100
60										84	84	85	85	86	86	86	87	87	88	88	88	89	89	90	90	90	91	91	92	92	92	93	93	94	94	94	95	95	96	96	96	97	97	98	98	98	99	99	100
59									83	84	84	84	85	85	86	86	86	87	87	88	88	89	89	89	90	90	91	91	91	92	92	93	93	93	94	94	95	95	95	96	96	97	97	98	98	98	99	99	100
58								82	83	83	84	84	84	85	85	86	86	87	87	87	88	88	89	89	90	90	90	91	91	92	92	92	93	93	94	94	95	95	95	96	96	97	97	97	98	98	99	99	100
57							82	82	82	83	83	84	84	85	85	85	86	86	87	87	88	88	88	89	89	90	90	91	91	91	92	92	93	93	94	94	94	95	95	96	96	97	97	97	98	98	99	99	100
56						81	81	82	82	82	83	83	84	84	85	85	85	86	86	87	87	88	88	89	89	89	90	90	91	91	92	92	93	93	93	94	94	95	95	96	96	96	97	97	98	98	99	99	100
55					80	80	81	81	82	82	82	83	83	84	84	85	85	86	86	87	87	87	88	88	89	89	90	90	91	91	91	92	92	93	93	94	94	95	95	96	96	96	97	97	98	98	99	99	100
54				79	79	80	80	81	81	82	82	83	83	83	84	84	85	85	86	86	87	87	88	88	89	89	89	90	90	91	91	92	92	93	93	94	94	94	95	95	96	96	97	97	98	98	99	99	100
53			78	78	79	79	80	80	81	81	82	82	83	83	84	84	84	85	85	86	86	87	87	88	88	89	89	90	90	91	91	92	92	92	93	93	94	94	95	95	96	96	97	97	98	98	99	99	100
52		77	77	78	78	79	79	80	80	81	81	82	82	83	83	84	84	85	85	86	86	87	87	88	88	88	89	89	90	90	91	91	92	92	93	93	94	94	95	95	96	96	97	97	98	98	99	99	100
51	76	76	77	77	78	78	79	79	80	80	81	81	82	82	83	83	84	84	85	85	86	86	87	87	88	88	89	89	90	90	91	91	92	92	93	93	94	94	95	95	96	96	97	97	98	98	99	99	100

Source: American Medical Association. Guides to the Evaluation of Permanent Impairment (4th ed). Chicago: American Medical Association, 1993;322–324.

CHAPTER 4

Neurotoxicity of Organic Solvents

Neil L. Rosenberg, M.D.

Among the ten leading work-related disorders and injury categories in the United States, four include problems commonly brought to the attention of a neurologist: musculoskeletal injuries, neurotoxic disorders, noise-induced hearing loss, and psychological disorders.[1] Neurotoxic disorders are apparently common because many industrial chemicals as well as other substances used in the environment have deleterious effects on the nervous system. One major group of industrial compounds, the organic solvents, have the potential to produce neurologic syndromes related to both acute and chronic overexposure. Since hundreds of organic compounds are commonly used in both the household and workplace environments, many potential toxic effects have been recognized. This is particularly true with the organic solvents, chemicals primarily used in the petrochemical and paint industries.

This chapter examines current information on the acute and chronic neurotoxic properties of selected organic solvents, principally those of interest to the petrochemical industry. Emphasis is on the neurobehavioral effects, since these are the most controversial. While most organic solvents possess acute narcotizing properties, few have been shown to induce chronic disease associated with pathologic changes in either the central or peripheral nervous systems. Although petrochemicals that have primarily peripheral nervous system (PNS) toxicity are discussed, this chapter focuses on the central nervous system (CNS) toxicity of selected petrochemicals and specifically on their neurobehavioral effects.

Statement of the Problem

Organic solvents are widely prevalent compounds and inadvertent exposure, primarily industrial, as well as volitional abuse occurs primarily by inhalation, with significantly less absorption occurring via skin or gastrointestinal routes. These compounds are highly lipophilic, which explains their distribution to organs rich in lipids (e.g., brain, liver, adrenal). In general, these lipid-soluble products are eliminated through the kidneys after several breakdown reactions to render them more water soluble. Additional compounds, sometimes more neurotoxic than the parent chemical, arise through these reactions.[2–6]

Although most organic solvents produce nonspecific effects (i.e., acute reversible encephalopathy) in extremely high concentrations, a few result in relatively specific neurologic syndromes with lower-level, chronic exposure. These include *n*-hexane and methyl-*n*-butyl ketone, which produce a peripheral neuropathy. Most of the early animal studies, which serve as the basis for the setting of tolerance levels in industry, emphasized the acute effects of high-level exposure, with determination of the degree of exposure needed to cause death. More recent clinical and experimental studies have focused on the chronic, lower-level exposures to solvents that have been reported to result in slowly developing PNS and CNS syndromes. Two major neurotoxic syndromes occur in individuals chronically exposed to organic solvents: a peripheral neuropathy and an encephalopathy. Less commonly, a cerebellar ataxic syndrome, parkinsonism, or a myopathy may occur alone or in combination with any of these clinical syndromes. In some instances, solvent mixtures with complicated chemical interactions and synergistic effects have been encountered, resulting in multifocal CNS and PNS damage.

Many organic solvents are capable of inducing an acute, reversible encephalopathy at high levels of exposure. Chronic, long-lasting, or irreversible changes in nervous system structure and/or function from organic solvents are being debated. For certain organic solvents with proven neurotoxic properties, the type of neurologic damage (i.e., PNS vs. CNS) is often closely related to the structure of the chemical agent, whereas the degree of impairment and the extent of reversibility are related to the potency, dose, and duration of exposure.[7] Examples of this principle include *n*-hexane and methyl-*n*-butyl ketone, both aliphatic hydrocarbons that produce peripheral neuropathy. Chronic inhalation abuse of toluene, on the other hand, produces an irreversible, multifocal CNS syndrome characterized by dementia, cerebellar ataxia, spasticity, and brain stem dysfunction, but such changes have not been found in workers exposed to toluene in the occupational setting.

In either the occupational or abuse setting, exposure to organic solvent mixtures is far more common than exposure to a single solvent. An estimated 49 million tons of organic solvents were produced in the United

States in 1984, exposing almost 10 million individuals in the workplace,[8] primarily to solvent mixtures.

The Psycho-Organic Syndrome

Investigators, primarily from Denmark and other Scandinavian countries, have alleged that chronic occupational exposure to organic solvents induces a pattern of irreversible changes in neurologic function that has been described by various terms, including psycho-organic syndrome (POS), neurasthenic syndrome, painter's syndrome, and chronic toxic encephalopathy. This syndrome is characterized by personality change, memory loss, fatigue, depression, and loss of interest in daily activities.

Most studies of the POS have used epidemiologic techniques to compare and contrast findings in solvent-exposed and unexposed reference groups. Methods applied have included self-administered questionnaires, neuropsychological tests, and clinical neurophysiologic and neuroimaging tests. Most reports consider that ten or more years of exposure is required to produce the POS, but one study has suggested that only 3 years may be needed.[9] Few papers, however, have even suggested either dose-effect[10] or duration-effect[11] relationships, critical issues in establishing a toxin-induced syndrome. Virtually all of the studies on this subject have been written by scientists and physicians from Denmark, Sweden, and Finland, who are of the opinion that organic solvents, as a class, have chronic neurotoxic properties. In these countries, permanent neurologic deficit of the type described as the POS is a recognized and compensable occupational disability. Scientists and physicians from other European countries and from North America generally have been less willing to recognize this entity and have instead attempted to understand the chronic effects of individual organic solvents.

Solvent exposure in the occupational setting more often involves various solvent mixtures than a single solvent. This makes elucidation of the neurotoxicity of individual solvents extremely difficult. How or if the individual components of these mixtures interact with each other to potentiate toxicity is not known. In addition, published studies lack information regarding exposure levels to these mixtures, so dose-response effects regarding neurotoxicity are not known.

Despite this lack of scientific information, because of the concerns of health professionals, industry, workers, and governments, an attempt was made to standardize the terminology used to describe this syndrome, in order that there be some consistency in reporting future studies. An international conference was convened, and those present (including representatives from industry, government, and the legal and medical professions) proposed a categorization of the POS by degree of impairment.[12] A similar categorization was previously proposed by the World Health Organization.[13] This can be summarized as follows:

Type 1: Symptoms only. Complaints of nonspecific symptoms; completely reversible if exposure discontinued; equivalent to "neurasthenic syndrome."

Type 2A: Sustained personality or mood change. Same as type 1, but symptoms are not reversible.

Type 2B: Impairment in intellectual function. Symptoms are accompanied by objective evidence of impairment on neuropsychological tests; "minor neurologic signs" may be seen and may not be reversible, synonymous with "psycho-organic syndrome" and "mild dementia."

Type 3: Dementia. Marked global deterioration in intellectual function; neurologic signs evident, poorly reversible, if at all, but is generally nonprogressive once exposure has ceased.

For those who use this type of categorization, it is generally believed that type 3 is only seen in situations of solvent abuse and is primarily due to high-level intermittent exposure. Types 1 and 2 would result from low-level, more sustained exposure and be more likely to occur in the occupational setting. Unfortunately, neither this nor other classifications take into account possible confounding factors regarding other conditions that may produce the same symptoms, and they do not consider duration of exposure.

The cornerstone of data collection in these studies has primarily been in the form of extensive neuropsychological testing in workers exposed to solvents at concentrations considered to be safe by current occupational standards. Those tests have recently been reviewed elsewhere.[14,15] Since the tests were not standardized among the various studies, comparison of results is difficult and in some cases impossible. Nevertheless, although the results of these studies have varied somewhat, they consistently suggest that chronic, low-level solvent exposure is associated with cognitive changes on tests of psychomotor function and perceptual speed, short-term memory, and occasionally visuoconstructive functions. Verbal and nonverbal reasoning are almost never affected.

In addition, current criteria for diagnosis of chronic toxic encephalopathy differ greatly among the various Nordic countries.[13] They all generally assume that if "typical" subjective symptoms are present and other examinations fail to reveal another organic or psychiatric disorder, then a chronic toxic encephalopathy is the cause of the individual's complaints. As will be shown, however, one can make this diagnosis on virtually any individual with subjective complaints who happened to have worked with solvents for any length of time. What are clearly difficult to assess are the degree and duration of exposure and what compounds are involved.

The various published studies do not provide the necessary information to assist in evaluating individuals with low-level solvent exposure.

They generally fail to include analysis of the compounds individuals have been exposed to and give crude (if any) estimates as to levels and duration of exposure. Other confounding factors, including alcohol and/or other drug use, nutrition, head trauma, psychiatric disorder, aging, and other diseases affecting the CNS are rarely considered in any detail. Other major problems are lack of knowledge about preexposure cognitive functioning and preexisting psychological dysfunction. Few provide an analysis of the solvent mixture to which the workers were exposed, and some studies were conducted on subjects experiencing the acute effects of the solvent mixture under study. Many of these studies failed to include an appropriate reference group. Finally, there are no neuropathologic studies of this syndrome and no appropriate animal models.

Many of these studies were done in a retrospective fashion on individuals already diagnosed as having chronic toxic encephalopathy, psychoorganic syndrome, or solvent poisoning.[16-20] The obvious difficulties inherent in any retrospective data analysis are compounded when individuals have been diagnosed as having the syndrome and, as is often the case, have been given disability pensions for this problem.

This syndrome has been reported in workers from various industries where exposure to solvent mixtures is common; these individuals include printers,[21] aviation fuel workers,[22-24] and painters.[21,25-35] Although the majority of reports have focused on symptoms and neuropsychological testing, uncontrolled reports have shown abnormalities on vestibular function testing,[36-38] electroencephalography (EEG),[16,39,40] electromyography and nerve conduction testing,[40,41] visual evoked potentials,[40,42] cerebral blood flow[43,44] pneumoencephalography,[45] and computed tomography (CT)[46] in both symptomatic and asymptomatic individuals.

A controlled study of patients with the diagnosis of chronic toxic encephalopathy, however, failed to show any difference in cerebral atrophy between patients and control subjects.[47] This study was done by assessing bifrontal horn, bicaudate, and third-ventricle–Sylvian fissure distance measurements on CT scans with all measurements adjusted for variation in skull diameter.[47] Also, in some epidemiologic group studies, no actual increase in the frequency of abnormal EEGs has been found in workers exposed to solvent mixtures.[48]

Other recent studies have begun to cast doubt as to whether long-term occupational exposure to solvents causes any permanent neurologic dysfunction.[14,49-53] A 1984 published literature review[14] concluded that with the exception of carbon disulfide exposure, where pathologic alterations in the CNS have been found, there is no evidence that long-term occupational solvent exposure leads to permanent structural or functional injury to the CNS or PNS.

A far more critical 1986 review of the Danish literature regarding organic solvents and the painter's syndrome concluded that these studies have not proved that occupational exposure to organic solvents produces a "presenile dementia."[49] These authors go so far as to state "that the papers are so ill-based scientifically, that they must be rejected as failing to qualify as medical research." They further state that two of the papers reviewed were sent to a statistician for analysis. One manuscript, though using relevant statistical methods, could not be considered of enough importance to help clarify the issue of organic solvent-induced CNS injury. The second paper was totally unacceptable from a statistical point of view.[49] This review also pointed out the problem related to premorbid intellectual function, "self-inflicted" injury, the effects of even low levels of alcohol consumption, and retrospective epidemiologic investigations based on questionnaires. Another research study, looking at the long-term effects of occupational exposure to toluene, found that the only parameter correlating with exposure to toluene was high alcohol consumption.[50]

Three recent studies merit more detailed review. In a large, retrospective study of 105 house painters and 53 control subjects (nonpainters) from the Federal Republic of Germany, no cases of clinically relevant chronic encephalopathy could be found.[51] In this study, house painters had been employed for at least 10 years (median 27 years, range 10–36 years) and controls were matched with regard to age, occupational training, and socioeconomic status. Care was taken to exclude individuals in both groups with excessive alcohol consumption and drug abuse, familial occurrence of neuropsychiatric conditions, and any prior or current process or medical condition that could affect CNS or PNS function. On the basis of these criteria, 19 painters (18%) and 14 nonpainters (26%) were excluded from further study. All further examinations were performed blind and took place after at least a 16- to 24-hour exposure-free interval to minimize the possible acute effects of organic solvent exposure. In neither group was there a single case of a clinically manifest polyneuropathy or encephalopathy. No abnormalities were seen on nerve conduction studies, EEG, or CT scans. On neurobehavioral tests, significant differences in the results were seen only on the subtests "change of personality" and "short-term memory capacity" in a subgroup of painters with repeated prenarcotic (i.e., acute effects) symptoms in the workplace. Therefore, the results of this well-controlled retrospective study failed to support findings from other studies on the existence of the POS. Although some of the differences may have been due to lower levels of exposure to solvents in the German painters, the care in properly selecting study groups and methods for selecting diagnostic tests probably played a much larger role in the results of this study.[51]

The second study deserving more detailed discussion comes from a group in Denmark who had previously reported the occurrence of a chronic toxic encephalopathy in 20 house painters.[52] Their initial studies, based on nonstandardized tests, did not contain control groups.[54,55] Testing consisted of neuropsychological tests, and on retesting 2 years after the initial study,[54] performance was unchanged. The 1988 study[52] compared the scores of the original group of 20 solvent-exposed individuals with the scores of 20 nonexposed control subjects. The control group was a subsample of 120 nonexposed controls who were individually matched to each of the 20 solvent-exposed patients on sex, age, and education. When compared with these controls, the previously reported solvent-exposed individuals had no evidence of intellectual impairment.

These results are similar to those of other studies in which control groups were matched on premorbid levels of intelligence,[56,57] or when statistical corrections are made for differences in intelligence.[58] These negative results are also consistent with results from cross-sectional psychometric studies of solvent-exposed workers and control subjects, where group differences have generally been small, acute effects of solvent exposure have not been anticipated, and dose-effect relations were not seen.[59]

Finally, a recently published study evaluated the neuropsychiatric effects of chronic low-level solvent exposure in 187 workers at two U.S. paint manufacturers where 13–15 years of exposure data were available.[60] This study is unique and of great importance in that a dose-response relationship between chronic low-level exposure to mixed solvents and the POS could be studied for the first time. This study failed to demonstrate an association or dose-response relationship between chronic low-level solvent exposure and symptoms suggestive of the POS. In a structured psychiatric interview, however, there were a greater number of positive responses to items characteristic of depression in the exposed group. This finding was not believed to be of clinical significance by the authors for several reasons, including the identification of recent life stressors in this group and the fact that none of the workers were "clinically depressed." Equally important is the fact that higher levels of exposure failed to produce more symptoms; some dose-effect relationships were actually opposite from those expected (i.e., the greater the exposure, the fewer symptoms reported). Overall, the results of this well-controlled study fail to support the association between chronic low-level solvent exposure and the POS.

In conclusion, current literature does not support previously published studies relating chronic occupational solvent exposure to any permanent CNS or PNS injury. In particular, there is no compelling evidence to suggest that chronic low-level exposure to solvent mixtures causes adverse neurobehavioral effects.

General Principles of Recognizing Organic Solvent-Induced Neurotoxic Illness

The nervous system may be affected at many levels by organic solvents as well as by other neurotoxic substances. As a general rule, resultant syndromes are diffuse in their manifestations.[61] Because of their nonfocal presentation, neurotoxic disorders may be confused with metabolic, degenerative, nutritional, or demyelinating disease.[61] This principle is illustrated in the setting of chronic toluene abuse, which may resemble the multifocal demyelinating disease, multiple sclerosis, in the findings on neurologic examination.[62–64] In addition, neurotoxic syndromes rarely have specific identifying features on diagnostic tests such as CT, magnetic resonance imaging (MRI), or nerve conduction studies.[61] As a result, mild cases of neurotoxic injury may be very difficult to diagnose. The most reliable information, in fact, comes from documented cases of massive exposure, and information concerning health effects from low-level exposure and presymptomatic diagnosis are vague at best.

Acute, high-level exposure to most, if not all, solvents will induce short-lasting effects on brain function. A few have been shown to exert chronic effects associated with neuropathologic changes. These solvents (e.g., methanol) probably act by producing secondary systemic effects such as cerebral hypoxia or a metabolic acidosis; none has been proved to induce a primary, irreversible functional abnormality. In general, both acute high-level and low-level exposure to organic solvents are associated with full reversibility and the acute toxicity with high-level exposure in no way predicts whether chronic low-level exposure will lead to chronic, irreversible neurologic disease.

Chronic high-level exposure to organic solvents occurs only in the inhalant abuse setting, where levels several thousandfold higher than the occupational setting occur frequently. For example, chronic CNS neurotoxic disease related to toluene abuse is slowly and incompletely reversible but does not progress after cessation of exposure.[63,64] Both acute and chronic neurotoxicity from organic solvents are predominantly related to the dose and duration of exposure.

There may be no relationship between the mechanism of acute neurotoxicity and the clinical manifestations of chronic neurotoxicity. For example, an acute effect of a particular organic solvent may be attributable to the parent compound, whereas a chronic effect may be associated with a metabolite of this compound. In addition, several solvents have been reported either to diminish or to potentiate the neurotoxic potency of a second solvent. For example, methyl ethyl ketone, normally not a neurotoxin, is known to potentiate the neurotoxic effect of methyl-*n*-butyl ketone (see the section on aliphatic hydrocarbons).

There is little or no apparent individual variability or altered susceptibility to the neurotoxic effects of either acute or chronic exposure to organic solvents. Unless subject to other toxic exposures or illnesses that also cause neurologic sequelae, individuals will develop a similar clinical picture when exposed to solvents at equivalent doses for equivalent durations of time.

Chemical structure does not always predict the neurotoxic effects. Two closely related compounds, 2,5-hexanedione (the toxic metabolite of *n*-hexane and methyl-*n*-butyl ketone) and 2,4-hexanedione provide an example. A fixed dose of 2,5-hexanedione produces a fixed amount of axonal degeneration in a particular species, but 2,4-hexanedione never produces these changes.

Compounds of Interest
ALCOHOLS
Methanol (Methyl Alcohol)*

OSHA PEL: TWA 200 ppm

ACGIH TLV: TWA 200 ppm; STEL 250 ppm (skin)

DFG MAK: 200 ppm (260 mg/m^3)

NIOSH REL: TWA 200 ppm; CL 800 ppm/15 minutes

Methanol, first identified in 1822 by Taylor[65] from wood distillation, has been widely used in industry as a solvent, as a component of antifreeze, and in the manufacture of paints, rubber, textiles, and dyes.[66] It has also been used as an adulterant to denature products containing ethanol. Synonyms include wood alcohol, wood spirits, methylol, carbinol, colonial spirits, and Columbian spirits.

Although methanol toxicity was noted as far back as 1855,[67] it was not until 1904 that Wood and Buller's[68] compilation of case histories of methanol poisoning identified methanol, and not contaminants in crude commercial products, as a cause of blindness and death.[68,69] Methanol's metabolic products, formaldehyde and formic acid, induce a severe acidosis and account for the neurotoxicity. Although ingestion is the main route of methanol poisoning,[70] both inhalation of fumes and absorption through the skin have been reported to cause serious or fatal intoxication.[66]

Toxic effects vary somewhat from individual to individual, and in some cases a protective effect appears to be related to concomitant ingestion of ethanol, which competes with alcohol dehydrogenase, the degrading enzyme shared by both. Competition by ethanol diminishes the rapid production of formaldehyde and formic acid, and more methanol is excreted unchanged by the kidney.

The clinical neurologic manifestations, which usually occur after a 12- to 24-hour latent period, characteristically involve vision and the CNS.[66,70] Visual disturbances are noted by most patients and vary from mild diminution of acuity to total blindness. CNS symptoms include headache, dizziness, and decreased level of consciousness. Severely intoxicated individuals may rapidly develop seizures, stupor, and coma. Gastrointestinal complaints are also common, especially anorexia and abdominal pain. A rare neurologic sequela is a parkinsonian syndrome characterized by bradykinesia, hypophonia, rigidity, and tremor,[71-74] with lesions seen on CT scan in the putamen and globus pallidus.[75,76]

Dementia has been reported after high-level exposure to methanol.[72] Other, mild neurobehavioral effects have not been described, although much less information is available on the health effects of long-term exposure to low levels of methanol. In one study, office workers exposed to

---

*For explanation of terms, see chapter appendix.

methanol levels in the range of 15–375 ppm developed frequent and recurrent headaches,[77] but no other symptoms were reported.

ALIPHATIC HYDROCARBONS: METHYL-*N*-BUTYL KETONE AND *N*-HEXANE

Both *n*-hexane and methyl-*n*-butyl ketone (MBK) are metabolized to the same neurotoxin, 2,5-hexanedione (2,5-HD), and produce a similar peripheral neuropathy.[78] 2,5-HD is responsible for most, if not all, of the neurotoxic effects that follow exposure to *n*-hexane or MBK.[79–81] As mentioned previously, methyl ethyl ketone (MEK) alone produces neither clinical nor pathologic evidence of a peripheral neuropathy in experimental animals.[82] MEK's importance is related to a synergistic effect between MEK and MBK and between MEK and *n*-hexane, which has been detected in experimental animals and probably in humans.[83–85] This potentiation of toxicity of one compound (MBK or *n*-hexane) by an otherwise nontoxic compound (MEK) underscores the difficulty in sorting out toxic effects of individual solvents within a mixture.

Methyl-n-Butyl Ketone (2-Hexanone)

OSHA PEL: TWA 100 ppm

ACGIH TLV: TWA 5 ppm (skin)

NIOSH REL: (Ketones) TWA 4 mg/m^3

MBK had limited industrial use until the 1970s, when it became more widely used as a paint thinner, a clearing agent in histology preparations, and a solvent for dye printing. Soon afterward, numerous outbreaks of polyneuropathy associated with chronic exposure to MBK were being reported.[86–90] Originally, MEK had been used as a solvent, followed by a mixture of MEK (90%) with methyl isobutyl ketone (10%). When the methyl isobutyl ketone was replaced by MBK (10%), reports of polyneuropathy began to appear in the literature. The route of exposure is usually inhalation, but contaminated food may be ingested in work areas, and skin absorption can also occur.

The clinical syndrome is characterized by the onset of an initially painless sensorimotor polyneuropathy, which begins several months after continued exposure. In some situations, the neuropathy may initially develop following cessation of exposure. The neuropathy may also continue to progress for up to 3 months following cessation of exposure.[86–90] In severe cases, an unexplained weight loss may be an early symptom. Sensory and motor disturbance begins in the hands and feet. Sensory loss is primarily small fiber (i.e., light touch, pinprick, temperature), with relative sparing of large-fiber sensation (i.e., position and vibration). Electrophysiologic studies reveal an axonal polyneuropathy, and pathologically, multifocal axonal degeneration, multiple axonal swellings, and neurofilamentous accumulation at paranodal areas are seen.[91] Overlying the axonal swellings, the myelin sheath is thinned. These findings are typical of a distal axonopathy or "dying-back" neuropathy as described with other toxic and metabolic causes of peripheral neuropathy. Prognosis for recovery correlates directly with the intensity of the neurologic deficit before removal from toxic exposure; mild to moderate residual neuropathy is seen in the most severely affected individuals up to 3 years after exposure.

In conclusion, PNS toxicity occurs in individuals chronically exposed to MBK. Neurobehavioral effects do not appear to be clinically relevant but have not been systematically studied.

N-Hexane

OSHA PEL: TWA 500 ppm

ACGIH TLV: TWA 50 ppm

N-Hexane is used in the printing of laminated products, in extraction of vegetable oils, as a diluent in the manufacture of plastics and rubber, in cabinet finishing, a solvent in biochemical laboratories, and as a solvent for glues and adhesives.

Cases of n-hexane polyneuropathy have been reported both after occupational exposure[92] and after deliberate inhalation of vapors from products that contain n-hexane, such as glues.[93–99] Clinically and pathologically, the neuropathy that occurs with n-hexane is that of a distal axonopathy,[100] indistinguishable from that associated with MBK.

When glues have been analyzed in past reports of polyneuropathy occurring after glue sniffing, n-hexane has been a major component of the products' composition (between 27 and 50% by weight). Another major component of these glues has been toluene, but polyneuropathy does not occur from inhalation of toluene alone and the neuropathy has not been reported to appear until the subject switched to a product containing n-hexane. In contrast to toluene, n-hexane does not usually induce significant signs of CNS dysfunction, except with high-level exposures, where an acute encephalopathy may occur.

Although clinical studies primarily show the peripheral effects, both clinical and experimental studies have shown evidence of CNS effects from n-hexane. Experimental animal studies have shown n-hexane to cause axonal degeneration in the CNS.[100,101] Clinically, cranial neuropathy, spasticity, and autonomic dysfunction occasionally occur.[83] Electrophysiologic tests of CNS function, including electroencephalography, visual evoked responses, and somatosensory evoked responses have shown abnormalities.[102,103] In spite of these observations, clinically the effect of chronic exposure to n-hexane is restricted to the PNS, with no adverse neurobehavioral effects. As with MBK, however, neurobehavioral effects have not been systematically studied.

AROMATIC HYDROCARBONS

Toluene (Methyl Benzene)

OSHA PEL: TWA 200 ppm; CL 300; peak 500/10M

ACGIH TLV: TWA 100 ppm; STEL 150 ppm

DFG MAK: 100 ppm (375 mg/m^3); BAT: blood end of shift 340 mg/dl

NIOSH REL: TWA 100 ppm; CL 200 ppm/10 minutes

Toluene is one of the most widely used solvents and is used as a paint and lacquer thinner, as a cleaning and drying agent in the rubber and lumber industries, and in the motor and aviation fuels and chemical industries. It is a major component in many paints, lacquers, glues and adhesives, inks, and cleaning liquids. As with other solvents, inhalation is the major route of entry, though some absorption occurs percutaneously. Of all the solvents, toluene seems to have the highest potential for abuse.[104]

In 1961, Grabski[105] reported the first patient with persistent neurologic consequences of chronic toluene inhalation. Since then, numerous reports of severe neurotoxicity have appeared.[106–120] Most have described either an acute intoxication or chronic high-level exposure, both generally occurring in the setting of inhalant abuse. Acute intoxication with toluene produces headache, euphoria, giddiness, and cerebellar ataxia. At lower levels (just over 200 ppm), fatigue, headache, paresthesias, and slowed reflexes appear.[121,122] Exposure to levels over 600 ppm causes an acute confusional state (delirium), and euphoric effects appear above 800 ppm. Although solvent abusers have favorite compounds (usually paints, adhesives, or other aerosol products), occasionally they use an unpredictable array of solvents.

Although the acute dose-related neurotoxicity of toluene is known,[121,122] the effects of chronic exposure are less well understood. Complete resolution of signs and symptoms has been reported after chronic abuse with prolonged abstinence and no significant treatment.[108,123] Syndromes describing severe and persistent neurotoxicity include cognitive dysfunction,[107,112,117–120,124–126] cerebellar ataxia,[64,105,106,108,11–113,117] optic neuropathy,[109–116] sensorineural hearing loss,[116] and an equilibrium disorder.[110] The most common syndrome is that of multifocal CNS involvement.[112,115,117–120] Despite the many instances of "persistent" neurologic deficits, in only one study was abstinence documented before clinical evaluation.[118] This point is of great importance, since it has already been noted that some individuals will completely remit with prolonged abstinence.[108,123]

In a study of 20 chronic abusers of spray paint, which almost entirely consisted of toluene, abstinence was documented for at least one month before evaluation.[118] In these 20 chronic solvent abusers, 65% showed neurologic impairment. This was a small and unselected sample, so the findings probably do not reflect the true prevalence of neurologic damage. The pattern of neurologic abnormality, however, was fairly consistent. As others have suggested, the CNS is selectively vulnerable. In fact, no peripheral neuropathy was found and there is no convincing evidence that pure toluene or other aromatic hydrocarbons cause peripheral neuropathy.

Neurologic abnormalities varied from mild cognitive impairment to severe dementia, associated with elemental neurologic signs such as cerebellar ataxia, corticospinal tract dysfunction, oculomotor abnormalities, tremor, deafness, and hyposmia. Cognitive dysfunction was the most disabling and frequent feature of chronic toluene toxicity and may be the earliest sign of permanent damage. Dementia, when present, was typically associated with cerebellar ataxia and other signs.[118]

Other investigators have found a similar syndrome after chronic exposure to toluene.[64,108,111,117] Although some emphasized the cerebellar disorder, most cases also demonstrated impairment in a variety of cerebral functions. One study found a similar pattern of cognitive impairment with neurologic abnormality, but the individuals were studied as soon as 3 days after the last exposure and there have been no other studies on long-term cognitive outcome after prolonged toluene abuse. It should be noted, however, that many chronic toluene abusers have had no persistent cognitive impairment, despite approximately calculated cumulative doses equivalent to those in individuals with cognitive impairment.[118,120] This suggests either that the abuse histories obtained were not accurate or that other factors possibly play a role in those individuals.

We found other neurologic dysfunction in many subjects, especially pyramidal and cerebellar signs,[118] but observed this pattern in only one patient who was not also cognitively impaired or demented. Oculomotor dysfunction, deafness, and tremor were seen only in severely affected individuals. Cranial nerve abnormalities were confined to olfactory and auditory dysfunction. Toluene-induced optic neuropathy, previously reported,[109] did not occur in our series.[118]

Our clinical data suggested that the cognitive, cerebellar, corticospinal, and brainstem signs are due to diffuse effects of toluene on the CNS. In one prior report of an autopsy of a chronic solvent abuser, there was prominent degeneration and gliosis of ascending and descending long tracts with cerebral and cerebellar atrophy.[127] Unfortunately, as in most reports of toluene neurotoxicity, this patient was abusing many solvents contained in several different mixtures, so the effects of individual solvents could not be determined.

We reported that chronic toluene abuse causes diffuse CNS white matter changes.[119] This was based on MRI findings in the brain in six individuals and neuropathologic changes in one abuser not studied by MRI. All individuals abused the same mixture, which contained primarily toluene (61%) and methylene chloride (10%). MRI revealed (1) diffuse cerebral, cerebellar, and brainstem atrophy; (2) loss of differentiation of the gray and white matter throughout the CNS; and (3) increased periventricular white-matter signal intensity on T2-weighted images. The brain of the individual studied pathologically revealed diffuse, ill-defined myelin pallor, which was maximal in the cerebellar, periventricular, and deep cerebral white matter.

Occasional, scant perivascular macrophage collections were seen, but neurons were preserved throughout, axonal swelling or beading was not seen, and gliosis was minimal. These findings suggest that toluene is a white-matter toxin; the mechanism of action, however, remains to be explained.

Another study attempted to correlate the severity of clinical involvement in 11 chronic toluene abusers and findings on brain stem–evoked responses (BAERs) and MRI.[120] Neurologic abnormalities were seen in four of the 11 individuals and included cognitive, pyramidal, cerebellar, and brain stem findings. MRI of the brain was abnormal in three of the 11, and all three also had abnormalities on neurologic examination. Abnormalities on MRI were the same as listed above.[119] BAERs were found to be abnormal (control mean + 3 standard deviations) in five of 11 individuals. As a group, the latency of wave V (p <0.01), the III-V interpeak (p <0.05), and the I-V interpeak latencies were prolonged compared to those of control subjects. These findings on BAERs were similar to those previously reported in toluene abusers.[115–117] Similar findings include normal wave I latency, after poorly defined waves II, III, and V, and prolonged wave I to wave V interpeak latency. All three individuals with abnormal MRI scans and neurologic examination also had abnormal BAERs. Two of five individuals with abnormal BAERs, however, had normal neurologic examinations and MRI scans. This study supported previous findings of diffuse white-matter involvement in chronic toluene abusers and suggests that BAERs may detect early CNS injury from toluene inhalation even at a time when neurologic examination and MRI scans are normal. This study suggests that BAERs may be a sensitive screening test to monitor individuals at risk from toluene exposure for early evidence of CNS injury.

Although an exact dose-effect relationship cannot be drawn yet for chronic toluene exposure, it is clear that all severely affected individuals have had heavy and prolonged exposure. The lack of correlation between the type or duration of exposure and neurologic impairment may be due to unreliable histories or other factors, such as genetic predisposition (unlikely) or hypoxemia due to "huffing" (placing a solvent-soaked rag directly over nose and mouth in order to inhale the vapors) or "bagging" (placing a solvent-soaked rag or solvent into a plastic bag, which is then placed directly over the nose and mouth in order to inhale the vapors). Nutritional factors and other concomitantly used substances may also be involved. The gradual resolution of acute toxicity and the absence of withdrawal symptoms were probably due to slow elimination of toluene from the CNS. We also have observed continued improvement in five patients who remained abstinent for 6 months or more, suggesting that continued recovery may proceed after toluene is cleared from the CNS.

Unlike the solvents that cause peripheral neuropathy, such as *n*-hexane, for which there are animal models of classic target organ neurotoxicity, no adequate animal model exists for toluene-induced neurotoxicity. Although several studies have addressed the behavioral effects of both acute and chronic toluene exposure in laboratory animals,[128–133] none have demonstrated either persistent effects or pathologic changes of the CNS. High-frequency hearing loss was noted after 5 weeks of exposure to 1,200 ppm or 1,400 ppm toluene.[133,134] This was reversible and was attributed to cochlear dysfunction rather than to the central conduction pathology found in the human studies noted above. The pharmacodynamics, distribution, and bioavailability of toluene and its metabolites have been barely investigated; however, there is no basis for comparing toluene's effects in experimental animals to those in humans.

Benzene

OSHA PEL: TWA 1 ppm/8 hours; peak 5 ppm/15 minutes

ACGIH TLV: TWA 10 ppm (suspected human carcinogen); BEI (total phenol in urine at end of shift) 50 mg/liter recommended as mean value

DFG TRK: 8 ppm (26 mg/m^3)

NIOSH REL: CL 1 ppm/60 minutes

Benzene is an important industrial toxin because of its widespread use primarily in the processing of rubber, motor fuel, munitions, leather, dyes, paints, lacquers, glues, and electric fittings. The major toxic effect of benzene is hematopoietic toxicity, an effect unique to benzene among the simple aromatic hydrocarbons. Unlike toluene (methyl benzene), which is very similar in structure, benzene has very little, if any, chronic effect on the CNS. Benzene poisoning usually occurs by inhalation of vapors in workers who clean or repair leaks in benzene tanks, but occasionally results from oral ingestion in suicide attempts.[135,136]

Acute intoxication produces euphoria, giddiness, nausea and vomiting, and a cerebellar ataxia. In severe intoxication, muscle twitching is followed by seizures, depressed level of consciousness, and terminal failure of respiration.

Chronic benzene intoxication is reported to affect the nervous system both directly and indirectly. Indirect CNS involvement with intracerebral hemorrhage has been reported in patients being treated with benzene for leukemia who develop aplastic anemia. Both the CNS and PNS have been noted to be affected in such patients, but it is unclear whether this involvement was directly caused by benzene. Poorly documented older reports claimed that chronic benzene intoxication causes peripheral neuropathy, pyramidal tract involvement, ataxia, visual loss from retrobulbar neuritis, and seizures.[135]

The most extensively studied neurologic complication of chronic benzene intoxication is peripheral neuropathy.[137] It is impossible, however, to attribute any of this involvement to benzene alone since most cases in which this effect was reported have involved a mixture of solvents, often containing toluene and *n*-hexane.

In conclusion, there is no convincing evidence that chronic exposure to benzene causes direct neurotoxic injury, including neurobehavioral effects.

Xylene

OSHA PEL: TWA 100 ppm

ACGIH TLV: TWA 100 ppm; STEL 150 ppm; BEI: methyl hippuric acids in urine at end of shift 1.5 g/g creatinine

NIOSH REL: (Xylene) TWA 100 ppm; CL 200 ppm/10 minutes

Xylene is used in the paint, rubber, and leather industries, and in paint solvents, glues and adhesives, varnishes, and printing inks. It is also widely used in histology laboratories as a clearing agent in tissue preparation.[138,139]

High-level, acute exposure to xylene can cause an acute confusional state and even death.[140] Neuropathologic study of a fatal case only demonstrated agonal changes, with cerebral anoxic changes being the most prominent.

In one study, a low-level, acute exposure did not seem to be associated with any CNS effects unless individuals exercised.[141] Another study of low-level exposure over several days suggested that both rapid adaptation and longer-term impairment are possible outcomes of xylene exposure.[142]

Chronic effects from exposure to xylene are poorly understood; however, in one epidemiogic study from the former Soviet Union and in a study of chronically exposed laboratory technicians, individuals reported problems with headache, irritability, and confusion reminiscent of the psycho-organic syndrome.[143,144] These uncontrolled studies should be interpreted with caution, and no convincing evidence exists that permanent neuropsychological impairment occurs from chronic xylene exposure.

Styrene (Vinyl Benzene)

OSHA PEL: TWA 100 ppm; CL 200 ppm

ACGIH TLV: TWA 50 ppm; STEL 100 ppm (skin); BEI: mandelic acid in urine at end of shift 1 g/liter styrene in mixed-exhaled air before shift 40 parts per billion (ppb), styrene in mixed-exhaled air during shift 18 ppb, styrene in blood at end of shift 0.55 mg/liter, styrene in blood before shift 0.02 mg/liter

DFG MAK: 100 ppm (420 mg/m^3)

NIOSH REL: (Styrene) TWA 50 ppm; CL 100 ppm

Styrene is a widely used solvent in the production of plastics and resins, rubber items, paints, adhesives, floor waxes and polishes, metal cleaners, and varnishes.[145] It is widely used in the boat-building industry, and many reports of the neurotoxicity of styrene have been in workers in the polyester-resin boat industry, in the manufacture of reinforced polyester plastic products, and in the styrene polymerization process.[146]

Acute short-term exposure to styrene has been well studied.[147,148] Individuals exposed to styrene vapor at approximately 50–375 ppm for up to several hours were symptom free until it reached 375 ppm.[147] At this level, headache, nasal and eye irritation, nausea, and CNS dysfunction appeared. These individuals also showed signs of impaired balance and manual dexterity. In another study, 30-minute exposure periods to 350 ppm styrene significantly slowed reaction times.[148] These studies of acute exposure to styrene occurred under controlled conditions. Similar studies looked at acute exposures in the work setting,[149,150] where workers were given a test of reaction time before and following a day's work. The mean exposure levels in these studies, ranging up to 101 ppm, did not cause impairment on tests of attention, reaction time, or short-term memory from preshift to postshift performance.

Chronic exposure to styrene has been reported to cause persistent problems that affect both the CNS and PNS.[151–163]

One study has reported PNS involvement.[151] On nerve conduction studies, styrene workers were found to have abnormalities that were believed to be consistent with a mild sensory neuropathy. These individuals were older men, however, who were asymptomatic for peripheral neuropathy, and no correlation was noted between exposure and degree of abnormality. The abnormality seen—small, dispersed sensory nerve action potentials—is also commonly seen with normal aging. These findings of peripheral neuropathy have not been replicated in animal studies.[152]

Although a few individuals have developed dramatic CNS involvement after exposure to styrene, [153,156] the majority of reports about CNS involvement after chronic exposure to styrene discuss asymptomatic disease with abnormalities noted on electroencephalography,[157,158] and increased reaction times.[157,159–163]

In conclusion, although acute, reversible neurobehavioral effects have been studied under controlled conditions, no convincing evidence of chronic, irreversible effects of styrene exposure has been presented.

CHLORINATED HYDROCARBONS

Trichloroethylene

OSHA PEL: TWA 100 ppm; CL 1,200 ppm

ACGIH TLV: TWA 50 ppm; STEL 200 ppm; BEI: trichloroethanol in urine at end of shift 320 mg/g creatinine, trichloroethylene in end-exhaled air before shift and at end of work week 0.5 ppm

DFG MAK: 50 ppm (260 mg/m³); BAT: blood end of work week and end of shift 500 mg/dl

NIOSH REL: (Trichloroethylene) TWA 250 ppm (waste anesthetic gases); CL 2 ppm/1 hour

Trichloroethylene (TCE) is an important organic solvent used extensively in industry in metal degreasing, extracting oils and fats from vegetable products, cleaning optical lenses and photographic plates, paints and enamels, and dry cleaning, and as an adhesive in the leather industry. Although its use in recent years has diminished somewhat because of concern that it could be a human carcinogen,[164] NIOSH estimates the total number of individuals exposed to TCE to be in excess of 3.5 million.[165]

Trichloroethylene has been recognized as an industrial hazard with neurotoxic properties for over 50 years.[166] It was once commonly used as an anesthetic agent despite early reports of toxicity.[167–170] Clinical experience suggested that it was safe in minimal concentrations, and at the time, it was one of the few nonexplosive agents that could supplement nitrous oxide and did not produce significant respiratory depression.[171,172] Trichloroethylene was abandoned as an anesthetic agent, apparently not because of its toxicity but because its anesthetic action was weak and eventually better agents became available.[171]

The major neurologic manifestation is related to a slowly reversible trigeminal neuropathy,[166–168, 173–176] although involvement of other cranial nerves and peripheral nerves has also been described.[166,177,178] The trigeminal neuropathy associated with TCE intoxication was recognized as characteristic, and for a time intentional exposure was considered a useful treatment of trigeminal neuralgia.[174] Cranial neuropathies after general anesthesia were noted with TCE over 40 years ago.[167,168,170] Of 13 cases of multiple cranial nerve palsies following general anesthesia, two were related to TCE anesthesia.[12] Paresthesias developed around the lips 24–48 hours after general anesthesia, which then spread to involve the entire trigeminal distribution bilaterally over the ensuing 2–3 days. Weakness also occasionally occurred in the trigeminal distribution, and the facial (VII), optic (II), and other lower cranial nerves also became affected.[166,167] Resolution of the trigeminal neuropathy occurred slowly in an "onion peel" distribution, believed to indicate segmental or nuclear trigeminal involvement.[166,178]

Most important, much of the earlier literature on the neurotoxicity of TCE includes observations that were most likely due to decomposition products (e.g., dichloroacetylene) rather than to TCE itself.[168,170,179–181] Dichloroacetylene, produced most prominently under alkali conditions, reacts violently with air to produce two noxious gases, phosgene and carbon monoxide.[180] Short-term exposure to narcotizing levels of TCE in the industrial setting has also been reported to induce a transverse myelopathy.[182] This report is of interest because it has also been shown that a transverse myelopathy can be experimentally induced in the rat with dichloracetate, which is a possible metabolite of TCE/dichloroacetylene.[183] Attempts to experimentally reproduce the neurotoxicity associated with the industrial use of TCE have not been successful using pure grades of TCE.[184–187] Based on the clinical and experimental data, it is unclear whether chemically pure TCE produces any chronic neurotoxic injury.

Few data are available on the neuropathologic changes after TCE exposure. A single autopsied case of an individual who died 51 days after industrial exposure to TCE and TCE decomposition products (probably dichloroacetylene) revealed bilaterally symmetric brainstem lesions.[173] These changes were most prominent in the fifth nerve nuclei, spinal tracts, and nerve roots. The fifth nerves showed extensive myelin and axonal degeneration, both within and outside the brainstem. Other neuropathologic changes were seen, but were less prominent. It has been suspected that this effect of TCE on the trigeminal nucleus results from activation of latent herpes simplex infection.[188]

Although the result of high-level exposures to TCE and its decomposition products are well described, reports of possible effects from chronic, low-level exposure occurring in the industrial setting are relatively few. These reports have focused on neuropsychiatric and behavioral effects including a neurasthenic syndrome with subjective complaints of dizziness, headache, nausea, fatigue, anxiety, and insomnia.[189–194] Although these disorders reportedly become more severe with length of employment and degree of exposure, the neurobehavioral and neuropsychological literature on the toxic effects of TCE is so fragmented and poorly documented that it is impossible to make any firm conclusions regarding the neurotoxic potential of low-level, chronic exposure to TCE.[195] Neurobehavioral disturbances following acute, high-level exposure have included severe psychiatric presentations.[196,197]

Several studies evaluated the behavioral effects of a single, short-term exposure to TCE.[193,198–201] These studies have indicated that, while fatigue and sleepiness occur in humans following exposure to concentrations above 100 ppm for 2 hours, no deterioration in performance or manual dexterity follows exposure to levels up to 300 ppm. In one study, adverse effects on performance were seen at 1,000 ppm, but no significant effects were seen at lower concentrations.[201] A frequently cited study found detrimental effects of 8 hours' exposure to 110 ppm TCE on performing tests of perception, complex reaction time, memory, and manual dexterity.[193] Others have been unable to replicate this study, however.[198,201] In a study in which subjects were exposed to 1,000 ppm TCE and optokinetic nystagmus was measured, minimal effects were seen and were found to persist for no more than 2 hours.[202] Effects are somewhat increased when ethanol ingestion is added to the TCE exposure;[199,200] it has been demonstrated that ethanol will inhibit metabolism of TCE to its breakdown products, trichloroethanol and trichloroacetic acid, thereby increasing TCE concentration in blood.[203] In general, however, studies have shown that the behavioral effects of ethanol are more pronounced than those of TCE.

In conclusion, there is no compelling evidence that either acute exposure to TCE at or below 300 ppm or chronic low-level exposure has adverse neurobehavioral effects.

Perchloroethylene (1,1,2,2-Tetrachloroethylene)

OSHA PEL: TWA 100 ppm; CL 200 ppm

ACGIH TLV: TWA 50 ppm (skin); STEL 200 ppm

DFG MAK: 50 ppm (345 mg/m³); BAT: blood 100 mg/dl

NIOSH REL: (Tetrachlorethylene) Minimize workplace exposure

Perchloroethylene (PCE) is a colorless, nonflammable liquid that has widely replaced TCE as a solvent in dry cleaning, and is also used as a degreasing agent and chemical intermediate. It is reported to produce similar neuropsychological effects to those of TCE, including a neurasthenic syndrome with long-lasting changes in personality and memory.[204] A single study examined 27 workers with daily PCE exposure who worked in dry cleaning operations.[205] Neurologic examination, including nerve conduction velocities, electromyography, and behavioral tests, was performed. Behavioral tests were administered both before and following each workshift (8 hours) over 5 consecutive days. This study failed to show acute neurobehavioral toxicity below exposures of 50 ppm of PCE.

Chronic neurologic effects have recently been reported in workers exposed to mixtures of TCE and PCE.[206,207] In these workers, trigeminal sensory defects, neurasthenic symptoms, and memory disturbances were noted. These were uncontrolled studies, however, with reporting of subjective symptoms only, and were therefore difficult to interpret. Although long-term exposures reportedly cause more serious effects, evidence in support of these claims has not been presented.

Methylene Chloride (Dichloromethane)

OSHA PEL: TWA 100 ppm; CL 200 ppm; peak 300/5 minutes/3 hours

ACGIH TLV: TWA 50 ppm; STEL 100 ppm (skin)

DFG MAK: 50 ppm (105 mg/m³)

Methylene chloride is widely used in industry for paint stripping, as a blowing agent for foam, as a solvent for degreasing, in the manufacture of photographic film, as the carrier in rapid-dry paints, and in aerosol propellants. It is also used in the diphasic treatment of metal surfaces, in the textile and plastics industry, and for extracting heat-sensitive edible fats and essential oils.[208] It is estimated that almost 100,000 individuals are exposed to methylene chloride in the workplace alone.[208]

As with other solvents, methylene chloride has CNS depressant properties at high levels of exposure and may lead rapidly to unconsciousness and death.[209–213] This has been reported both in industrial settings[209,211] and as a result of solvent inhalation abuse.[212,213]

Methylene chloride has generally been considered safer than other chlorinated hydrocarbons and has not been carefully studied as a possible cause of chronic CNS dysfunction. It is metabolized to carbon monoxide[214–217] and therefore it has potential hypoxic effects that must be considered when assessing its CNS depressant effects. Carbon monoxide at high levels and other forms of cerebral hypoxia are known to cause permanent neurologic sequelae.

The acute effects of exposure to methylene chloride have been studied in controlled experiments in humans.[218–220] In one study, 11 healthy nonsmokers were exposed to levels of methylene chloride up to 1,000 ppm for 1 to 2 hours.[218] Inhalation of methylene chloride at 500–1,000 ppm for this length of time was followed by a sustained (at 24 hours' postexposure) elevation of carboxyhemoglobin, but these levels never exceeded 10% saturation. Visual evoked responses in the three subjects tested showed an increase in peak-to-peak amplitudes after 2 hours of exposure, and returned to baseline 1 hour after termination of exposure. No untoward subjective symptoms occurred at levels of exposure below 1,000 ppm. At exposure to concentrations of 1,000 ppm, two of three subjects reported "mild light-headedness" that promptly resolved after cessation of exposure.

The effects of methylene chloride exposure on three tests of cognitive function (reaction time, short-term memory, calculation ability) were tested in 14 normal subjects.[219] Repeated tests at exposures to 870, 1,740, 2,600, and 3,470 mg/m³ methylene chloride showed no statistically significant impairment in performance of these tests, although at the highest exposure levels, a greater variation in the responses was obtained for reaction time than under control conditions.

Controlled exposure of normal volunteers for up to 24 hours to various concentrations (up to 800 ppm) of methylene chloride in five separate studies showed the following abnormalities: After 2.5 hours of exposure to 500 ppm, complaints of "general uneasiness" were noted. After 4 hours of exposure to 300 and 800 ppm, in only one experiment were mood rating scales noted to be significant for depression. There was no impairment of cognitive performance as measured by tests of short-term memory and calculation ability in any of these studies after 2.5 hours of exposure to methylene chloride at levels up to 1,000 ppm. Some impairment was noted in psychomotor performance and vigilance after 3–4 hours of exposure to 800 ppm.

Overall, studies of controlled human exposure to methylene chloride do not show effects of CNS toxicity, except at higher levels of exposure, and even then, the effects are minimal and rapidly reversible.

There have been few attempts to address the issue of chronic exposure and permanent neurologic sequelae to methylene chloride. A group of 46 men who worked in a factory making acetate film reported an excess of neurologic symptoms when compared to a nonexposed referent group.[221] These individuals were exposed to a methylene chloride–methanol (9 to 1) mixture; however, methylene chloride concentrations were below 100 ppm. Although neurologic symptoms were increased in the exposed group, no abnormalities were detected on neuropsychological tests. No evidence was found of long-term damage that could be attributed to exposure to methylene chloride. In a larger study to assess the potential chronic health effects of methylene chloride, no increase in the number of expected deaths due to diseases of the nervous system were seen among 1,013 workers chronically exposed to methylene chloride.[222]

In conclusion, the evidence suggests that methylene chloride does not produce permanent neurologic sequelae except with massive acute exposures, which are associated with hypoxic encephalopathy. No evidence exists that chronic low-level exposure causes adverse neurobehavioral effects.

1,1,1-Trichloroethane

OSHA PEL: TWA 350 ppm

ACGIH TLV: TWA 350 ppm; STEL 450 ppm

DFG MAK: 200 ppm (2,080 mg/m^3); BAT: blood 55 mg/dl

NIOSH REL: (1,1,1-Trichlorethane) CL 350 ppm/15 minutes

1,1,1-Trichloroethane is widely used as an industrial degreasing solvent and is considered to be relatively less toxic than other solvents, although several reports of severe toxicity and deaths exist in the literature.[223–226] Its acute toxicity has made it unsuitable as a volatile anesthetic and its use as a carrier in aerosols was abandoned in the United States in 1973.

In those cases in which postmortem examination of the brain was undertaken, the pathologic changes suggested cerebral hypoxia related either to a primary CNS depressant effect,[223] or secondary to cardiac or respiratory arrest.[223,226] The possible mechanisms of the effects of 1,1,1-trichloroethane have been postulated to be related either to its effect on the autonomic nervous system[227] or to central sleep apnea.[228] Chronic cardiac toxicity and possible sensitization to other inhalation anesthetics have also been suggested as possible mechanisms of 1,1,1-trichloroethane toxicity.[229]

There are several reports of acute behavioral and neuropsychological changes after voluntary exposure of humans to 1,1,1-trichloroethane.[230–233] No impairment was seen on a series of psychomotor tests following several days of exposure to 500 ppm, however.[230] In another study, no behavioral effects were seen after two 4.5-hour exposures to 450 ppm.[231] Two additional studies demonstrated some performance deficits.[232,233] In one study, after 3.5 hours of exposure to 0, 175, and 350 ppm of 1,1,1-trichloroethane, abnormalities were seen on some behavioral tests, most notably those concerned with attention and concentration and those concerned with analysis of grammatical statements.[233] Overall, these studies suggest only mild acute effects, if any, of exposure to levels of trichloroethane up to 500 ppm.

With regard to chronic exposure, a clinical neurophysiologic and behavioral study of female workers chronically exposed to this agent at levels of 110–990 ppm found no differences when compared to a reference solvent-unexposed group.[234]

In conclusion, it appears that 1,1,1-trichloroethane is not associated with acute or chronic neurotoxicity at levels below 990 ppm, and that the only permanent neurologic sequelae are related to cerebral hypoxia after massive exposure.

MISCELLANEOUS COMPOUNDS

Hydrogen Sulfide

OSHA PEL: CL 20 ppm

ACGIH TLV: TWA 10 ppm; STEL 15 ppm

NIOSH REL: (Hydrogen sulfide) CL 15 mg/m^3/10 minutes

Hydrogen sulfide is a colorless, flammable gas found naturally in volcanic gases, decaying matter, and intestines as a result of normal bacterial flora action. It has been identified as a leading cause of death in the workplace in the petrochemical and chemical industries, the production of fibers and sheets from viscose syrup, sewage treatment, and fishing.[235] Hydrogen sulfide is known to be a leading cause of death in the workplace, and brief high-level exposures have been known to have adverse effects on the eyes (conjunctivitis and keratitis) and respiratory system. Death can occur rapidly from respiratory failure with brief, high-level exposures.[236]

Hydrogen sulfide, technically not an organic solvent, is discussed here because of its association with the petrochemical industry as well as its common association with carbon disulfide (see below). Reports rarely mention hydrogen sulfide exposure, but exposure to both carbon disulfide and hydrogen sulfide is common and hydrogen sulfide may increase the hazard of exposure to carbon disulfide.[237] Both hydrogen sulfide and hydrogen cyanide are thought to act through a mechanism termed "histotoxic hypoxia," even though there may be an adequate supply of oxygen to peripheral tissues. The peripheral PO$_2$ is often normal or even greater than normal, but the cells are unable to use oxygen, probably by inhibition of cytochrome oxidase.[56,238]

Although adverse effects from acute high-level exposure are well documented, no conclusive reports have demonstrated adverse effects from chronic, low-level exposure to hydrogen sulfide. Chronic, low-level exposure to carbon disulfide, with concurrent presence of hydrogen sulfide, has been reported to cause neurologic sequelae, but possible synergistic effects of these two compounds have not been thoroughly investigated.

Two reports have suggested persistent neurologic effects of exposure to hydrogen sulfide.[239,240] In one of these articles,[239] widely quoted as showing persistent neurologic sequelae, it is really unclear what problems became persistent. First, all individuals with neurologic symptoms recovered, usually within 6 weeks. Virtually all of these individuals suffered multiple low-level exposures. Finally, the transient neurologic problems consisted of neurasthenic symptoms and not dementia or a seizure disorder, as is often implied.[239]

Another widely cited paper about permanent neurologic sequelae to hydrogen sulfide exposure described a high-level exposure in a community surrounding a recycling and sulfur-recovery plant, where 320 persons were hospitalized and 22 died.[240] Of the 320 survivors of this massive exposure, four were believed to have suffered permanent neurologic sequelae. Two "experienced dysarthria as evidenced by lingual difficulty," and one epileptic patient had an increase in his seizure frequency. It is not clear if these four individuals actually suffered any structural CNS changes or if they had any permanent neurologic sequelae, since details of their examinations were not discussed.

A more recent paper reviewed 221 cases of exposure to hydrogen sulfide in the petrochemical industry of Alberta, Canada, over a 5-year period.[241] Neurologic symptoms occurring acutely were common and 75% of individuals had a period of unconsciousness. Long-term adverse effects were not apparent in any of the survivors, however.

In conclusion, it does not appear that permanent neurologic sequelae result from hydrogen sulfide exposure, except in individuals who experience high-level exposures that result in hypoxic encephalopathy. No evidence suggests that chronic, low-level exposure to hydrogen sulfide is associated with adverse neurobehavioral effects.

Carbon Disulfide

OSHA PEL: TWA 20 ppm; CL 30 ppm

ACGIH TLV: TWA 10 ppm (skin)

DFG MAK: 10 ppm (30 mg/m³)

NIOSH REL: TWA 1 ppm; CL 10 ppm/15 minutes

Carbon disulfide is used in the rubber and rayon industries (viscose rayon), in grain and soil fumigation, in certain insecticides, as an ingredient in organic solvents and adhesives, and in the production of carbon tetrachloride. Although inhalation of the vapor is the major route of entry, it can also be absorbed through skin contact and by the gastrointestinal tract in its liquid form. Carbon disulfide is among the few organic solvents clearly shown to be a chronic human neurotoxicant based on its production of a uniform pattern of neurologic dysfunction and the ability to reproduce this pattern in experimental animals. Carbon disulfide intoxication has been associated with the following clinical syndromes: (1) acute and chronic encephalopathy (often with prominent psychiatric manifestations), (2) polyneuropathy (both peripheral and cranial), (3) parkinsonism, and (4) asymptomatic CNS and PNS dysfunction.

An acute encephalopathy occurs as the result of high-level exposure. It is nonspecific and consists of an acute confusional state and seizures, with the frequent sequela of mental impairment.[243] Symptoms first begin to appear at 300 ppm after several hours. The encephalopathy will occur progressively faster with higher levels of exposure, such that 2,000–3,300 ppm leads to narcosis in 30 minutes, and concentrations of 5,000 ppm will cause death in 30 to 60 minutes. Reports of these high levels of exposure are uncommon; most reports concern lower-level chronic exposure.

Most reports of carbon disulfide neurotoxicity are in viscose rayon workers,[243–250] but several more recent reports are in grain storage workers.[251,252] Although carbon disulfide neurotoxicity was once common in the viscose rayon industry, with improvement in factory ventilation, only intermittent and chronic, insidious neurologic syndromes are now seen.[253,254] Higher levels may still be found in developing countries, but in industrialized countries, levels average 10–30 ppm. These levels meet the legal limits for human occupational exposure set in the United States.

Peripheral neuropathy related to carbon disulfide is usually mild and is characterized by distal paresthesias and painful cramps in the calf muscles.[243,245,246,248,249] In more severe cases reported in the past, difficulty in walking, diminished reflexes, and motor weakness were seen.[246] Neurophysiologic studies have shown slowing of nerve conduction velocities and electromyographic abnormalities consistent with chronic partial denervation.[248,249,255–258]

Electrophysiologic studies have also suggested spinal cord and neuromuscular junction involvement.[256] Cranial nerve abnormalities consist of a diminished or absent corneal reflex, with preserved facial sensation and a reduced pupillary light reflex. Visual abnormalities occur in 10% of exposed workers and consist of enlarged blind spots and blurring of the disk margins.

Historically, acute high-level exposures resulted in a toxic psychosis with an agitated delirium and frequently permanent mental impairment.[247] The more frequent chronic syndrome involves the development of progressive cognitive impairment with associated parkinsonism, and peripheral and cranial neuropathy. The parkinsonian syndrome reported in association with carbon disulfide exposure consists of cogwheel rigidity, decreased associated movements, tremor, and bradykinesia.[245,246,251,252] It is atypical in that it virtually always occurs in combination with other findings of intoxication including neuropsychiatric changes and peripheral neuropathy.

In a study comparing clinically affected individuals, an exposed asymptomatic group, and unexposed individuals, statistically significant differences were found among the groups on tests of speed, vigilance, manual dexterity, and intelligence.[247] Individuals in the "latent" group showed traits indicative of depressive mood, mild motor impairment, and intellectual impairment, whereas the clinically symptomatic group displayed more severe disturbances.[247]

A more recent study of neuropsychological function in 131 viscose rayon workers exposed for at least 1 year to carbon disulfide levels generally below 20 ppm failed to show any significant differences between exposed and unexposed individuals,[250] although exposed individuals did have a higher incidence of neurasthenic symptoms. Similar studies of chronic exposure to presumably safe levels of carbon disulfide report the gradual onset of behavioral abnormalities, including a neurasthenic syndrome, irritability, insomnia, and depression.[254,258–261] Subclinical peripheral neuropathy has also been described.[57,257,262]

Pathologic changes occur in both the CNS and PNS, but neither the levels nor durations of exposure required for the development of these adverse effects are known in humans. Human cases are few, but experimental animal studies have produced similar pathologic changes.[263,264] CNS pathology consists of neuronal degeneration diffusely throughout the cerebral hemispheres but maximally in the frontal regions. Cell loss is also noted in the globus pallidus, putamen, and cerebellar cortex, with loss of Purkinje cells. Vascular abnormalities have also been seen with endothelial proliferation of arterioles, sometimes associated with focal necrosis or demyelination. PNS changes have consisted primarily of myelin swelling and fragmentation and large focal axonal swellings characteristic of a distal axonopathy.

In conclusion, both the abundant human and experimental animal data are sufficient to place carbon disulfide as one of the proven human neurotoxicants. Both CNS and PNS involvement can be seen, but toxic levels of exposure are not known.

Major Issues in Future Studies

Many of the problems with the prior studies on the neurotoxicity, and specifically on the neurobehavioral effects, of organic solvents have already been discussed. These and other issues merit further discussion, however, in relation to both past and future studies in this area.

CONTROLLED STUDIES

Future studies will need to focus on using appropriate control groups. The validity of uncontrolled studies in this area was seriously questioned by a Danish study cited previously.[52] In their original study, these investigators rated 16 of 20 solvent-exposed workers as mildly to moderately demented, 3 of 20 as possibly demented, and 1 of 20 as unimpaired. This rating was obtained without adequate controls and was based on a combination of symptoms, test results, and clinical impression. After reanalysis and the addition of proper controls (age-, sex-, and education-matched), none of the 20 solvent-exposed individuals were rated as intellectually impaired. To date, the evidence is unconvincing that a chronic, irreversible neurobehavioral CNS disorder occurs among spray painters or among workers chronically exposed to jet fuel or other mixed solvents. The use of statistical manipulation of grouped data obtained by interviews, questionnaires, and neuropsychological tests lacks validity and reliability, especially when inadequate controls are used.

DOSE-EFFECT RELATIONSHIP

There is an almost complete lack of understanding of what solvent mixtures (and at what dose) will cause structural damage to the nervous system. It is known, though, that many toxins associated with structural damage to the nervous system produce a consistent pattern of disease, strongly linked to the dose and duration of exposure.[61] At the present time, only five solvents have been shown to have neurotoxic properties: carbon disulfide, *n*-hexane, methyl–butyl ketone, toluene (in abusers only), and impure trichloroethylene.[7] However, even among these solvents, dose-effect relationships regarding chronic neurotoxicity are not well known. Past studies of solvent mixtures have not even vaguely suggested what degree of exposure individuals have had over the years. The composition of the solvent mixtures is often not known. Future studies will need to provide an analysis of the solvent mixture and attempt to quantify the degree of exposure more accurately.

SOLVENT ABUSE IN OCCUPATIONAL SETTINGS

Most studies on the subject of solvent abuse focus on adolescents.[63,64,265] It has been observed that adults at risk for solvent abuse include those whose work brings them into contact with these substances. Among this group are shoemakers, painters, individuals who work in gas stations, individuals involved in the refinement of petrochemicals, and others.[266] However, few attempts have been made to identify the prevalence of solvent abuse in industry.

One study reviewed industrial accidents due to exposure to chlorinated hydrocarbons. Of 384 cases of industrial accidents due to either trichloroethylene, perchloroethylene, or 1,1,1-trichloroethane, nine (2.3%) were in individuals identified as habitual solvent abusers by the person investigating the accident.[267] Though 2.3% seems to be a small number, one needs to consider that the number may be much higher, especially in those industries where solvents with higher abuse potential (e.g., toluene) are used, such as the paint industry. In addition, considering the millions of individuals exposed to solvents in the workplace, even 2.3% represents a large number of people.

Finally, when discussing abuse in industry, one needs to consider issues of personal protection. It is our opinion that if a worker is instructed on the proper use of protective devices (respirators) on the particular job being performed, and that individual chooses not to comply, the injury should be considered self-inflicted (i.e., abuse) rather than occupational injury, provided the employer has observed its part of the rules and instructions in force. This last issue has been ignored in the occupational literature but needs to be addressed in a critical manner in future studies.

ALCOHOL ABUSE

The effects of acute and chronic alcohol abuse on the CNS and PNS are well known to those in the field of occupational medicine. Nevertheless, few studies on the neurotoxicity of organic solvents pay sufficient attention to the effects of alcohol on cognitive function.[49,268] When investigators pay careful attention to alcohol consumption, interesting results may be seen.[50,51] In one study, the only variable correlated with solvent exposure was excessive alcohol consumption.[50] In a cross-sectional epidemiologic study of house painters and control subjects, several individuals from both groups had to be excluded because of excessive alcohol consumption.[51] Future studies will need to address the issue of alcohol abuse in solvent-exposed individuals more critically and quantifiably in order to control for this factor.

Summary

Organic solvents are the most prevalent group of industrial compounds with neurotoxic potential. Despite their wide distribution in the workplace, and the numerous studies that have focused on neurotoxicity, many questions remain unanswered. With the exception of those five solvents with proven human neurotoxicity at relatively high levels of exposure, low-level exposure to most solvents and solvent mixtures remains unproven as human neurotoxicants. Physicians need to be wary of claims of neurotoxic effects of solvents and to evaluate workers with these claims carefully for possible explanations of their symptoms.

References

1. Leading work-related diseases and injuries—United States. MMWR 1983;32:24–26.
2. Allen N. Solvents and Other Industrial Organic Compounds. In PJ Vinken, GW Bruyn (eds), Handbook of Clinical Neurology. New York: Elsevier, 1979;36:361–389.
3. Goetz CG. Organic Solvents. In CG Goetz (ed), Neurotoxins in Clinical Practice. Jamaica, NY: Spectrum, 1985;65–90.
4. Spencer PS, Schaumburg HH. Experimental and Clinical Neurotoxicology. Baltimore: Williams & Wilkins, 1980.
5. O'Donoghue JL. Neurotoxicity of Industrial and Commercial Chemicals. Vol. I. Boca Raton, FL: CRC Press, 1985.
6. O'Donoghue JL. Neurotoxicity of Industrial and Commercial Chemicals. Vol. II. Boca Raton, FL: CRC Press, 1985.
7. Spencer PS, Schaumburg HH. Organic solvent neurotoxicity: facts and research needs. Scand J Work Environ Health 1985;11(Suppl 1):53–60.
8. Organic solvents in the workplace. MMWR 1987;36:282–283.

9. Flodin U, Edling C, Axelson O. Clinical studies with psychoorganic syndromes among workers with exposure to solvents. Am J Ind Med 1984;5:287–295.
10. Gregersen P, Angelso B, Elmo Nielson T, Norgaard B, Vldal C. Neurotoxic effects of organic solvents in exposed workers: an occupational, neurophysiological, and neurological investigation. Am J Ind Med 1984;5:201–225.
11. Lindstrom K. Changes in psychological performances of solvent-exposed workers. Am J Ind Med 1980;1:69–84.
12. Report of the workshop session on clinical and epidemiological topics: human aspects of solvent neurobehavioral effects. Neurotoxicology 1987;7:54–55.
13. World Health Organization/Nordic Council of Ministers. Chronic effects of organic solvents on the central nervous system and diagnostic criteria. Copenhagen: WHO, 1985.
14. Grasso P, Sharratt M, Davies DM, Irvine D. Neurophysiological and psychological disorders and occupational exposure to organic solvents. Food Chem Toxicol 1984;10:819–852.
15. Hartman DE. Neuropsychological Toxicology: Identification and Assessment of Human Neurotoxic Syndromes. New York: Pergamon, 1988.
16. Seppalainen AM, Linstrom K, Martelin T. Neurophysiological and psychological picture of solvent poisoning. Am J Ind Med 1980;1:31–42.
17. Flodin U, Edling C, Axelson O. Clinical studies of psychoorganic syndromes among workers with exposure to solvents. Am J Ind Med 1984;5:287–295.
18. Juntunen J, Hupli V, Hernberg S, Luisto M. Neurological picture of organic solvent poisoning in industry: a retrospective clinical study of 37 patients. Int Arch Occup Environ Health 1980;46:219–231.
19. Gregersen P, Klausen H, Elsnab CV. Chronic toxic encephalopathy in solvent-exposed painters in Denmark 1976–1980: clinical cases and social consequences after a 5 year follow-up. Am J Ind Med 1987;11:399–417.
20. Axelson O, Hane M, Hogstedt C. A case-referent study on neuropsychiatric disorders among workers exposed to solvents. Scand J Work Environ Health 1976;2:14–20.
21. Iregren A. Effects of psychological test performance of workers exposed to a single solvent (toluene)—a comparison with effects of exposure to a mixture of organic solvents. Neurobehav Toxicol Teratol 1982;4:695–701.
22. Knave B, Persson HE, Goldberg M, Westerholm P. Long-term exposure to jet fuel. An investigation on occupationally exposed workers with special reference to the nervous system. Scand J Work Environ Health 1976;2:152–164.
23. Knave B, Mindus P, Struwe G. Neurasthenic symptoms in workers occupationally exposed to jet fuel. Acta Psychiatr Scand 1979;60:39–49.
24. Knave B, Anshelm-Olson BA, Eloffson S, Gamberale F, Isaksson A, Mindus P, Persson HE, Struwe G, Wennberg A, Westerholm P. Long-term exposure to jet fuel II. A cross-sectional epidemiologic investigation on occupationally exposed industrial workers with special reference to the nervous system. Scand J Work Environ Health 1978;4:19–45.
25. Hanninen H, Eskelinen L, Husman K, Nurminen M. Behavioral effects of long-term exposure to a mixture of organic solvents. Scand J Work Environ Health 1976;4:240–255.

26. Hane M, Axelson O, Blume J, Hogstedt C, Sundell L, Ydreborg B. Psychological function changes among house painters. Scand J Work Environ Health 1977;3:91–99.
27. Linz DH, deGarmo PL, Morton WE, Wiens AN, Coull BM, Maricle RA. Organic solvent-induced encephalopathy in industrial painters. J Occup Med 1986;28:119–129.
28. Baker EL, Letz RE, Eisen EA, Pothier LJ, Plantamura DL, Larson M, Wolford R. Neurobehaviroal effects of solvents in construction painters. J Occup Med 1988;30:166–123.
29. Husman K, Karli P. Clinical neurological findings among car painters exposed to a mixture to organic solvents. Scand J Work Environ Health 1980;6:33–39.
30. Husman K. Symptoms of car painters with long-term exposure to a mixture of organic solvents. Scand J Work Environ Health 1980;6:19–32.
31. Elofsson G, Gamberale F, Hindmarsh T et al. Exposure to organic solvents: a cross-sectional epidemiologic investigation on occupationally exposed car and industrial spray painters with special reference to the nervous system. Scand J Work Environ Health 1980;6:239–273.
32. Linstrom K, Wickstrom G. Psychological function changes among maintenance house painters exposed to low levels of organic solvent mixtures. Acta Psychiatr Scand 1983;67(Suppl 3030):81–91.
33. Orbaek P, Risberg J, Rosen I et al. Effects of long-term exposure to solvents in the paint industry. Scand J Work Environ Health 1985;11(Suppl 2):1–28.
34. Valciukas JA, Lilis R, Singer RM et al. Neurobehavioral changes among shipyard painters exposed to solvents. Arch Environ Health 1985;40:47–52.
35. Fidler AT, Baker EL, Letz RE. The neurobehaviroal effects of occupational exposure to organic solvents among construction painters. Br J Ind Med 1987;44:292–308.
36. Arlien-Soborg P, Zilstorff K, Grandjean B, Pedersen LM. Vestibular dysfunction in occupational chronic solvent intoxication. Clin Otolaryngol 1981;6:285–290.
37. Binaschi S, Cantu L. Vestibular Function in Solvent Exposure: Clinical Criteria. In R Gilioli, MG Cassitto, V Foa V (eds), Neurobehavioral Methods in Occupational Health. Oxford: Pergamon, 1983;205–210.
38. Hodgson MJ, Furman J, Ryan C, Durrant J, Kern E. Encephalopathy and vestibulopathy following short-term hydrocarbon exposure. J Occup Med 1989;31:51–54.
39. Seppalainen AM. Neurotoxic effects of industrial solvents. Electroencephalogr Clin Neurophysiol 1973;34:702–703.
40. Seppalainen AM. Neurophysiological findings among workers exposed to organic solvents. Acta Neurol Scandinav 1982;66(Suppl 92):109–116.
41. Mutti A, Cavatorta A, Lommi G, Lotta S, Franchini I. Neurophysiological effects of long-term exposure to hydrocarbon mixtures. Arch Toxicol 1982;5:120–124.
42. Elofsson SA, Gamberale F, Hindmarsch T, Iregren A et al. En epidemiologisk undersokning av yrkesmassigt exponerade bil-och industrilackerare. Lakartidn 1979;46:4127–4148.
43. Hagstadius S, Risberg J. Regional Cerebral Blood Flow in Subjects Occupationally Exposed to Organic Solvents. In R Gilioli, MG Cassitto, V Foa (eds), Neurobehaviroal Methods in Occupational Health. Oxford: Pergamon, 1983;211–217.

44. Arlien-Soborg P, Henriksen L, Gade A, Glydensted C, Paulson OB. Cerebral blood flow in chronic toxic encephalopathy in house painters exposed to organic solvents. Acta Neurol Scandinav 1982;66:34–41.

45. Juntunen J, Hernberg S, Eistola P, Hupli V. Exposure to industrial solvents and brain atrophy: a retrospective study of pneumoencephalographic findings among 37 patients with exposure to industrial solvents. Eur Neurol 1980;19:366–375.

46. Jensen PB, Nielsen P, Nielsen NO, Olivarius B de F, Hansen JH. Chronic toxic encephalopathy following occupational exposure to organic solvents. The course after cessation of exposure illustrated by a neurophysiological follow-up investigation. Ugeskr Laeger 1984;146:1387–1390.

47. Orbaek P, Lindgren M, Olivecrona H, Haeger-Aronsen B. Computed brain tomography and psychometric test performances in patients with solvent induced chronic toxic encephalopathy and healthy controls. Br J Ind Med 1987;44:175.

48. Seppalainen AM, Husman K, Martenson C. Neurophysiological effects of long-term exposure to a mixture of organic solvents. Scand J Work Environ Health 1978;4:304–314.

49. Errebo-Knudsen EO, Olsen F. Organic solvents and presenile dementia (the painters' syndrome). A critical review of the Danish literature. Sci Total Environ 1986;48:45–67.

50. Juntunen J, Matikainen E, Antti-Poika M et al. Nervous system effects of long-term occupational exposure to toluene. Acta Neurol Scand 1985;72:512–517.

51. Triebig G, Claus D, Csuzda I et al. Cross-sectional epidemiological study on neurotoxicity of solvents in paints and lacquers. Int Arch Occup Environ Health 1988;60:233–241.

52. Gade A, Mortensen EL, Bruhn P. "Chronic painter's syndrome." A reanalysis of psychological test data in a group of diagnosed cases, based on comparisons with matched controls. Acta Neurol Scand 1988;77:293–306.

53. Errebo-Knudsen, Olsen F. Solvents and the brain: explanation of the discrepancy between the number of toxic encephalopathy reported (and compensated) in Denmark and other countries. Br J Ind Med 1987;44:71–72.

54. Arlien-Soborg P, Bruhn P, Gyldensted C, Melgaard B. Chronic painters' syndrome: chronic toxic encephalopathy in house painters. Acta Neurol Scand 1979;60:149–156.

55. Bruhn P, Arlien-Soborg P, Gyldensted C, Christensen EL. Prognosis in chronic toxic encephalopathy: a two-year follow-up study in 26 house painters with occupational encephalopathy. Acta Neurol Scand 1981;64:259–272.

56. Smith L, Kruszyna H, Smith RP. The effect of methemoglobin on the inhibition of cytochrome c oxidase by cyanide, sulfide and azide. Biochem Pharmacol 1977;26:2247–2250.

57. Knave B, Kolmodin-Hedman B, Persson HE, Goldberg JM. Chronic exposure to carbon disulfide: effects on occupationally exposed workers with special reference to the nervous system. Work Environ Health 1974;11:49–58.

58. Cherry N, Hutchins H, Pace T, Waldron HA. Neurobehavioral effects of repeated occupational exposure to toluene and paint solvents. Br J Ind Med 1985;42:291–300.

59. Gamberale F. Use of behavioral performance tests in the assessment of solvent toxicity. Scand J Work Environ Health 1985;11(Suppl 1):65–74.

60. Bolla KI, Schwartz BS, Agnew J, Ford PD, Bleecker ML. Subclinical neuropsychiatric effects of chronic low-level solvent exposure in US paint manufacturers. J Occup Med 1990;32:671–677.
61. Schaumburg HH, Spencer PS. Recognizing neurotoxic disease. Neurology 1987;37:276–278.
62. Lazar RB, Ho SU, Melen O et al. Multifocal central nervous system damage caused by toluene abuse. Neurology 1983;33:1337–1340.
63. Hormes JT, Filley CM, Rosenberg NL. Neurologic sequelae of chronic solvent vapor abuse. Neurology 1986;36:698–702.
64. Fornazzari L, Wilkinson DA, Kapur BM et al. Cerebellar, cortical and functional impairment in toluene abusers. Acta Neurol Scand 1983;67:319–329.
65. Taylor P. On pyroligneous aether. Philos Mag J 1822;60:315–317.
66. Schneck SA. Methyl Alcohol. In PJ Vinken, GW Bruyn (eds), Handbook of Clinical Neurology. New York: Elsevier, 1979;36:351–360.
67. MacFarlan JF. On methylated spirits, and some of its preparations. Pharm J Trans 1855;15:310–315.
68. Wood CA, Buller F. Cases of death and blindness from Columbian spirits and other methylated preparations. JAMA 1904;43:972–977, 1058–1062.
69. Wood CA. Death and blindness as a result of poisoning by methyl, or wood alcohol and its various preparations. Int Clin 1906;16:68–78.
70. Bennett IL Jr, Cary FH, Mitchell GL Jr, Cooper MN. Acute methyl alcohol poisoning: a review based on experiences in an outbreak of 323 cases. Medicine 1953;32:431–463.
71. Crook JE, McLaughlin JS. Methyl alcohol poisoning. J Occup Med 1965;6:467–470.
72. McLean DR, Jacobs H, Mielke BW. Methanol poisoning: a clinical and pathological study. Ann Neurol 1980;8:161–167.
73. Erlanson P, Fritz H, Hagstam KE et al. Severe methanol intoxication. Acta Med Scand 1965;177:393–408.
74. Guggenheim MA, Couch JR, Weinberg W. Motor dysfunction as a permanent complication of methanol ingestion. Arch Neurol 1971;24:550–554.
75. Rosenberg NL. Methylmalonic acid, methanol, metabolic acidosis, and lesions of the basal ganglia. Ann Neurol 1987;22:96–97.
76. Aquilonius SM, Bergstrom K, Enoksson P et al. Cerebral computed tomography in methanol intoxication. J Comput Assist Tomogr 1980;4:425–428.
77. Kingsley WH, Hirsch FG. Toxicologic considerations in direct process spirit duplicating machines. Compen Med 1954;40:7–8.
78. DiVincenzo GD, Kaplan CJ, Dedinas J. Characterization of the metabolites of methyl n-butyl ketone, methyl iso-butyl ketone and methyl ethyl ketone in guinea pig serum and their clearance. Toxicol Appl Pharmacol 1976;36:511–522.
79. Spencer PS, Couri D, Schaumburg HH. N-Hexane and Methyl N-Butyl Ketone. In PS Spencer, HH Schaumburg (eds), Experimental and Clinical Neurotoxicology. Baltimore: Williams & Wilkins, 1980;456–475.
80. Perbellini L, Brugnone F, Gaffuri E. Neurotoxic metabolites of "commercial hexane" in the urine of shoe factory workers. Clin Toxicol 1981;18:1377–1385.
81. Graham DG, Carter Anthony D, Boekelheide K. In vitro and in vivo studies of the molecular pathogenesis of n-hexane neuropathy. Neurobehav Toxicol Teratol 1982;4:629–634.

82. Spencer PS, Schaumburg HH, Sabri MI, Veronesi B. The enlarging view of hexacarbon neurotoxicity. Crit Rev Toxicol 1980;3:279–356.
83. Altenkirch H, Wagner HM, Stoltenburg-Didinger G, Steppat R. Potentiation of hexacarbon-neurotoxicity by methyl-ethyl-ketone (MEK) and other substances: clinical and experimental aspects. Neurobehav Toxicol Teratol 1982;4:623–627.
84. Altenkirch H, Mager J, Stoltenburg G et al. Toxic polyneuropathies after sniffing a glue thinner. J Neurol 1977;214:137–152.
85. Saida K, Mendell JR, Weiss HS. Peripheral nerve changes induced by methyl n-butyl ketone and potentiated by methyl ethyl ketone. J Neuropathol Exp Neurol 1976;35:207–225.
86. Menkes JH. Toxic polyneuropathy due to methyl n-butyl ketone. Arch Neurol 1976;33:309.
87. Billmaier D, Yee HT, Allen N, Craft B, Williams N, Epstein S, Fontaine R. Peripheral neuropathy in a coated fabrics plant. J Occup Med 1974;16:665–671.
88. McDonough JR. Possible neuropathy from methyl n-butyl ketone. N Engl J Med 1974;290:695.
89. Allen N, Mendell JR, Billmaier DJ, Fontaine RE, O'Neill J. Toxic polyneuropathy due to methyl n-butyl ketone: an industrial outbreak. Arch Neurol 1975;32:209–218.
90. Mallov JS. MBK neuropathy among spray painters. JAMA 1976; 235:1455–1457.
91. Spencer PS, Schaumburg HH, Raleigh RL, Terhaar CJ. Nervous system degeneration produced by the industrial solvent methyl n-butyl ketone. Arch Neurol 1975;32:219–222.
92. Herskowitz A, Ishii N, Schaumburg H. N-hexane neuropathy: a syndrome occurring as a result of industrial exposure. N Engl J Med 1971;285:82–85.
93. Gonzalez EG, Downey JA. Polyneuropathy in a glue sniffer. Arch Phys Med Rehabil 1972;53:333–337.
94. Shirabe T, Tsuda T, Terao A, Araki S. Toxic polyneuropathy due to glue-sniffing: report of two cases with a light and electron-microscopic study of the peripheral nerves and muscles. J Neurol Sci 1974;21:101–113.
95. Goto I, Matsumura M, Inove N et al. Toxic polyneuropathy due to glue sniffing. J Neurol Neurosurg Psychiatry 1974;37:848–853.
96. Prockop LD, Alt M, Tison J. "Huffer's" neuropathy. JAMA 1974;229:1083–1084.
97. Korobkin R, Asbury AK, Sumner AJ, Nielsen SL. Glue-sniffing neuropathy. Arch Neurol 1975;32:158–162.
98. Oh SJ, Kim JM. Giant axonal swelling in "huffer's" neuropathy. Arch Neurol 1976;33:583–586.
99. Towfighi J, Gonatas NK, Pleasure D, Cooper HS, McCree L. Glue sniffer's neuropathy. Neurology 1976;26:238–243.
100. Schaumburg HH, Spencer PS. Degeneration in central and peripheral nervous systems produced by pure n-hexane: an experimental study. Brain 1976;99:183–192.
101. Frontali N, Amantini MC, Spagnolo A, Guarcini AM, Saltari MC. Experimental neurotoxicity and urinary metabolites of the C5-C7 aliphatic hydrocarbons used as glue solvents in shoe manufacture. Clin Toxicol 1981;18:1357–1367.

102. Seppalainen AM, Raitta C, Huuskonen MS. *N*-hexane induced changes in visual evoked potentials and electroretinograms of industrial workers. Electroencephalogr Clin Neurophysiol 1979;47:492–498.
103. Mutti A, Ferri F, Lommi G, Lotta S, Lucertini S, Franchini I. *N*-Hexane-induced changes in nerve conduction velocities and somatosensory evoked potentials. Int Arch Occup Envion Health 1982;51:45–54.
104. Press E, Done AK. Solvent sniffing: physiologic effects and community control measures. Pediatrics 1967;39:451–461, 611–622.
105. Grabski DA. Toluene sniffing producing cerebellar degeneration. Am J Psych 1961;118:461–462.
106. Kelly TW. Prolonged cerebellar dysfunction associated with paint-sniffing. Pediatrics 1975;56:605–606.
107. Knox JW, Nelson JR. Permanent encephalopathy from toluene inhalation. N Engl J Med 1966:275:1494–1496.
108. Boor JW, Hurtig HI. Persistent cerebellar ataxia after exposure to toluene. Ann Neurol 1977;2:440–442.
109. Keane JR. Toluene optic neuropathy. Ann Neurol 1978;4:390.
110. Sasa M, Igarashi S, Miyazaki T, Miyazaki K, Nakano S, Matsuoka I. Equilibrium disorders with diffuse brain atrophy in long-term toluene sniffing. Arch Otorhinolaryngol 1978;221:163–169.
111. Malm G, Lying-Tunell U. Cerebellar dysfunction related to toluene sniffing. Acta Neurol Scandinav 1980;62:188–190.
112. Streicher HZ, Gabow PA, Moss AH, Kono D, Kaehny WD. Syndromes of toluene sniffing in adults. Ann Intern Med 1981;94:758–762.
113. Takeuchi Y, Hisanaga N, Ono Y, Ogawa T, Hamaguchi Y, Okamoto S. Cerebellar dysfunction caused by sniffing of toluene-containing thinner. Indust Health 1981;19:163–169.
114. King MD. Neurological sequelae of toluene abuse. Human Toxicol 1982;1:281–287.
115. Metrick SA, Brenner RP. Abnormal brainstem auditory evoked potentials in chronic paint sniffers. Ann Neurol 1982;12:553–556.
116. Ehyai A, Freemon FR. Progressive optic neuropathy and sensorineural hearing loss due to chronic glue sniffing. J Neurol Neurosurg Psychiatry 1983;46:349–351.
117. Lazar RB, Ho SU, Melen O, Daghestani AN. Multifocal central nervous system damage caused by toluene abuse. Neurology (Cleveland) 1983;33:1337–1340.
118. Hormes JT, Filley CM, Rosenberg NL. Neurologic sequelae of chronic solvent vapor abuse. Neurology 1986;36:698–702.
119. Rosenberg NL, Kleinschmidt-DeMasters BK, Davis KA, Dreisbach JN, Hormes JT, Filley CM. Toluene abuse causes diffuse central nervous system white matter changes. Ann Neurol 1988;23:611–614.
120. Rosenberg, NL, Spitz, MC, Filley CM, Davis KA, Schaumburg HH. Central nervous system effects of chronic toluene abuse—clinical, brainstem evoked response and magnetic resonance imaging studies. Neurotoxicol Teratol 1988;10:489–495.
121. Benignus VA. Health effects of toluene: a review. Neurotoxicology 1981;2:567–588.
122. Von Oettingen WF, Neal PA, Donahue DD et al. Toxicity and potential dangers of toluene with special reference to its maximal permissible concentration. US Pub Health Serv Bull 1942;279:1–50.

123. Wiedmann KD, Power KG, Wilson JTL, Hadley DM. Recovery from chronic solvent abuse. J Neurol Neurosurg Psychiatry 1987;50:1712–1713.
124. Berry JG, Heaton RK, Kirby MW. Neuropsychological Deficits of Chronic Inhalant Abusers. In B Rumack, A Temple (eds), Management of the Poisoned Patient. Princeton, NJ: Science Press, 1977;9–31.
125. Channer KS, Stanley S. Persistent visual hallucinations secondary to chronic solvent encephalopathy: case report and review of the literature. J Neurol Neurosurg Psychiatry 1983;46:83–86.
126. Tsushima WT, Towne WS. Effects of paint sniffing on neuropsychological test performance. J Abnorm Psychol 1977;86:402–407.
127. Escobar A, Aruffo C. Chronic thinner intoxication: clinico-pathologic report of a human case. J Neurol Neurosurg Psychiatry 1980;43:986–994.
128. Miyake H, Ikeda T, Maehara N, Harabuchi I, Kishi R, Yokota H. Slow learning in rats due to long-term inhalation of toluene. Neurobehav Toxicol Teratol 1983;5:541–548.
129. Lorenzana-Jimenez M, Salas M. Neonatal effects of toluene on the locomotor behavioral development of the rat. Neurobehav Toxicol Teratol 1983;5:295–299.
130. Pryor GT, Dickinson J, Howd RA, Rebert CS, Neurobehavioral effects of subchronic exposure of weanling rats to toluene or hexane. Neurobehav Toxicol Teratol 1983;5:47–52.
131. Wood RW, Rees DC, Laties VG. Behavioral effects of toluene are modulated by stimulus control. Toxicol Applied Pharmacol 1983;68:462–472.
132. Rees DC, Knisely JS, Jordan S, Balster RL. Discriminitive stimulus properties of toluene in the mouse. Toxicol Applied Pharmacol 1987;88:97–104.
133. Pryor GT, Dickinson J, Howd RA, Rebert CS. Transient cognitive deficits and high-frequency hearing loss in weanling rats exposed to toluene. Neurobehav Toxicol Teratol 1983;5:53–57.
134. Rebert CS, Sorenson SS, Howd RA, Pryor GT. Toluene-induced hearing loss in rats evidenced by the brainstem auditory-evoked response. Neurobehav Toxicol Teratol 1983;5:59–62.
135. Lehman KB, Flury F. Toxicology and Hygiene of Industrial Solvents. Baltimore: Williams & Wilkins, 1943.
136. Andrews LS, Snyder R. Toxic Effects of Solvents and Vapors. In CD Klaassen, MO Amdur, J Doull (eds), Toxicology: The Basic Science of Poisons. New York: Macmillan, 1986;3:636–668.
137. Baslo A, Aksoy M. Neurologic abnormalitites in chronic benzene poisoning. Environ Res 1982;27:457–465.
138. National Institute for Occupational Safety and Health. Criteria for a recommended standard: occupational exposure to xylene. DHEW Publication No. (NIOSH) 75-168. Washington, DC, 1975.
139. Kilburn KH, Seidman BC, Warshaw R. Neurobehavioral and respiratory symptoms of formaldehyde and xylene exposure in histology technicians. Arch Environ Health 1985;40:229–233.
140. Morley R, Eccleston DW, Douglas CP, Greville WEJ, Scott DJ, Anderson J. Xylene poisoning—a report on one fatal case and two cases of recovery after prolonged unconsciousness. Br Med J 1970;3:442–443.
141. Gamberale F, Annwall G, Hultengren M. Exposure to xylene and ethylbenzene. III. Effects on central nervous system functions. Scand J Work Environ Health 1978;4:204–211.

142. Savolainen K, Riihimaki V, Linnoila M. Effects of short-term xylene exposure on psychophysiological functions in man. Int Arch Occup Environ Health 1979;44:201–211.
143. Hippolito RN. Xylene poisoning in laboratory workers: case reports and discussion. Lab Med 1980;11:593–595.
144. Sukhanova VA, Makareva LM, Boiko VI. Investigation of functional properties of leukocytes of workers engaged in the manufacture of xylene. Hyg Sanit 1969;34:130–132.
145. U.S. Department of Health and Human Services. Occupational exposure to styrene. DHHS (NIOSH) Publication No. 83–119. Washington, DC, 1983.
146. Tossavainen A. Styrene use and occupational exposure in the plastics industry. Scand J Work Environ Health 1978;4(Suppl 2):7–13.
147. Stewart RD, Dodd HC, Baretta ED, Schaffer AW. Human exposure to styrene vapor. Arch Environ Health 1968;16:656-662.
148. Gamberale F, Hultengren M. Exposure to styrene. II. Psychological functions. Work Environ Health 1974;11:86–93.
149. Gamberale F, Lisper HO, Olson BA. The Effect of Styrene Vapour on the Reaction Time of Workers in the Plastic Boat Industry. In N Horvath, E Frantik (eds), Adverse Effects of Environmental Chemicals and Psychotropic Drugs. Amsterdam: Elsevier, 1976:135–148.
150. Cherry N, Waldron HA, Wells GG, Wilkinson RT, Wilson HK, Jones S. An investigation of the acute behavioral effects of styrene on factory workers. Br J Ind Med 1980;37:234–240.
151. Rosen I, Haeger-Aronsen B, Rehnstrom S, Welinder H. Neurophysiological observations after chronic styrene exposure. Scand J Work Environ Health 1978;4(Suppl 2):184–194.
152. Politis MJ, Schaumburg HH, Spencer PS. Neurotoxicity of Selected Chemicals. In PS Spencer, HH Schaumburg (eds), Experimental and Clinical Neurotoxicology. Williams & Wilkins, 1980;613–630.
153. Stepien T. Two cases of lesions of the organ of vision with chemicals used in certain branches of industry and in agriculture. Klin Oczna 1973;43:169–172.
154. Barsotti M, Parmeggiani L, Sassi C. Observations on occupational pathology in a polystyrene factory. Med Lav 1952;43:418–424.
155. Pratt-Johnson JA. Case report. Retrobulbar neuritis following exposure to vinyl benzene (styrene). Can Med Assoc J 1964;90:975.
156. Araki S, Abe A, Ushio K, Fujino M. A case of skin atrophy, neurogenic muscular atrophy and anxiety reaction following long exposure to styrene. Jpn J Ind Health 1971;13:427.
157. Harkonen H, Lindstrom K, Seppalainen AM, Sisko A, Hernberg S. Exposure-response relationship between styrene exposure and central nervous system functions. Scand J Work Environ Health 1978;4:53–59.
158. Seppalainen AM. Neurotoxicity of styrene in occupational and experimental exposure. Scand J Work Environ Health 1978;4(Suppl 2):181–183.
159. Gamberale F, Kjellberg A. Behavioral Performance Assessment as a Biological Control of Occupational Exposure to Neurotoxic Substances. In R Gilioli, MG Cassitto, V Foa (eds), Neurobehavioral Methods in Occupational Health. New York: Pergamon, 1982;111–121.
160. Mutti A, Mazzucchi A, Rustichelli P, Frigeri G, Arfini G, Franchini I. Exposure-effect and exposure-response relationships between occupational

exposure to styrene and neuropsychological functions. Am J Ind Med 1984;5:275–286.

161. Cherry N, Rodgers B, Venables H, Waldron HA, Wells GG. Acute behavioral effects of styrene exposure: a further analysis. Br J Ind Med 1981;38:346–350.

162. Edling C, Ekberg K. No acute behavioral effects of exposure to styrene: a safe level of exposure? Br J Ind Med 1985;42:301–304.

163. Lindstrom K, Harkonen H, Hernberg S. Disturbances in psychological functions of workers occupationally exposed to styrene. Scand J Work Environ Health 1976;3:129–139.

164. Lloyd JW, Moore RM, Breslin P. Background information on trichloroethylene. J Occup Med 1975;17:603–605.

165. National Institute for Occupational Safety and Health. Special occupational hazard review with control recommendations: Trichloroethylene. DHEW Publication No. 78–130. Washington, DC, 1978.

166. Feldman RG. Trichloroethylene. In PJ Vinken, GW Bruyn (eds), Handbook of Clinical Neurology. Vol. 36. Intoxications of the Nervous System, Part I. Amsterdam: North-Holland, 1979;457–464.

167. Humphrey JH, McClelland M. Cranial-nerve palsies with herpes following general anesthesia. Br Med J 1944;1:315–318.

168. McClelland M. Some toxic effects following trilene decomposition products. Proc Royal Soc Med 1944;37:526–528.

169. Enderby GEH. The use and abuse of trichlorethylene. Br Med J 1944;2:300–302.

170. Firth JB, Stuckey RE. Decomposition of trilene in closed circuit anaesthesia. Lancet 1945;1:814–816.

171. Atkinson RS. Trichlorethylene anesthesia. Anesthesiology 1960;21:67–77.

172. Hewer CL. Further observations on trichlorethylene. Proc Royal Soc Med 1943;36:463–465.

173. Buxton PH, Hayward M. Polyneuritis cranialis associated with trichloroethylene poisoning. J Neurol Neurosurg Psychiatry 1967;30:511–518.

174. Glaser MA. Treatment of trigeminal neuralgia with trichlorethylene. JAMA 1931;96:916–920.

175. Defalque RJ. The "specific" analgesic effect of trichlorethylene upon the trigeminal nerve. Anesthesiology 1961;22:379–384.

176. Mitchell ABS, Parsons-Smith BG. Trichloroethylene neuropathy. Br Med J 1969;1:422–423.

177. Gwynne EI. Trichloroethylene neuropathy. Br Med J 1969;2:315.

178. Feldman RG, Mayer RM, Taub A. Evidence for peripheral neurotoxic effect of trichloroethylene. Neurology 1970;20:599–606.

179. Defalque RJ. Pharmacology and toxicology of trichloroethylene: a critical review of the world literature. Clin Pharmacol Ther 1961;2:665–688.

180. Waters EM, Gerstner HB, Huff JE. Trichloroethylene. I. An overview. J Toxicol Environ Health 1977;2:671–707.

181. Schaumburg HH, Spencer PS, Thomas PK. Disorders of Peripheral Nerves (2nd ed). Philadelphia: FA Davis, 1992.

182. Sagawa K. Transverse lesion of the spinal cord after accidental exposure to trichloroethylene. Int Arch Arbeitsmed 1973;31:257–264.

183. Spencer PS, Bischoff MC. Spontaneous remyelination of spinal cord plaques in rats orally treated with sodium dichloroacetate. J Neuropathol Exp Neurol 1982;41:373.

184. Adams EM, Spencer HC, Rowe VK, McCollister DD, Irish DD. Vapor toxicity of trichloroethylene determined by experiments on laboratory animals. Arch Ind Hyg Occup Med 1951;3:469–481.
185. Utesch RC, Weir FW, Bruckner JV. Development of an animal model of solvent abuse for use in the evaluation of extreme trichloroethylene inhalation. Toxicology 1981;19:169–182.
186. Tucker AN, Sanders VM, Barnes DW, Bradshaw TJ, White KL Jr, Sain LE, Borselleca JF, Munson AE. Toxicology of trichloroethylene in the mouse. Toxcol Appl Pharmacol 1982;62:351–357.
187. Dorfmueller MA, Henne SP, York RG, Bornschein RL, Manson JM. Evaluation of teratogenicity and behavioral toxicity with inhalation exposure of maternal rats to trichloroethylene. Toxicology 1979;14:153–166.
188. Cavanagh JB, Buxton PH. Trichloroethylene cranial neuropathy: is it really a toxic neuropathy or does it activate latent herpes virus? J Neurol Neurosurg Psychiatry 1989;52:297–303.
189. Andersson A. Health dangers in industry from exposure to trichloroethylene. Acta Med Scand 1957;157(Suppl 323):7–220.
190. Bardodej Z, Vyskocil J. Trichloroethylene metabolism and its effects on the nervous system as a means of hygienic control. Arch Ind Health 1956;13:581–592.
191. Grandjean E, Murchinger R, Turrian V, Haas PA, Knoepfel H-K, Rosenmund H. Investigations into the effects of exposure to trichloroethylene in mechanical engineering. Br J Ind Med 1955;12:131–142.
192. Lilis R, Stanescu D, Muica N, Roventa A. Chronic effects of trichloroethylene exposure. Med Lav 1969;60:595–601.
193. Salvini M, Binaschi S, Riva M. Evaluation of the psychophysiological functions in humans exposed to trichloroethylene. Br J Ind Med 1971;28:293–295.
194. Smith GF. Investigations of the mental effects of trichloroethylene. Ergonomics 1970;13:580–586.
195. Annau Z. The neurobehavioral toxicity of trichloroethylene. Neurobehav Toxicol Teratol 1981;3:417–424.
196. Todd J. Trichloroethylene poisoning with paranoid psychosis and Lilliputian hallucination. Br Med J 1954;7:439–440.
197. Harenko A. Two peculiar instances of psychotic disturbance in trichloroethylene poisoning. Acta Neurol Scand 1967;31(Suppl):139–140.
198. Stewart RD, Dodd HC, Gay HH, Erley DS. Experimental human exposure to trichloroethylene. Arch Environ Health 1970;20:64–71.
199. Ferguson RK, Vernon RJ. Trichloroethylene in combination with CNS drugs: effects on visual-motor tests. Arch Environ Health 1970;20:462–467.
200. Winneke G. Acute behavioral effects of exposure to some organic solvents—psychophysiological aspects. Acta Neurol Scand 1982;66(Suppl 92):117–129.
201. Vernon RJ, Ferguson RK. Effects of trichloroethylene on visual-motor performance. Arch Environ Health 1969;18:894–900.
202. Kylin B, Axell K, Samuel HE, Lindborg A. Effect of inhaled trichloroethylene on the CNS: as measured by optokinetic nystagmus. Arch Environ Health 1967;15:49–52.
203. Muller G, Spassowski M, Henschler D. Metabolism of trichloroethylene in man. III. Interaction of trichloroethylene and ethanol. Arch Toxicol 1975;33:173–189.

204. Gold JH. Chronic perchloroethylene poisoning. Can Psychiatr Assoc J 1969;14:627–630.
205. Tuttle TC, Wood GB, Grether CB, Johnson BL, Xintaras C. A behavioral and neurological evaluation of dry cleaners exposed to perchloroethylene. DHEW Publication No. 77–214. Washington, DC, 1977.
206. Antti-Poika M. Prognosis of symptoms in patients with diagnosed chronic organic solvent intoxication. Int Arch Occup Environ Health 1982;51:81–89.
207. Juntunen J, Antti-Poika M, Tola S, Partanen T. Clinical prognosis of patients with diagnosed chronic solvent intoxication. Acta Neurol Scand 1982;65:488–503.
208. National Institute for Occupational Safety and Health. Criteria for a recommended standard. Occupational exposure to methylene chloride. DHEW Publication No. 76-138. Cincinnati, 1976.
209. Moskowitz S, Shapiro H. Fatal exposure to methylene chloride vapor. Arch Ind Hyg Occup Med 1952;6:116–123.
210. Winek CL, Collum WD, Esposito F. Accidental methylene chloride fatality. Forensic Sci Int 1981;18:165–168.
211. Tariot PN. Delirium resulting from methylene chloride exposure: case report. J Clin Psychiatry 1983;44:340–342.
212. Sturmann K, Mofenson H, Caraccio T. Methylene chloride inhalation: an unusual form of drug abuse. Ann Emerg Med 1985;14:903–905.
213. Horowitz BZ. Carboxyhemoglobinemia caused by inhalation of methylene chloride. Am J Emerg Med 1986;4:48–51.
214. Stewart RD, Fisher TN. Carboxyhemoglobin elevation after exposure to dichloromethane. Science 1972;176:295–296.
215. Kubic VL, Andres MW, Engel RR, Barlow CH, Caughey WS. Metabolism of dihalomethanes to carbon monoxide. I. In vivo studies. Drug Metabol Disp 1974;2:53–57.
216. Ratney RS, Wegman DH, Elkins HB. In vivo conversion of methylene chloride to carbon monoxide. Arch Environ Health 1974;28:223–226.
217. Astrand I, Ovrum P, Carlsson A. Exposure to methylene chloride I. Its concentration in alveolar air and blood during rest and exercise and its metabolism. Scand J Work Environ Health 1975;1:78–94.
218. Stewart RD, Fisher TN, Hosko MJ, Peterson JE, Baretta ED, Dodd HC. Experimental human exposure to methylene chloride. Arch Environ Health 1972;25:342–348.
219. Gamberale F, Annwall G, Hultengren M. Exposure to methylene chloride. II. Psychological Functions. Scand J Work Environ Health 1975;1:95–103.
220. Winneke G. The neurotoxicity of dichloromethane. Neurobeh Toxicol Teratol 1981;3:391–395.
221. Cherry N, Venables H, Waldron HA, Wells GG. Some observations on workers exposed to methylene chloride. Br J Ind Med 1981;38:351–355.
222. Hearne FT, Grose F, Pifer JW, Friedlander BR, Raleigh RL. Methylene chloride mortality study: dose-response characterization and animal model comparison. J Occup Med 1987;29:217–228.
223. Jones RD, Winter DP. Two case reports of deaths on industrial premises atributed to 1,1,1-trichloroethane. Arch Environ Health 1983;38:59–61.
224. Silverstein MA. Letter to the editor. Arch Environ Health 1983;38:252.

225. McCarthy TB, Jones RD. Industrial gassing poisonings due to trichlorethylene, perchlorethylene, and 1,1,1-trichloroethane, 1961–80. Br J Ind Med 1983;40:450–455.
226. Gresham GA, Treip CS. Fatal poisoning by 1,1,1-trichloroethane after prolonged survival. Forensic Sci Int 1983;23:249–253.
227. Kobayashi H, Hobara T, Kawamoto T, Sakai T. Effect of 1,1,1-trichloroethane inhalation on heart rate and its mechanism: a role of autonmomic nervous system. Arch Environ Health 1987;42:140–143.
228. Wise MG. Trichloroethane (TCE) and central sleep apnea: a case study. J Toxicol Environ Health 1983;11:101–104.
229. McLeod AA, Marjot R, Monaghan MJ, Hugh-Jones P, Jackson G. Chronic cardiac toxicity after inhalation of 1,1,1-trichloroethane. Br Med J 1987;294:727–729.
230. Stewart RD, Gay HH, Schaffer AW, Erley DS, Rose VK. Experimental human exposure to methyl chloroform vapor. Arch Environ Health 1969;19:467–472.
231. Salvini M, Binaschi S, Riva M. Evaluation of the psychophysiological functions in humans exposed to the 'threshold limit value' of 1,1,1-trichloroethane. Br J Ind Med 1971;28:286–292.
232. Gamberale F, Hultengren M. Methylchloroform exposure. II. Psychophysiological functions. Work Environ Health 1973;10:82–92.
233. Mackay CJ, Campbell L, Samuel AM, Alderman KJ, Idzikowski C, Wilson HK, Gompertz D. Behavioral changes during exposure to 1,1,1-trichloroethane: time-course and relationship to blood solvent levels. Am J Ind Med 1987;11:223–239.
234. Maroni M, Bulgheroni C, Cassitto G, Merluzzi F, Gilioli R, Foa V. A clinical, neurophysiological and behavioral study of female workers exposed to 1,1,1-trichlorethane. Scand J Work Environ Health 1977;3:16–22.
235. National Institute for Occupational Safety and Health. Criteria for a recommended standard: Occupational exposure to hydrogen sulfide. DHEW (NIOSH) Publication No. 77-158. Cincinnati, 1977;1–149.
236. Stine RJ, Slosberg B, Beacham BE. Hydrogen sulfide intoxication. Ann Intern Med 1976;85:756–758.
237. Bittersohl G. On relationships in action between carbon disulfide and hydrogen sulfide. Med Lav 1971;62.
238. Smith RP. Toxic Responses of the Blood. In CD Klaassen, MO Amdur, J Doull (eds), Toxicology: The Basic Sciences of Poisons (3rd ed). New York: Macmillan, 1986;223–244.
239. Ahlborg G. Hydrogen sulfide poisoning in shale oil industry. AMA Arch Ind Hyg Occup Med 1951;3:247–266.
240. McCabe LC, Clayton GD. Air pollution by hydrogen sulfide in Poza Rica, Mexico. Arch Ind Hyg Occup Med 1952;6:199–213.
241. Burnett WW, King EG, Grace M, Hall WF. Hydrogen sulfide poisoning: review of 5 years' experience. CMA Journal 1977;117:1277–1280.
242. Seppalainen AM, Haltia Matti. Carbon Disulfide. In PS Spencer, HH Schaumburg (eds), Experimental and Clinical Neurotoxicology. Baltimore: Williams & Wilkins, 1980;356–373.
243. Lewey FH. Neurological, medical and biochemical signs and symptoms indicating chronic industrial carbon disulfide absorption. Ann Intern Med 1941;15:869–883.

244. Gordy ST, Trumper M. Carbon disulfide poisoning: report of 21 cases. Ind Med 1940;9:231–234.
245. Vigliani EC. Clinical observations on carbon disulfide intoxication in Italy. Ind Med Surg 1950;19:240–242.
246. Vigliani EC. Carbon disulfide poisoning in viscose rayon factories. Br J Ind Med 1954;11:235–244.
247. Hanninen H. Psychological picture of manifest and latent carbon disulfide poisoning. Br J Ind Med 1971;28:374–381.
248. Corsi G, Maestrelli P, Picotti G, Manzoni S, Negrin P. Chronic peripheral neuropathy in workers with previous exposure to carbon disulfide. Br J Ind Med 1983;40:209–211.
249. Johnson BL, Boyd J, Burg JR, Lee ST, Xintaras C, Albright BE. Effects on the peripheral nervous system of workers' exposure to carbon disulfide. Neurotoxicology 1983;1:53–66.
250. Putz-Anderson V, Albright BE, Lee ST, Johnson BL, Chrislip DW, Taylor BJ, Brightwell WS, Dickerson N, Culver M, Zentmeyer D, Smith P. A behavioral examination of workers exposed to carbon disulfide. Neurotoxicology 1983;1:67–78.
251. Peters HA, Levine RL, Matthews CG, Sauter SL, Rankin JH. Carbon disulfide-induced neuropsychiatric changes in grain storage workers. Am J Ind Med 1982;3:373–391.
252. Peters HA, Levine RL, Matthews CG, Chapman LJ. Extrapyramidal and other neurologic manifestations associated with carbon disulfide fumigant exposure. Arch Neurol 1988;45:537–540.
253. Fajen J, Albright B, Leffingwell SS. A cross-sectional medical and industrial hygiene survey of workers exposed to carbon disulfide. Scand J Work Environ Health 1981;7(Suppl 4):20–27.
254. Tuttle TC, Wood GD, Grether CB. Behavioral and neurological evaluation of workers exposed to carbon disulfide (CS2). Final report for National Institute for Occupational Safety and Health. DHEW (NIOSH) Publication No. 77–128. Cincinnati, 1976
255. Manu P, Lilis R, Lancranjan I, Ionescu S. Vasilescu I. The value of electromyographic changes in the early diagnosis of carbon disulphide peripheral neuropathy. Med Lav 1970;61:102–108.
256. Seppalainen AM, Tolonen M, Karli P, Hanninen H, Hernberg S. Neurophysiological findings in chronic carbon disulfide poisoning: a descriptive study. Work Environ Health 1972;9:71.
257. Vasilescu C. Sensory and motor conduction in chronic carbon disulphide poisoning. Eur Neurol 1976;14:447–457.
258. Hanninen H, Nurminen M, Tolonen M, Martelin T. Psychological tests as indicators of excessive exposure to carbon disulfide. Scand J Psychol 1978;19:163–174.
259. Wood R. Neurobehavioral toxicity of carbon disulfide. Neurobehav Toxicol Teratol 1981;3:397–405.
260. Cassitto MG, Bertazzi PA, Camerino D, Bulgheroni C, Cirla AM, Gilioli R, Graziano C, Tomasini M. Subjective and objective behavioral alterations in carbon disulfide workers. Med Lav 1978;69:144–150.
261. Gilioli R, Bulgheroni C, Bertazzi PA, Cirla AM, Tomasini M, Cassitto MG, Jacovone MT. Study of neurological and neurophysiological impairment carbon disulfide workers. Med Lav 1978;69:130–143.

262. Seppalainen AM, Tolonen M. Neurotoxicity of long-term exposure to carbon disulfide in the viscose rayon industry: a neurophysiological study. Work Environ Health 1974;11:145–153.
263. Alpers BJ, Lewy FH. Changes in the nervous system following carbon disulfide poisoning in animals and in man. Arch Neurol Psychiatry 1940;44:725–739.
264. O'Donoghue JL. Carbon Disulfide and Organic Sulfur-Containing Compounds. In JL O'Donoghue (ed), Neurotoxicity of Industrial and Commercial Chemicals. Vol. II. Boca Raton, FL: CRC Press, 1985;39–60.
265. Ron MA. Volatile substance abuse: a review of possible long-term neorological, intellectual and psychiatric sequelae. Br J Psychiatry 1986;148:235–246.
266. Westermeyer J. The psychiatrist and solvent-inhalant abuse: recognition, assessment, and treatment. Am J Psychiatry 1987;144:903–907.
267. Cherry N, McArthy TB, Waldron HA. Solvent sniffing in industry. Human Toxicol 1982;1:289–292.
268. Juntunen J. Alcoholism in occupational neurology: diagnostic difficulties with special reference to the neurological syndromes caused by exposure to organic solvents. Acta Neurol Scandinav 1982;66(Suppl 92):89–108.

Appendix to Chapter 4: Glossary

OSHA	Occupational Safety and Health Act of 1970
OSHA PEL	OSHA air contaminant standards
TWA	time-weighted average. Levels to which workers can be exposed for a normal 8-hour day, 40-hour week, without ill effects
CL	ceiling limit
ACGIH	American Conference of Governmental Industrial Hygienists
ACGIH TLV	ACGIH threshold limit value
STEL	short-term exposure limit. Usually a 15-minute time-weighted average, which should not be exceeded
DFG	German Research Society
DFG MAK	DFG maximum allowable concentration value
BAT	biological tolerance value
NIOSH	National Institute for Occupational Safety and Health
NIOSH REL	Indicates that a NIOSH criteria document recommending a certain occupational exposure has been published
BEI	Biological exposure indices. Set to provide a warning level of biological response to the chemical or warning levels of that chemical or its metabolic products in tissues, fluids, or exhaled air of exposed workers

CHAPTER 5

Neurobehavioral Disorders in Workers

Christopher M. Filley, M.D.

The physician who is asked to evaluate a worker who has symptoms or signs of a neurobehavioral disorder faces a challenging task. Not only are workers subject to all the neurologic illnesses that commonly affect behavior, but they are also at risk for a variety of conditions that are relatively specific to the workplace. Neurotoxic disorders comprise one of the ten leading work-related disease and injury categories in the United States[1] (see Chapter 1), and many of these intoxications impair cognition and emotional functioning through their actions on the central nervous system (CNS). In addition, psychiatric disorders are frequently encountered in the workplace,[1] leading to considerable diagnostic confusion, as these conditions often complicate or mimic the effects of neurotoxic syndromes.

This chapter provides a clinically useful approach to the recognition and treatment of significant neurobehavioral disorders. These conditions may arise independent of the work environment or be directly related to it. Attention is also devoted to conditions of psychological distress in which CNS effects from a workplace toxin are alleged but unproven, in part to illustrate the relative paucity of useful data in this emerging area.

Two neurobehavioral syndromes are most relevant to the work environment: the acute confusional state and dementia. These are discussed in general terms, since detailed descriptions of specific neurotoxic states affecting behavior are found elsewhere in this book. Throughout the discussion, the issue of psychological dysfunction appears, and guidelines for distinguishing CNS disease from psychiatric disorders will be developed. In particular, the role of neuropsychological testing is considered, as many cases revolve primarily around these data.

Acute Confusional State

The acute confusional state is a neurobehavioral syndrome familiar to physicians treating a wide spectrum of medical and neurologic disease. A useful definition describes an acute confusional state as a rapidly developing condition of altered arousal, inattention, and incoherent thought.[2] Two forms are commonly encountered: an agitated, hyperactive state with hallucinations, delusions, and autonomic overactivity, and a lethargic, withdrawn condition with somnolence and apathy. Less florid examples between these extremes are also seen and may involve a wide variety of alterations in intellect, personality, and behavior. The psychiatric description for such patients is delirium, and the internist is inclined to use the term *toxic-metabolic encephalopathy*, but terminology should not obscure the recognition of this common disorder.

Fundamentally, an acute confusional state implies that neuronal systems in the brain subserving arousal and attention have been acutely disrupted.[2] Because these fundamental systems are disturbed, all higher functions of the brain may be affected, so that, in addition to altered sleep-wake cycles and gross inattention, memory, language, visuospatial skills, and complex cognition may also be impaired.[2] In most instances, fortunately, this disturbance is due to a toxic or metabolic insult that can be corrected; structural damage to the brain is less common.

In the workplace, toxic exposure of any sort is clearly the leading cause of the acute confusional state. Table 5.1 lists the agents most often implicated in this setting. As can be seen, drugs—prescription and nonprescription—make up a large category of these toxins. Many clinicians are accustomed to dealing with drug-induced confusional states, particularly in the elderly,[3] and anticholinergic drugs[4] and sedative-hypnotics[5] appear to be the most common culprits. Intoxication with recreational drugs needs little elaboration; typical inebriation with alcohol is in fact an acute confusional state, and a variety of illicit drugs produce a similar condition.[6] Heavy metals,[7] carbon monoxide,[8] organic solvents,[9] and pesticides[10] may also cause acute confusional states with intense exposure. Other causes of this syndrome appear in Table 5.2. Metabolic disturbances, traumatic brain injury, CNS infections, and cerebrovascular disease must be considered.

Diagnosis of an acute confusional state is usually not difficult, although differentiation from dementia, aphasia, and the psychoses (schizophrenia and mood disorders) must be made. Table 5.3 lists diagnostic tests that may be helpful. These tests should be used as indicated to identify the causative problem(s) as promptly as possible.

Treatment of the acute confusional state depends on the cause of the disorder. As most instances involve a toxic or metabolic insult, removal of the toxin or correction of the metabolic derangement is, of course, critical. Treatment of infections, stroke, and the like are also obvious. Less appar-

TABLE 5.1
Toxins Capable of Causing Acute Confusional State

Prescription drugs	**Pesticides**
Sedative-hypnotics	Organophosphates
Anticholinergic compounds	Carbamates
Neuroleptics	Organochlorines
Anticonvulsants	Paraquat
Antidepressants	**Gases**
Lithium	Carbon monoxide
Nonprescription drugs	Ethylene oxide
Alcohol	
Amphetamines	
Cocaine	
Opiates	
Phencyclidine	
Marijuana	
LSD	
Industrial chemicals	
Metals	
Lead	
Mercury	
Arsenic	
Manganese	
Thallium	
Solvents	
Toluene	
Carbon disulfide	
Styrene	
Xylene	
Trichloroethylene	
Perchloroethylene	
Methyl chloride	
Methyl alcohol	
Carbon tetrachloride	

ent but equally important is attention to environmental manipulations that assist recovery; reassurance, frequent orientation, provision of adequate sleep, and judicious tranquilization can all be very gratifying.[2]

Dementia

Dementia is a problem of enormous magnitude and one that increasingly preoccupies both the medical community and the public imagination. The rapid emergence of Alzheimer's disease (AD)[11] has resulted in a growing concern about dementia in general. Workers in industrial settings are particularly alarmed that dementia may ensue from a chronic low-level intox-

TABLE 5.2
Nontoxic Causes of Acute Confusional State

Metabolic disturbances	Central nervous system infections
Hypoxia	Meningitis
Hypoglycemia	Encephalitis
Uremia	Abscess
Hepatic disease	**Cerebrovascular disease**
Electrolyte disturbances	Stroke
Endocrinopathies	Subarachnoid hemorrhage
Traumatic brain injury	**Epilepsy**
Concussion	Ictal states
Contusion	Postictal states
Subdural hematoma	Complex partial and absence status
Epidural hematoma	epilepticus

TABLE 5.3
Diagnostic Tests for Acute Confusional State

Chemistry survey	Thyroid function tests
Complete blood count	B_{12} and folate levels
Computed tomography or magnetic res-	Lumbar puncture
onance imaging scan of the brain	Electroencephalography
Chest roentgenogram	24-hour urine for heavy metals
Arterial blood gases	Carboxyhemoglobin
Urinalysis	Plasma cholinesterase
Toxicology screen	

ication. Because complaints of memory loss and cognitive dysfunction are so common, a major part of this chapter is devoted to a consideration of this menacing syndrome.

A standard definition of dementia holds that it is an acquired, persistent impairment in intellectual functioning, with deficits in at least three of the following five areas: memory, language, visuospatial function, complex cognition, and emotion or personality.[12] Memory loss, although not the only deficit in dementia, assumes primary importance in the workplace since both AD and the toxic dementias involve significant disturbances of new learning and recall. As in any other context, the physician's major role is to establish whether or not an irreversible dementia is present. Once this question is answered, the condition can either be specifically treated—in the fortunate few—or dealt with intelligently and sensitively as an illness that will not allow recovery. Despite the fact that most dementias are irreversible,[13] failure to detect and treat a reversible condition is a serious error.

Table 5.4 provides a differential diagnosis of the dementias. AD leads the list because of the well-recognized observation, from both clinical[14] and pathologic[15] series, that at least 50% of dementias in later life are a

TABLE 5.4
Differential Diagnosis of Dementia in the Workplace

Alzheimer's disease	Central nervous system infections
Multi-infarct dementia	Metabolic disorders
Prescription drugs	Vasculitides
Nonprescription drugs	Posttraumatic dementia
Toxins	Postanoxic dementia
Neoplasms	Parkinson's disease
Subdural hematoma	Huntington's disease
Normal-pressure hydrocephalus	

TABLE 5.5
Industrial Chemicals Implicated in the Etiology of Dementia

Metals	**Pesticides**
Arsenic	Organophosphates
Lead	Carbamates
Mercury	Organochlorines
Manganese	Paraquat
Aluminum	**Gases**
Thallium	Carbon monoxide
Solvents	Ethylene oxide
Toluene	
Carbon disulfide	
Styrene	
Xylene	
Trichloroethylene	
Perchloroethylene	
Methyl chloride	
N-hexane	
Methyl butyl ketone	
Methylene chloride	
Methyl alcohol	
Carbon tetrachloride	
Ethylene glycol	

result of this devastating disease. Vascular dementia, with its many subtypes, forms the second most common cause.[16] Drugs and toxins then become prominent, since workers are at risk for intoxications to which the rest of the population is less prone. Other entities in the table are familiar from standard textbooks of neurology and internal medicine.

Table 5.5 lists the major industrial chemicals that have been implicated in the causation of dementia. Some, such as lead[17] and toluene,[18] are well-known CNS toxins with observable clinical and pathologic features, whereas many others are less clearly culpable. Among the metals, aluminum and silicon deserve special consideration because of their putative link with AD.

TABLE 5.6
Tests to Evaluate Dementia in the Workplace

Computed tomography or magnetic resonance imaging of the brain	Erythrocyte sedimentation rate
Chemistry survey	Lumbar puncture
Complete blood count	Electroencephalography
Thyroid function tests	24-hour urine for heavy metals
Syphilis serology	Carboxyhemoglobin
Human inmmunodeficiency virus	Plasma cholinesterase
B_{12} and folate levels	

Since AD is still an idiopathic illness, concerns about the possibility of toxic causes are real. For the most part, environmental toxins have been excluded in this regard. A case control study of 98 patients and 162 control subjects found no increased risk of AD in individuals who had ever had exposure to organic solvents or lead.[19] In another such study, with 116 patients and 97 controls, no association of AD was found with any of eight occupation categories, ranging from factory worker to professional.[20]

Aluminum, however, remains an intriguing possibility. This metal has been strongly implicated in the pathogenesis of dialysis dementia, a progressive encephalopathy that was encountered before dialysate was rid of aluminum.[21] In addition, laboratory animals exposed to high levels of aluminum develop neurofibrillary tangles.[22] However, much evidence suggests that aluminum is not a significant agent in the etiology of AD. First, dialysis dementia patients do not develop neurofibrillary tangles.[23] Second, tangles in laboratory animals are morphologically distinct from those in AD patients.[24] Third, aluminum levels in brain,[25] cerebrospinal fluid,[26] and serum[27] may be normal in AD patients. Silicon, like aluminum, is found in neuritic plaques and neurofibrillary tangles, but its significance in terms of causation remains only speculative.

Table 5.6 lists a standard group of tests that can be performed in the evaluation of a demented patient. Several points deserve emphasis. A careful history, including occupational history, and examination, as discussed in Chapter 2, are crucial, both to determine whether dementia is in fact present and to identify symptoms and signs that might give clues to causation. Next, a cerebral imaging procedure is mandatory, either computed tomography (CT) or magnetic resonance imaging (MRI), so that a structural lesion such as a subdural hematoma or meningioma can be promptly detected. In addition, MRI can disclose cases of severe toluene intoxication,[28] which to date is the only example of a toxic CNS injury with a relatively specific MRI appearance. Loss of gray/white matter differentiation and increased periventricular white matter signal intensity on T2-weighted images have been noted in chronic toluene abusers.[28] In the occupational context, special attention must be given to workplace factors that might be relevant, such as exposure to prolonged high levels of solvent vapor or

TABLE 5.7
Treatment of Dementia

Reversible cases
    Elimination of toxin
    Treatment of causative illness
Irreversible cases
    Informed and sympathetic counseling
    Consideration of tacrine (Cognex) for probable Alzheimer's disease
    Cautious trial of antidepressant if depression is significant
    Appropriate sedation for agitation, wandering, inappropriate behavior

---

inadvertent intoxication with carbon monoxide or heavy metals. The remainder of the tests in Table 5.6 can be obtained as indicated by this historical information.

Treatment of dementia obviously relies on the cause of the impairment. Removal from the source of intoxication is clearly indicated if such a source exists. Other reversible or potentially reversible causes can be addressed by appropriate medical or surgical therapy. More difficult are the irreversible cases, and much skill may be required to provide the best advice and guidance for such individuals and their families. Table 5.7 gives more detail on this important topic.

Psychiatric Disorders

For purposes of this discussion, a psychiatric disorder is one in which structural disease of the nervous system is either absent or equivocal, and the presenting syndrome involves emotional and sometimes cognitive dysfunction. As with neurobehavioral syndromes, psychiatric disorders may arise in workers irrespective of the work setting or as a result of it. A detailed account of all psychiatric conditions that may afflict the worker is beyond the scope of this chapter, but some general guidelines for the physician evaluating such patients may be helpful.

The most perplexing problem is that of diagnosis. In many instances the presenting complaints suggest intoxication of the nervous system to patient, examiner, or both, but no objective signs of disease are present. Symptoms such as forgetfulness, poor concentration, irritability, and fatigue are common but so nonspecific as to imply diverse syndromes such as depression, anxiety, or dementia. Considerable confusion is also introduced by deliberate (i.e., malingering) or unintentional (i.e., somatoform disorder) attempts to magnify symptoms for compensatory or psychological reasons. In such cases, referral to a skilled psychiatrist is often very helpful. In general, the absence of objective findings on neurologic examination and appropriate laboratory tests leads to consideration of a psychiatric diagnosis, although further research may reveal that we simply lack the proper instruments in many cases to detect subtle CNS involvement. In all cases, firm diagnosis of a psychiatric disorder requires clear psychiatric evidence, not only the exclusion of neurologic disease.

The occurrence of psychiatric disorder related to the workplace brings up the problem of occupational stress. The concept of stress has defied definition, but stress in workers appears to involve a perception that demands at work may exceed response capability and lead to important negative consequences.[29] It is generally recognized that stress plays a role in the development of work-related anxiety, depression, and substance abuse.[29] Data are accumulating to suggest that certain occupations, primarily those involving blue-collar employees such as assembly line workers and machine operators, are more likely to be associated with psychological disorders.[30] In contrast, white-collar professionals appear to be less vulnerable to occupational stress.[30] It is apparent that workplace stressors can contribute to clear psychiatric states such as posttraumatic stress disorder[31] and panic disorder.[32] Mass psychogenic illness in an industrial setting has also been reported and appears to occur among workers experiencing substantial psychosocial stress.[33]

Psychiatric referral is, of course, appropriate for all workers with psychiatric disorders. When stress in the workplace is deemed to play a significant role, a comprehensive approach to stress management is recommended, involving the worker, the employer, and the health professional. Individual counseling and organizational restructuring may both have beneficial effects.[29]

Psycho-Organic Syndrome

A particularly puzzling diagnostic entity has been described in Scandinavian countries. The psycho-organic syndrome,[34] also known as the painter's syndrome,[35] highlights many of the difficulties inherent in the evaluation of neurobehavioral symptoms in the workplace: Is there any objective impairment? Does a workplace toxin damage the CNS? How much do compensation and psychological factors influence these cases? This syndrome is also discussed in detail in Chapter 3.

The psycho-organic syndrome consists primarily of neurobehavioral complaints: fatigue, difficulty with concentration, poor memory, and personality changes.[36] An unresolved controversy has been sparked by the assertion that chronic, low-level solvent exposure causes dementia in some painters exposed to mixed solvents on a daily basis.[37] Objective data have been more difficult to acquire than patients with symptoms, and many studies have suffered from inadequate control groups, nonstandardized assessment techniques, and failure to identify the culpable toxin or toxins.[38] Indeed, some studies, particularly those including proper control groups, have not found significant neurobehavioral impairment.[39,40]

TABLE 5.8
Terminology of Solvent Exposure Syndromes

Mild
    Neurasthenic syndrome
    Organic affective syndrome
    Type 1 exposure syndrome
Moderate
    Psycho-organic syndrome
    Mild chronic toxic encephalopathy
    Type 2A exposure syndrome
    Type 2B exposure syndrome
Severe
    Dementia
    Severe chronic toxic encephalopathy
    Type 3 exposure syndrome

Similarly, neuropathologic mechanisms and dose-response relationships have not been established in this postulated syndrome.[41] One problem in addressing this issue stems from a lack of consensus on the nomenclature describing the psycho-organic syndrome and related states. Table 5.8 gives a sample of various terms that have been given to solvent exposure syndromes of varying degrees of severity.[42,43] Typically, elemental neurologic deficits are not found in these cases, and the diagnosis rests primarily on the use of neuropsychological evaluation. The nosologic uncertainty of this area is, in part, related to this reliance on relatively subjective testing, and, at least in mild and moderate exposure cases, questions about the validity of neuropsychological testing may arise. Less ambiguity is likely to attend severe cases in which "type 3" exposure has occurred.

It is possible, therefore, that many cases of the psycho-organic syndrome actually represent psychiatric disorders. Most likely among these would be somatoform disorder, compensation neurosis, malingering, and factitious disorder.[44] It is of interest that in Denmark, where solvent exposure syndrome is a legitimate diagnostic entity, a worker who claims this as a disability is assumed disabled until the state proves otherwise.[45] The potential secondary gain in such a system is apparent. Until clear evidence of CNS damage on objective testing is available, the more reasonable position may be to assume that no damage has in fact occurred. Exceptions to this rule might be cases of severe or chronic exposure causing obvious dementia, or more subtle impairment that can clearly be shown to represent a decline in neuropsychological function.

The neurologist, therefore, must not dismiss all cases of subtle neurobehavioral impairment as psychiatric. Significant exposures do occur, and massive exposure to certain agents clearly causes serious results. Objective data should be sought vigorously in suspected toxic cases; for example, as mentioned above, cerebral MRI scanning will often be abnormal in significant toluene exposure.[28] Comprehensive neuropsychological testing, using standardized assessment methods and careful personality evaluations, can often generate very useful information. In a more general sense, neurotoxic disease can be more confidently diagnosed if the syndrome is commensurate with the dose and duration of exposure and if effects appear immediately or very soon after exposure occurs.[46]

Neuropsychological Testing

It should be clear from the foregoing account that considerable ambiguity complicates the evaluation of neurobehavioral disorders in workers. The obvious cases of massive exposure to toxin prove to be exceptional; more often, workers present with questionable syndromes that may or may not reflect significant workplace exposure. Unrelated disease, drug or medication effects, and psychiatric disorders all pose diagnostic problems. Because many syndromes are so perplexing, the clinician naturally turns to more detailed means of testing to gather useful data. Neuropsychological testing is one such option, and appropriate use of this service is critical.

A number of short mental status examinations have been presented in an effort to provide convenient, standardized tools to assess neurobehavioral impairment. Two of the most popular such instruments are the Mini-Mental State Examination (MMSE[47]) and the Information-Memory-Concentration (IMC) test;[48,49] a somewhat longer measure that has gained acceptance is the Dementia Rating Scale (DRS).[50] While offering a readily attainable score of overall cognitive status, these tests suffer from significant drawbacks. The MMSE, for example, is heavily weighted toward language and is unlikely to be sensitive to the predominantly nonlinguistic deficits in neurotoxic syndromes. In general, these tests were all developed using elderly populations and subjects with degenerative CNS disease and are most useful for longitudinal follow-up study of patients with diagnosed dementing illness.[51] It is important to realize that they have not been validated in the evaluation of occupational disorders and specifically not been tested in occupational neurotoxic disorders. As diagnostic tools, these tests will frequently be inadequate for detecting less obvious impairment, and more extensive neuropsychological testing will usually be required.

Neuropsychology is a young but very active area of clinical neuroscience, and its role in the understanding of brain-behavior relationships is already well established. In the area of neurotoxicology, however, some caution is advisable when interpreting neuropsychological results. Since many syndromes are subtle, evidence of CNS involvement may be quite equivocal and indeed may only reflect poor motivation or other psychological factors. In addition, test batteries differ widely in their composition and comprehensiveness and may not all be equally sensitive to neurotoxic disease.[52] Nevertheless, careful neuropsychological testing by a qualified neuropsychologist can suggest brain injury in the absence of other objective data.

TABLE 5.9
Neuropsychological Functions Commonly Assessed in Neurotoxicity Evaluations

General intellectual ability
Attention and concentration
Reaction time
Memory
Visuospatial skills
Executive function
Personality
Mood
Motor speed
Coordination

Neuropsychologists can be loosely grouped into two philosophical camps: those favoring a fixed battery of tests that are administered in a standardized fashion and those using a "flexible" battery in which tests are given in individualized ways that elucidate a patient's specific pattern of impairment. Advantages can be seen with each approach, and, in practice, most neuropsychologists blend the two together. Ideally, a useful evaluation should not only compare an individual's performance with that of a large sample of normals, as a fixed battery approach aims to do, but also identify the person's particular strengths and weaknesses in a sensitive manner, as a flexible battery attempts. This goal is as desirable in neurotoxic cases as in any other neurobehavioral syndrome.

The selection of tests used remains diverse mainly because there is no single test or set of tests that reliably identifies specific syndromes or diseases. Instead, neuropsychologists generate an impression based on a pattern that emerges from the tests that are administered. Thus, for example, a picture of significant memory loss may appear in one case, while in another attentional disturbance may be prominent. The validity of the results depends to a large extent on the skill and experience of the examiner. Despite the fact that no single test or set of tests can identify specific neurotoxic syndromes, a consensus is developing as to what specific functions should be included in a comprehensive neuropsychological evaluation.[53,54] These functions are listed in Table 5.9. Most of the standard neuropsychological domains are included, but language function is not on the list since no toxic syndrome seems to involve prominent language disturbance. It should be emphasized that these areas are included only because they appear to be most often affected by neurotoxic states; further experience may well add to or delete from this list.

Summary

This chapter has dealt with the issues raised by workers who have primarily neurobehavioral complaints. The physician assessing such cases should proceed in a systematic way to make the diagnosis as accurately as possible. Standard neurologic and medical evaluations form the foundation of this process, and many cases may be clear examples of massive or significant exposure to a toxin, unrelated neurologic disease, drug or medication toxicity, or psychiatric disorder. For those cases in which the situation remains unclear, careful testing by a competent neuropsychologist can be most helpful.

Ultimately, the determination of whether a neurobehavioral syndrome is related to a toxic agent rests with the physician who directs the neurobehavioral evaluation. A balanced judgment, made in light of certain reasonably well-established principles, can best be made when all the data are viewed as a whole. Even as neurobehavioral toxicology advances toward becoming a more objective discipline, clinical judgment will remain the best final arbiter.

References

1. Leading work-related disease and injuries—United States. MMWR 1983;32:24–26.
2. Strub RC. Acute Confusional State. In DF Benson, D Blumer (eds), Psychiatric Aspects of Neurologic Disease. Vol 2. New York: Grune & Stratton, 1982.
3. Vestal RE. Drug use in the elderly: a review of problems and special considerations. Drugs 1978;16:358–382.
4. Blazer DG, II, Federspiel CF, Ray WA, Schaffner W. The risk of anticholinergic toxicity in the elderly: a study of prescribing practices in two populations. J Gerontol 1983;38:31–35.
5. Bergman H, Borg S, Holm L. Neuropsychological impairment and exclusive abuse of sedatives or hypnotics. Am J Psychiatry 1980;137:215–217.
6. Strub RL, Black FW. Toxic Substances. In RL Strub, FW Black (eds), Neurobehavioral Disorders: A Clinical Approach. Philadelphia: FA Davis, 1988.
7. Goetz CG, Klawans HL, Cohen MM. Neurotoxic Agents. In AB Baker, LH Baker (eds), Clinical Neurology. New York: Harper & Row, 1981.
8. Garland H, Pearce J. Neurological complications of carbon monoxide poisoning. Q J Med 1967;144:445–455.
9. Gregerson P, Angelso B, Nielsen TE et al. Neurotoxic effects of organic solvents in exposed workers: an occupational, neuropsychological, and neurological investigation. Am J Ind Med 1984;5:201–225.
10. Grob D. The manifestations and treatment of poisoning due to nerve gas and organic phosphate anticholinesterase compounds. Arch Intern Med 1956;98:221–239.
11. Katzman R. Alzheimer's disease. N Engl J Med 1986;314:964–973.
12. Cummings JL, Benson DF. Dementia: A Clinical Approach. Boston: Butterworth-Heinemann, 1992;1–3.
13. Clarfield AM. The reversible dementias: do they reverse? Ann Intern Med 1988;109:476–486.

14. Marsden CD, Harrison MJG. Outcome of investigation of patients with presenile dementia. Br Med J 1972;2:249–252.
15 Tomlinson BE, Blessed G, Roth M. Obsevations on the brains of demented old people. J Neurol Sci 1970;11:205–242.
16. Garcia JH, Brown GG. Vascular dementia: neuropathologic alterations and metabolic brain changes. J Neurol Sci 1992;109:121–131.
17. Valpey R, Sumi SM, Copass MK, Goble GJ. Acute and chronic progressive encephalopathy due to gasoline sniffing. Neurology 1978;28:507–510.
18. Hormes JT, Filley CM, Rosenberg NL. Neurologic sequelae of chronic solvent vapor abuse. Neurology 1986;36:698–702.
19. Shalat SL, Seltzer B, Baker EL. Occupational risk factors and Alzheimer's disease: a case-control study. J Occup Med 1988;30:934–936.
20. Amaducci LA, Fratiglioni L, Rocca WA et al. Risk factors for clinically diagnosed Alzheimer's disease: a case-control study of an Italian population. Neurology 1986;36:922–931.
21. Alfrey AC, LeGendre GR, Kaehny WD. The dialysis encephalopathy syndrome: possible aluminum intoxication. N Engl J Med 1976;294:184–188.
22. Klatzo I, Wisniewski H, Streicher E. Experimental production of neurofibrillary degeneration. I. Light microscopic observations. J Neuropathol Exp Neurol 1965;24:187–199.
23. Burks JS, Alfrey AC, Huddlestone J, Norenberg MD, Lewin E. A fatal encephalopathy in chronic hemodialysis patients. Lancet 1976;1:764–768.
24. Terry RD, Pena C. Experimental production of neurofibrillary degeneration. 2. Electron microscopy, phosphatase histochemistry and electron probe analysis. J Neuropathol Exp Neurol 1965;24:200–210.
25. McDermott JR, Smith AI, Iqbal K, Wisniewski H. Aluminum and Alzheimer's disease. Lancet 1977;2:710–711.
26. Delaney JF. Spinal fluid aluminum levels in patients with Alzheimer's disease. Ann Neurol 1979;5:580–581.
27. Shore D, Millson M, Holtz JL et al. Serum aluminum in primary degenerative dementia. Biol Psychiatry 1980;15:971–977.
28. Filley CM, Heaton RK, Rosenberg NL. White matter dementia in chronic toluene abuse. Neurology 1990;40:532–534.
29. Baker DB. Occupational Stress. In BS Levy, DH Wegman (eds), Occupational Health (2nd ed). Boston: Little, Brown, 1988.
30. Leading work-related diseases and injuries. MMWR 1986;35:613–621.
31. Schottenfeld RS, Cullen MR. Occupation-induced posttraumatic stress disorder. Am J Psychiatry 1985;142:198–202.
32. Dager SR, Holland JP, Cowley DS, Dunner DL. Panic disorder precipitated by exposure to organic solvents in the workplace. Am J Psychiatry 1987;144:1056–1058.
33. Murphy LR, Colligan MJ. Mass psychogenic illness in a shoe factory. A case report. Int Arch Occup Environ Health 1979;44:133–138.
34. Flodin U, Edling C, Axelson O. Clinical studies of psychoorganic syndromes among workers with exposure to solvents. Am J Ind Med 1984;5:287–295.
35. Arlien–Soberg P, Bruhn P, Gyldensted C, Melgaard B. Chronic painters' syndrome: chronic toxic encephalopathy in house painters. Acta Neurol Scand 1979;60:149–156.
36. Baker EL, Smith TJ, Landrigan PJ. The neurotoxicity of industrial solvents: a review of the literature. Am J Ind Med 1985;8:207–217.

37. Grasso P, Sharratt M, Davies DM, Irvine D. Neuropsychological and psychological disorders and occupational exposure to organic solvents. Fd Chem Toxic 1984;22:819–852.
38. Errebo-Knudsen ED, Olsen F. Solvents and the brain: explanation of the discrepancy between the number of toxic encephalopathy reported (and compensated) in Denmark and other countries. Br J Ind Med 1987;44:71–72.
39. Gade A, Mortenson EL, Bruhn P. "Chronic painter's syndrome." A reanalysis of psychological test data in a group of diagnosed cases, based on comparisons with matched controls. Acta Neurol Scand 1988;77:293–306.
40. Hooisma J, Hanninen H, Emmen HH, Kulig BM. Behavioral effects of exposure to organic solvents in Dutch painters. Neurotoxicol Teratol 1993;15:397–406.
41. Baker EL, Fine LS. Solvent neurotoxicity: the current evidence. J Occup Med 1986;28:126–129.
42. Hartman DE. Neuropsychological Toxicology: Identification and Assessment of Human Neurotoxic Syndromes. New York: Pergamon, 1988;112–114.
43. Baker EL, Seppaleinen AM. Human aspects of solvent neurobehavioral effects. Neurotoxicology 1987;7:43–56.
44. American Psychiatric Association. Diagnostic and Statistical Manual of Mental Disorders (3rd ed, revised). Washington, DC: American Psychiatric Press, 1987.
45. Hartman DE. Neuropsychological Toxicology: Identification and Assessment of Human Neurotoxic Syndromes. New York: Pergamon, 1988:270.
46. Schaumburg HH, Spencer PS. Recognizing neurotoxic disease. Neurology 1987;37:276–278.
47. Folstein MF, Folstein SF, McHugh PR. "Mini-Mental State": a practical method for grading the cognitive state of patients for the clinician. J Psychiatr Res 1975;12:189–198.
48. Blessed G, Tomlinson BE, Roth M. The association between quantitative measures of dementia and of senile change in the cerebral grey matter of elderly subjects. Br J Psychiatry 1968;114:797–811.
49. Fuld PA. Psychological Testing in the Differential Diagnosis of Dementias. In R Katzman, RD Terry, KL Bick (eds), Alzheimer's Disease: Senile Dementia and Related Disorders. New York: Raven, 1978;185–193.
50. Mattis S. Dementia Rating Scale. Odessa, FL: Psychological Assessment Resources, 1989.
51. Salmon DP, Thal LS, Butters N, Heindel WC. Longitudinal evaluation of dementia of the Alzheimer type: a comparison of 3 standardized mental status examinations. Neurology 1990;40:1225–1230.
52. Hawkins KA. Occupational neurotoxicology: some neuropsychological issues and challenges. J Clin Exp Neuropsychol 1990;12:664–680.
53. Feldman RG, Ricks NL, Baker EL. Neuropsychological effects of industrial toxins: a review. Am J Ind Med 1980;1:211–227.
54. Lezak MD. Neuropsychological assessment in behavioral toxicology—developing techniques and interpretative issues. Scand J Work Environ Health 1984;10(Suppl 1):25–29.

CHAPTER 6

Paroxysmal Disorders and Occupational Neurology

Steven J. Gulevich, M.D.

Edward Lewin, M.D.

Neil L. Rosenberg, M.D.

Paroxysmal disorders present an unusual problem in the workplace. Rather than having a fixed deficit around which employment can be structured, a worker is faced with a neurologic deficit that may be absent for weeks or months and then develop unpredictably, resulting in a situation that endangers the worker and those around him or her. With a paroxysmal disorder, the patient exhibits few or no symptoms of disability until an attack occurs. The spectrum ranges from seizures that involve loss of consciousness and motor control to mildly disabling headaches. Epilepsy and migraine are the two classic paroxysmal disorders, but several sleep disorders are also considered paroxysmal, and sleep problems in general are considered here.

Of the paroxysmal neurologic disorders, those like epilepsy that can result in impairment of consciousness put the greatest restrictions on the workplace.[1] Tailoring the workplace to the needs of a patient with such problems poses a serious challenge to both worker and employer.

Although it is distinctly uncommon for epilepsy to find its cause in the workplace, sleep problems and headache disorders are often associated with occupational factors. The link between shift work and sleep complaints is well established, and certain headaches are probably exacerbated by working conditions.

TABLE 6.1
Abridged Seizure Classification

I. Generalized seizures (bilaterally symmetric, no local onset)
   A. Tonic-clonic, tonic, clonic, and aclonic
   B. Myoclonic
   C. Absence
II. Partial seizures (begin locally)
   A. Simple partial (consciousness not impaired)
      1. Motor
      2. Sensory
      3. Autonomic
   B. Complex partial (impairment of consciousness)
   C. Partial with secondary generalization

Epilepsy

The term *epilepsy* refers to a broad range of neurologic disorders characterized by recurrent seizures. Table 6.1 shows an abridged seizure classification.[2] Epilepsy may follow head trauma or other brain injury, but the etiology underlying most seizure disorders remains unknown.

In epilepsy, seizure type and frequency determine the degree of impairment. Seizure type (generalized, partial, partial complex) gives an approximate indication of seizure severity. Generalized seizures, by definition, result in loss of consciousness. In adults they are most frequently tonic-clonic, accompanied by involuntary rhythmic clonic movements of all four limbs. Partial seizures cause involuntary movements without impairment of consciousness. Partial complex seizures cause impairment, but not loss, of consciousness. These lapses of awareness may be preceded by olfactory hallucinations, epigastric sensations, or other cognitive or psychological disturbances, or may occur without warning. A brief period of postictal confusion may also occur.

In addition to seizure type, seizure frequency determines the degree to which epilepsy impairs a patient's ability to work. A patient who experiences daily partial complex seizures will have a greater work limitation than one who has a yearly generalized tonic-clonic seizure. Anticonvulsant medications, by markedly decreasing seizure frequency for most epileptic patients, have greatly improved their ability to work productively.

Work Restrictions

Most adult seizure patients are under good control; finding suitable employment for those individuals who continue to have seizures despite optimum medical management poses a major challenge. The generalized and partial complex epilepsies of adulthood are perhaps the most occupationally limiting of all paroxysmal disorders. In particular, the complex partial (e.g., temporal lobe, psychomotor) seizures are the largest group of incompletely controlled seizures in adults. For an airline pilot or deep-sea diver, a seizure will nearly always end a career. For those who operate heavy machinery, even a single seizure can pose severe limitations.

Driving an automobile is the most significant occupational (and recreational) restriction for most patients who have had one or more seizures. Most states impose restrictions on driving an automobile in patients with epilepsy. These restrictions apply even to single seizures provoked by clearly identifiable nonrecurrent events (head injury, drug intoxication). Twelve states require no seizure-free period before relicensing; the remainder require 3–24 months since the last seizure before renewing a driver's license. Most states also require proof of periodic medical follow-up examination to maintain a license after a seizure, but three do not. Finally, in six states, doctors must report seizures to the licensing bureau; laws are often unclear as to whether initial and recurrent seizures require notification. In addition to seizures, the laws are generally interpreted to include any disorder that impairs consciousness or sometimes even has a possibility of affecting the patient's ability to drive an automobile.

A recent population-based retrospective cohort study was designed to look at the effects of epilepsy and diabetes mellitus on traffic safety.[3] This study concluded that drivers with epilepsy or diabetes mellitus had a slightly higher risk of being involved in traffic accidents than did healthy control subjects. The risks; however, were smaller than what had been reported previously, and suggest that further restrictions on driving privileges in these populations are not warranted. Thus, while all physicians need to familiarize themselves with the epilepsy/impaired consciousness driving laws in their state, many of these laws may be unnecessarily restrictive.

The demands of most workplaces differ substantially from those of driving. Although no laws or guidelines for seizures in the workplace exist, a reasonable one might be that the patient with epilepsy not be placed in any situation that would endanger him or her or others should the patient have a seizure. Such a restriction would remain in effect until the probability of a seizure occurring approximates that of the general population, and may not be necessary in pure partial epilepsy, in which consciousness is not affected. With counseling and medical supervision, most epileptics adapt successfully to the workplace.[4]

Persons with well-controlled seizures and no other disability should be able to obtain and hold any kind of employment for which they are qualified, with the exceptions of certain occupations where the safety of the general public is at stake. For instance, an individual with epilepsy will generally be denied enlistment in the armed forces, although personnel who develop seizures while already on active duty are retained if they remain under satisfactory control. Not surprisingly, a convulsive disorder is a medical disqualification for a commercial pilot's license. However, persons with well-controlled seizure disorders should be able to follow almost all career opportunities consistent with their interests and talents. Nevertheless, epilepsy continues to be a major cause of denial or loss of employment, resulting in permanent disability for these individuals.

UNEMPLOYMENT IN PATIENTS WITH EPILEPSY

Unemployment among individuals with convulsive disorder is said to be two to three times the national average.[5] Although attitudes toward the prospective employee with epilepsy are improving,[6] employer conceptions concerning epilepsy remain the major identified reason for the difficulty that persons with epilepsy experience in finding employment.[7] The expectations of employers for workers with convulsive disorder include high accident rates, excessive absenteeism, and poor productivity.[6–8] In addition, employers are concerned that anxiety will develop in other employees, particularly if a seizure should occur in the workplace. Performance records, however, do not support these assumptions. Udel[8] studied the work records of 77 people with epilepsy employed by four companies. In three of the four companies, these employees had lost no time because of accidents, and in the fourth, loss was confined to the accident day. The job performance of these workers was rated as better than fellow employees in one company and equal in the other three. MacIntyre[9] surveyed 177 patients employed in the United Kingdom by a variety of industries. Of these, 158 (89%) had no difficulty with their jobs. Only 18 accidents were attributed to epilepsy over a 10-year period. The accident rate of employees with seizures was one-third that of nonepileptics. Hicks and Hicks,[7] in an investigation involving 31 employers in the San Francisco Bay area, found that accident rates, absenteeism, and productivity were similar in employees with and without epilepsy. Dasgupta et al.[10] found no difference in accident rate or performance when comparing 45 workers with epilepsy to a control group at the Teesside Division of the British Steel Corporation.

Some information is available concerning the loss of jobs by patients with seizures. In 20 people studied by Fraser et al.,[11] only one dismissal resulted from a seizure in the workplace. MacIntyre's series[9] included 13 individuals who had been "sacked." Only one was a result of a seizure at work.

Several characteristics have been associated with persons with seizures who have been successful in obtaining and keeping employment. Such individuals tend to be free of neurologic impairment other than epilepsy and also do not have psychiatric disorders or addiction problems.[11,12] Not surprisingly, persons with successful work histories were better able to find employment. Poor seizure control was correlated with poor occupational adjustment.[13] Finally, an applicant with a driver's license was more likely to secure employment.

The studies described above are largely dependent on employee disclosure of epilepsy. Yet, of 40 employees questioned by Scrambler and

Hopkins,[14] 21 had not informed their employers of their disorder, and only two of the remaining 19 had made their epilepsy known before obtaining employment. Fraser[5] indicates that he advises omission of any reference to epilepsy on the initial job application, although he suggests disclosure subsequently. As Fraser recognizes, it is difficult to advise applicants to provide a prospective employer with information that may have a negative impact on their application. However, in many states, disclosure is necessary before starting work in order that the employer be afforded secondary injury fund protection.

An often-stated reason for denying employment to applicants with epilepsy is the fear that workers' compensation premiums will rise. This fear is unfounded. Premiums are frequently "class rated"—that is, based on a group of companies in a specific class. Larger employers may be individually rated, in which case premiums are based on the accident rate experienced during a prior period. In either case, workers with epilepsy could increase premiums only by manifesting an excessive accident rate, and, as noted earlier, the frequency of accidents in the workplace in workers with epilepsy is similar to that in nonepileptics.

All 50 states and the District of Columbia have second injury funds or similar special funds. These funds limit the liability of an employer to that due directly to an injury on the job and exclude preexisting disability. The difference in compensation is paid by the fund rather than by the employer. If a seizure is directly responsible for an injury that otherwise would not have occurred, the employer may be completely reimbursed for benefits paid. Since most states require that the employer be aware of the employee's epilepsy when he or she is hired, employees would have to disclose their disorder to the employer before starting work.

PRECIPITATING FACTORS FOR SEIZURES

Precipitating factors that may provoke seizures in susceptible individuals should be screened from the workplace of the patient with epilepsy. Two major precipitants of seizures, missed medications and intercurrent infections, would not ordinarily occur in most occupations. A third major precipitant, sleep deprivation, can pose a serious problem in patients with epilepsy. Shift work or rotating shifts that force alternating sleep habits frequently lead to insomnia and sleep deprivation. Some patients with seizure disorders will prove unable to tolerate rotating shifts.

In addition to sleep deprivation, excessive sleepiness may be a concern in the patient with epilepsy. In this population, anticonvulsant medications are the principal cause of daytime somnolence. Although somnolence is most frequently attributed to therapeutic levels of barbiturates and benzodiazepines, the other commonly used anticonvulsants (phenytoin, carbamazepine) can also produce sleepiness and incoordination when levels exceed the therapeutic range.[15] Most patients achieve complete or near complete control of their seizures with anticonvulsant medications; for them, drug side effects may become the most limiting factor in their daily lives. Fortunately, most of these side effects can be managed successfully by judicious selection and monitoring of antiepileptic drugs.

RESOURCES AVAILABLE TO THE WORKER WITH EPILEPSY

Vocational rehabilitation agencies are established in all 50 states and the District of Columbia and can assist the person with epilepsy. The common objective of vocational rehabilitation ("voc rehab") is to provide services that will enable persons previously considered unemployable because of disability to obtain suitable employment. These services may include counseling, vocational training, on-the-job experience, sheltered workshops, and education aimed at improving job-seeking skills. Specific information can be obtained from state departments of labor or divisions of vocational rehabilitation.

An additional major resource available to individuals with epilepsy who are seeking employment is the Training and Placement Service (TAPS) of the Epilepsy Foundation of America. This program was founded in 1976 and initially served clients in five cities. Currently, 14 cities have TAPS programs (Atlanta, Boston, Cleveland, Denver, Kansas City, Los Angeles, Miami, Mobile, Portland [Maine], Portland [Oregon], Saint Paul, San Antonio, Trenton, and Washington) supported by grants from the Department of Labor and the Coelho Fund. In addition, almost twice as many similar programs, which are locally funded, have been established around the country by affiliates of the Epilepsy Foundation. These programs work both with prospective employees and potential employers. Employees are helped to set realistic employment goals consistent with their abilities, interests, and the nature of their seizure disorders. Such assistance is provided individually and through workshops and job clubs. Follow-up after placement is also carried out to deal with problems arising on the job. Potential employers are provided with information regarding epilepsy, restrictions on type of work if indicated, stress in the workplace, workers' compensation, medication side effects, and other relevant matters. This program reports a success rate of over 70%.

EVALUATION OF THE WORKER WHO DEVELOPS EPILEPSY

Although several workplace factors affect epilepsy, it is much less common for a workplace exposure to account for the illness. Since a wide range of etiologies may be linked to the onset of epilepsy, a neurologic history must be obtained to exclude other possibilities; head imaging is also necessary to identify an intracranial abnormality capable of producing a seizure. Even with a thorough neurologic evaluation, however, it may not be possible to distinguish seizures related to occupational exposure from those with unrelated causes.

TABLE 6.2
Toxins Associated with Seizures

Metals	Gases
Aluminum (chronic)	Carbon monoxide
Antimony (acute)	Hydrogen sulfide
Arsenic	Methyl chloride
Lead	**Environmental toxins**
Mercury	Camphor
Thallium	Chlordane
Solvents	Hexachlorophene
Benzene	Organophosphates
Carbon tetrachloride	Picrotoxin
Ethylene glycol	Strychnine
Methanol	

A number of industrial toxins and metals can produce seizures as a result of acute exposure (Table 6.2). Acutely, the presence of toxic substances in blood or urine is usually detectable, often with a characteristic metabolic disturbance. Generally, symptoms of toxic exposure progress as toxic load increases, with convulsions representing the extreme end of severity. Toxic exposure seldom produces seizures in the absence of systemic signs or symptoms. Accordingly, the diagnosis of acute toxin-induced seizure is seldom difficult to make.

The ability of toxins to produce recurrent seizures following acute or prolonged exposure is less certain. In the absence of an acute toxic effect, the underlying mechanism would be neuroglial damage. Therefore, other signs of brain injury should be present in order to entertain the diagnosis of toxin-induced seizure disorder. Epilepsy caused by toxin exposure without concurrent neurologic damage is extremely uncommon, and the clinician should approach this diagnosis with utmost caution.

Sleep Disorders

Sleep complaints are common, occurring in 25% of all workers.[16] The most frequent sleep complaints are insomnia and excessive sleepiness. Although not strictly paroxysmal, they are considered here because of their great impact on the workplace. Industrial accidents and lost productivity are frequently attributed to worker fatigue or inattention. The occupational physician may be asked to determine the relationship between the job and a chronically sleepy worker.

The interaction between the workplace and disorders of sleep has seen considerable study, particularly regarding the effects of shift work.[17] Ordinarily, the circadian rhythm regulates the daily cycle of sleep and wakefulness, aided by external cues such as light, noise, and activity level. Persistently conflicting cues—activity at night and light during the day—

occur as a consequence of shift work and cause disruption of the circadian rhythm. Patients then complain of fatigue, loss of appetite, and impaired job performance.[18]

A number of approaches have been put forth to remedy the symptoms of the night worker. Initial attempts at altering mealtimes and other similar cues of the circadian cycle met with limited success. Hypnotics have proved useful to produce adequate daytime sleep.[19] Probably the best remedy, however, is exposure to a period of bright light at night followed by light deprivation during the day. In most night workers, bright light exposure can temporarily align the circadian rhythm to the work schedule and is probably the most effective single remedy for the night worker.[20]

In those who are not long-term night shift workers, bright light exposure is probably not practical. To avoid excessive daytime sleepiness in these workers, occupational physicians advise limiting night shifts to one per week.

In addition to shift work, industrial chemical exposures may produce somnolence and sleep disturbance. Unlike seizures, which may represent a late manifestation of toxin exposure, sleepiness may present after minimal exposure. Somnolence has been reported to follow exposure to solvents and metals, generally followed by other symptoms, such as gait imbalance, nausea, and incoordination. In a workplace where solvents are used, the development of persistent somnolence in a worker should raise the possibility of toxin exposure. Since fatigue is a nonspecific symptom of many illnesses, however, a clear history of exposure, along with associated signs and symptoms, is necessary for diagnosis.

Sleep apnea and narcolepsy, the classic paroxysmal sleep disorders, also deserve mention as they relate to the workplace. A variety of factors (airway abnormality, obesity) combine with the decreased muscle tone present during sleep to cause periods of apnea. The patient then experiences episodic awakening and consequent unsatisfactory sleep and excessive daytime sleepiness. Although rare toxins can produce sleep apnea,[21] this condition is of importance to the occupational physician mainly as a consideration in the excessively sleepy patient.

Narcolepsy-cataplexy syndrome refers to the tetrad of cataplexy, excessive daytime sleepiness, sleep paralysis, and visual hallucinations while falling asleep.[22] It usually begins between ages 15 and 25 (80% by age 35) and occurs at a rate of 4 per 10,000. Although the exact cause has not yet been determined, the clinical phenomena are explained by the uncontrolled onset of rapid eye movement sleep. Because the cataplexy (sudden involuntary loss of motor tone) is often triggered by stressful events such as noises, anger, and anxiety, patients with untreated narcolepsy seldom achieve gainful employment. Furthermore, involuntary behaviors develop in some patients with narcolepsy-cataplexy syndrome. These may last several minutes to an hour and usually occur in association with routine motor movements such as writing, typing, or conversing.

TABLE 6.3
Abridged Headache Classification

---

1. Vascular headaches, migraine type
   a. Classic and common migraine
   b. Cluster headache
   c. Hemiplegic and ophthalmoplegic migraine
2. Muscle contraction headache
3. Mixed vascular/muscle contraction headache
4. Psychogenic headache
5. Vascular headache, nonmigraine type: secondary to systemic disorders that affect cranial arteries (e.g., hypoxia, caffeine withdrawal, nitrates, carbon monoxide).
6. Inflammatory headache (e.g., meningitis, subarachnoid hemorrhage, arteritis)
7. Traction headache
   a. Intracerebral mass (tumor, hematoma, abscess)
   b. Post–lumbar puncture headache
   c. Pseudotumor cerebri

Fortunately, most of the symptoms of narcolepsy-cataplexy can be successfully treated. Patients whose narcolepsy is under treatment can usually work, but the possibility of a cataplectic attack necessitates restrictions similar to those of patients with epilepsy.

Headache Disorders

The interaction between headache and the workplace is a major branch of occupational neurology. Headaches are among the most frequent reason for consulting a physician; they also are responsible for many days of missed work. Headache, like excessive sleepiness, is a nonspecific symptom with numerous possible causes, some work-related, most not, and distinguishing the occupational from the incidental headache often requires considerable skill.

Since the 1960s, headaches have been basically classified into "vascular" (migraine), "tension" (muscle contraction), and "other" categories, as shown in Table 6.3.[23] Although recent thinking has blurred the distinction between migraine and tension headaches, the classification still retains clinical usefulness. Regardless of the headache type, the frequency, severity, and duration of the headaches determine the consequent level of disability. Additional considerations for the occupational physician are precipitating factors, since modification of these in the workplace can ameliorate the headache disorder and decrease the need for headache medications.

Although it is generally assumed that work-related stress can produce headaches, particularly of the muscle contraction type, evidence for this view is difficult to accumulate. An epidemiologic survey of 975 men and women in various occupations identified no significant difference in the prevalence of headaches across occupational categories or education levels.[24] Men, on the other hand, but not women, reporting "stress on the job" had twice the frequency of both muscle contraction and migraine headaches. Furthermore, men in managerial positions had significantly more headaches than those who were not managers. A reasonable conclusion is that occupational factors aggravate headache disorders but do not cause them.

The best predictors of headache occurrence remain age, sex, and personality type.[25] Ultimately, a patient who is headache-prone is best advised to select a job carefully, with an understanding of its particular stresses and how to manage them effectively.

Underlying headache disorder explains most work-related headaches, although exposure to certain substances can cause headaches that mimic the common headache syndromes.[26] Clues that headaches are occupational include timing of arrival at work to onset of headache, headache-free periods when away from the job, and the presence of significant levels of chemicals in the workplace. Although few controlled studies explore the relationship between solvents and headache, the vasoactive properties of some solvents imply their capability of producing headaches. In order to precipitate a headache, a toxin must affect either the cerebral vasculature, the meninges, or the structures overlying the scalp. Since delivery of the chemical occurs via blood vessels, and other structures receive considerably less blood flow, virtually all true chemical-induced headaches are of the vascular type. The headaches may throb, are moderate to severe, and resolve with removal of the offending chemical, although certain substances (e.g., caffeine) can produce headaches during withdrawal. The principal solvents and gases implicated in occupational headache are toluene (present in many forms of glue), acetone, and amyl alcohol. Headache may also be a symptom of heavy metal intoxication, although again, other symptoms are usually predominant.

Many people report headaches following exposure to "fumes" (e.g., gasoline, paint). The amounts of solvents present in casually inhaled fumes do not enter the circulation in sufficient quantities to provoke a vascular headache. These headaches are probably attributable to secondary muscle contraction.

Other Paroxysmal Disorders

SYNCOPE

The term *syncope* is applied to the loss of consciousness that occurs when blood flow to the brain is interrupted. Syncope may be produced by cardiac dysrhythmia, aortic stenosis, carotid sinus syndrome, intravascular volume depletion, forceful coughing, micturition, and other situations such as the Valsalva maneuver that increase vagal tone. Another important entity is neurocardiogenic syncope. This benign condition occurs in the absence of underlying pathology, and always from the standing position.[27] It may recur with certain stresses, such as prolonged standing. Prolonged standing has been curtailed in many occupations (e.g., soldiers, bellhops) because it can precipitate syncope even in healthy people. Although uncommon, intractable syncope will generally exclude an employee from the workplace. The guidelines in such cases resemble those for seizure disorders.

EPISODIC VERTIGO

Vertigo must first be distinguished from dizziness, a nonspecific symptom of many disorders. Vertigo is the hallucination of movement and is related to disease in the inner ear, vestibular nerve, brainstem, or cerebellum. Although a lesion anywhere along this axis can produce vertigo, the principal episodic causes of vertigo are disorders of the inner ear: benign positional vertigo and Ménière's disease.

Patients with benign positional vertigo episodically become vertiginous with change in head position. The vertigo is usually mild and controllable with exercise and antihistamines. Ménière's syndrome, on the other hand, is characterized by recurrent sudden attacks of severe, disabling vertigo.[28] The syndrome is attributed to accumulation of endolymphatic fluid and thus is accompanied by the symptoms of tinnitus and hearing loss.

Whatever the cause, episodic vertigo can prove dangerous in many situations. Those who work with heavy equipment or on ledges (e.g., construction workers) must be protected from these situations until their vertigo is under control.

Summary

The challenge of paroxysmal disorders in occupational medicine is to understand the relationship between the disorder and the occupation and to tailor the treatment and the workplace appropriately. Cases of paroxysmal disorders that can be traced to the workplace are exceedingly uncommon. Occupational factors, however, may exacerbate epilepsy, migraine, and other episodic illnesses. Identifying such factors will ease the management of these conditions. Moreover, a temporal relationship of symptoms to work schedule should prompt an inquiry into occupational exposure.

Although not truly paroxysmal, certain sleep disorders may have an occupational cause, particularly when related to shift work. With attention to the needs of these workers, sleep complaints can usually be treated satisfactorily.

In spite of treatment, some patients will continue to experience spells. For them, the occupational physician may be asked to provide an impairment rating. As noted in this chapter and emphasized in the guidelines of the American Medical Association (AMA),[29] impairment from episodic neurologic disorders depends on the frequency, duration, and severity of attacks. The AMA guidelines are based mainly on activities of daily living and only minimally on ability to work. A person whose epilepsy is controlled at two seizures per year would receive a low impairment rating. Driving privileges would be curtailed or eliminated, and he or she would be barred from certain occupations. The AMA *Guides* does not define work restrictions imposed by medical conditions. Making this judgment becomes an important task for the occupational physician.

Paroxysmal disorders in general, and convulsive disorders in particular, remain a major cause of unemployment among potentially productive individuals. The majority of seizure disorders in adults are under good control, and these people should be able to be successfully employed in any field in which they are interested and qualified. For individuals who continue to have seizures on optimal therapy, some restrictions understandably exist, but a multitude of career opportunities are available to this group as well. Available data indicate that individuals with seizure disorders have an accident rate, a rate of absenteeism, and a record of productivity equal to or better than those of their nonepileptic coworkers. Employers who hire epileptic employees should not anticipate any increase in workers' compensation premiums, and "second injury" or similar funds limit the liability of an employer and exclude preexisting disability. The employee with a paroxysmal neurologic disorder is protected against discrimination because of this disorder by federal and state legislation, although using this protection may involve lengthy civil rights commission proceedings and court action. Resources available to the individual with epilepsy who is seeking employment include the Training and Placement Service of the Epilepsy Foundation of America and similar programs affiliated with local chapters of this foundation and with all 50 states.

References

1. Dikmen S, Morgan SF. Neuropsychological factors related to employability and occupational status in persons with epilepsy. J Nerv Ment Dis 1980;168(4):236–240.
2. Commission on Classification and Terminology of the International League Against Epilepsy. Proposal for revised clinical and electroencephalographic classification of seizures. Epilepsia 1981;22:489–501.
3. Hansotia P, Broste SK. The effect of epilepsy or diabetes mellitus on the risk of automobile accidents. N Engl J Med 1991;324:22–26.
4. Sorel L. The epileptic worker in the construction industry. Epilepsia (Amst) 1972;13:57–62.
5. Fraser RT. Epilepsy. Annu Rev Rehabil 1981;2:147–172.

6. Holmes DA, McWilliams JM. Employers' attitudes toward hiring epileptics. J Rehabil 1981;47:20–21.
7. Hicks RA, Hicks MJ. The attitude of major companies toward the employment of epileptics: an assessment of two decades of change. Am Correct Ther J 1978;32:180–182.
8. Udel MM. The work performance of epileptics in industry. Arch Environ Health 1960;1:257–264.
9. MacIntyre I. Epilepsy and employment. Community Health (Bristol) 1976;1:195–204.
10. Dasgupta AK, Saunders M, Dick DJ. Epilepsy in the British Steel Corporation: an evaluation of sickness, accident, and work records. Br J Ind Med 1982;39:145–148.
11. Fraser RT, Clemmons D, Trejo W, Tenkin NR. Program evaluation in epilepsy rehabilitation. Epilepsia 1983;24:737–746.
12. Rodin EA, Rennick P, Denerll RD. Vocational and educational problems of epileptic patients. Epilepsia 1972;13:149–160.
13. Agustine EA, Novelly RA, Mattson RH. Occupational adjustment following neurosurgical treatment of epilepsy. Ann Neurol 1984;15:68–72.
14. Scambler G, Hopkins A. Social class, epileptic activity, and disadvantage at work. J Epidemiol Community Health 1980;34:129–133.
15. Engel J. Seizures and Epilepsy. Philadelphia: FA Davis, 1989.
16. Partinen M, Eskelinen L, Tuomi K. Complaints of insomnia in different occupations. Scand J Work Environ Health 1984;10:467–469.
17. Kogi K. Sleep problems in night and shift work. J Hum Ergol 1982;11(Suppl):217–231.
18. Akerstedt T. Sleepiness as a consequence of shift work. Sleep 1988;11:17–34.
19. Walsh JK, Muehlbach MJ, Schweitzer PK. Acute administration of triazolam for the daytime sleep of rotating shift workers. Sleep 1984;7(3):223–229.
20. Czeisler CA, Johnson MP, Duffy J, Brown EN, Ronda JM, Kronauer RE. Exposure to bright light and darkness to treat physiologic maladaption to night work. N Engl J Med 1990;322(18):1253–1308.
21. Leznoff A, Haight JS, Hoffstein V. Reversible obstructive sleep apnea caused by occupational exposure to guar gum dust. Am Rev Respir Dis 1986;133:935–936.
22. Dement W, Reichschaffen A, Gulevich G. The nature of the narcoleptic sleep attack. Neurology 1966;16:18–3.
23. Ad Hoc Committee on Headache Classification. JAMA 1962;169:717–18.
24. Tobiasz–Adamcyk B, Flak E, Jedrychowski WA. Impact of psychosocial factors on the prevalence of headaches in the industrial setting. Neuroepidemiology 1985;4:86–95.
25. Davis RA, Wetzel RD, Kashiwagi T, McClure JN. Personality, depression, and headache type. Headache 1976;246:4–16.
26. Goetz CG. Neurotoxins in Clinical Practice. New York: Spectrum, 1985.
27. Barron SA. Vagal cardiovascular reflexes in young persons with syncope. Ann Intern Med 1993;118: 943–946.
28. Wilmot TJ. Ménière's disorder. Clin Otolaryngol 1979;4:131–143.
29. American Medical Association. Guides to the Evaluation of Permanent Impairment (3rd ed, revised). Chicago: American Medical Association, 1990.

CHAPTER 7

Movement Disorders

John P. Hammerstad, M.D.
Julie H. Carter, R.N., M.N., A.N.P.

The term *movement disorders* is applied to a variety of abnormalities of motor function in which weakness is not the reason for the disordered movement. In contrast to the weakness and spasticity that are the hallmarks of lesions in the motor cortex and the corticospinal (pyramidal) pathway, movement disorders result from dysfunction in the basal ganglia and cerebellum, producing abnormalities in motor function that can range from a slowness in initiating or executing movement (e.g., bradykinesia in Parkinson's disease) to an excess of movement (e.g., chorea in Huntington's disease). The one exception to this pathologic anatomy of movement disorders is myoclonus, which can be generated at many different sites in the nervous system. Most movement disorders are associated with a degeneration of specific neuronal systems of unknown (e.g., idiopathic Parkinson's disease) or hereditary (e.g., Huntington's disease) cause. However, other pathologic processes affecting basal ganglia or cerebellum, such as stroke, tumor, trauma, or toxic-metabolic insults, may produce a movement disorder.

Several movement disorders are associated with known or suspected occupational exposures (Table 7.1). Also, a variety of movement disorders may result from head trauma, which may be a risk to workers in some occupations, but most civilian head injuries result from motor vehicle accidents, and head trauma will not be considered further except for a brief description of the chronic encephalopathy suffered by boxers. A controversy receiving more attention recently—the possibility that movement disorders, especially dystonia, are triggered by trauma to a limb or the neck—will be discussed in more detail.

It is not surprising that substances that are toxic to the central nervous system should also damage motor systems and give rise to movement disorders. However, toxins are seldom selective, and neurologic

143

TABLE 7.1
Movement Disorders Associated With Known,
Suspected, or Potential Occupational Exposures

Parkinsonism	Movement disorders of brain stem-cerebellar origin: tremor, ataxia, intention myoclonus, opsoclonus
Toxins	
Carbon disulfide[5]	Toxins
Manganese[23]	Mercury [132]
Carbon monoxide[32,33]	Chlordecone (Kepone)[145]
MPTP[36,38]	Acrylamide[128]
Methanol[166]	Toluene[144,146]
Carbon tetrachloride[6,167]	Methyl bromide[148]
Cyanide[168]	Trauma[114]
Head trauma	High-pressure neurologic syndrome[149]
Late sequela of acute trauma[169,170]	
Pugilistic encephalopathy[84]	
Dystonia	
Toxins	
Manganese[23]	
Dioxin[171]	
Head trauma[170]	
Peripheral trauma[170]	
"Overuse" syndromes[172]	

MPTP = 1-methyl-4-phenyl-1,2,3,6-tetrahydropyridine.

symptoms and signs of more diffuse injury are usually present and betray that the disorder is not the idiopathic disease. A notable exception is the neurotoxin 1-methyl-4-phenyl-1,2,3,6-tetrahydropyridine (MPTP), which selectively damages the substantia nigra, producing a syndrome virtually indistinguishable from idiopathic Parkinson's disease. Although industrial toxins known to cause parkinsonian signs produce other neurologic damage not associated with the idiopathic disease, the experience with MPTP has rekindled interest in the possibility that Parkinson's disease may be caused by an exogenous toxin associated with the rise of industrialization. A related development is the epidemiologic evidence that ingestion of a cycad nut indigenous to the western Pacific islands may be responsible for the neurodegenerative disease, most prevalent on the island of Guam, that combines features of amyotrophic lateral sclerosis, Parkinson's disease, and dementia. Because of the potential implications for occupational medicine, the evidence for and against the environmental toxin hypothesis is reviewed.

Finally, the last section of this chapter departs from the traditional discussion of the hazards of the workplace that expose workers to the risk of neurologic damage and focuses on the impact certain movement disorders have on the workplace and how an understanding of the limitations imposed by the disease can lead to a realistic plan to accommodate to the workers' needs and prolong their productivity.

Table 7.2
Parkinsonism Caused by Documented or
Potential Occupational Exposure to Toxins

Toxin	Industry/Occupation
Definite association	
Carbon disulfide	Viscose rayon workers[2–4]
	Grain storage workers[5]
Manganese	Miners[18]
	Foundry workers[14]
MPTP	Pharmaceutical chemists[36]
Possible association	
Carbon monoxide	Use of gasoline-powered tools
	Utility workers[30,32]
Carbon tetrachloride	Grain storage workers[6]
	Chemists[167]
Potential association	
Cyanide	Suicide attempt
Methanol	Intentional ingestion

Parkinsonism

The causes of a parkinsonian syndrome that can be attributed to occupational exposure are listed in Table 7.2. The cardinal features of resting tremor, bradykinesia, rigidity, and postural instability are present in various degrees of severity and combinations, but other neurologic deficits occur as well and differentiate these forms of secondary or "pseudoparkinsonism" from primary or idiopathic parkinsonism (IP). For example, cerebellar, corticospinal signs and peripheral neuropathy are also present in viscose rayon and grain storage workers exposed to carbon disulfide. Dementia and corticospinal signs as well as parkinsonian signs are features of pugilistic encephalopathy. The clinical differences mirror the difference in pathology of idiopathic and secondary parkinsonism. In IP the primary lesion is the degeneration of pigmented neurons in the substantia nigra, locus ceruleus, and dorsal vagal nucleus. A cytoplasmic inclusion in the degenerating neurons, the Lewy body, is considered the pathologic hallmark of the idiopathic disease. By contrast, the lesions in secondary parkinsonism are usually more widespread, and the lesion responsible for the parkinsonian features is often in the striatum (caudate and putamen) or globus pallidus rather than the substantia nigra itself. Also, Lewy bodies are seldom found in the secondary forms. The only exception is MPTP, which produces a pure syndrome by virtue of its selective toxicity to the substantia nigra, and Lewy body–like inclusions have now been described in aged squirrel monkeys given MPTP.[1]

INDUSTRIAL TOXINS
Carbon Disulfide

Carbon disulfide (CS_2) has been recognized as a neurotoxin for over 60 years, when a neuropsychiatric syndrome was described in workers using CS_2 in the production of viscose rayon fibers for the textile industry.[2] Parkinsonian signs have been described in up to approximately 60% of viscose rayon workers.[3,4] CS_2 is also used in other industrial applications, including the production of pesticides, cellophane films for packaging, flotation agents, and the extraction of oil from olives.[5] In 1985, following reports of a neurobehavioral syndrome in grain storage workers similar to that seen in viscose rayon workers, the United States Environmental Protection Agency banned the use of CS_2 in fumigants used to treat grain to control insects during storage.[6]

Peters et al.[6,7] carefully studied 16 grain storage workers with high exposure, two inspectors with intermediate exposure, and four laboratory workers with lower exposures from handling and analyzing grain samples. Ninety percent of the storage workers and inspectors had cogwheeling, 80% had decreased associated movements, 47% had resting tremor, 44% had retropulsion, and 20–25% had bradykinesia. A wide variety of other neuropsychiatric symptoms and signs included, in decreasing order of frequency, hearing loss, sensory neuropathy, neurasthenic symptoms (weakness, headaches, dizziness, decreased memory), intention tremor, gait ataxia, extensor plantar responses, and hyperreflexia in at least 15% of the high-exposure group. Even two of the four "low-exposure" laboratory workers had intention tremor, cogwheeling, and resting tremor. Tremorographic transducer recordings increased the yield to 74% with tremor while four workers had manifest parkinsonism. Symptoms progressed after leaving grain storage work and five of seven evaluated later showed progression.[8]

The parkinsonian features can be explained by lesions of the globus pallidus and the zona reticulata of the substantia nigra as demonstrated by the classic neuropathologic study of Richter[9] of four monkeys exposed to CS_2 by inhalation for 12–21 months. The corticospinal signs and peripheral neuropathy are most likely due to an axonopathy in spinal cord and peripheral nerves thought to be due to disruption of neurofilaments and axonal transport as seen in experimental animal models.[10]

Manganese

Chronic manganese intoxication has been recognized as an occupational hazard for over a century in manganese miners in several countries (e.g., Russia, India, Chile, Cuba, Morocco)[11] and more recently in ore-crushing plants and steel foundries in the United States and Taiwan.[12–16] The inhaled manganese dust is swallowed and the absorbed trace metal preferentially concentrated in mitochondria-rich organs, such as the liver, which regulates the body burden by excreting the excess in the bile.[17] The accumulation and turnover of manganese in the brain is slow. In a study of Chilean miners, Mena and colleagues[18] found that manganese overload was present only during exposure and was not in parallel to the presence of extrapyramidal symptoms, unlike Wilson's disease, in which the concentration of brain copper parallels the severity of the symptoms and removal of the copper by chelation alleviates the symptoms. As predicted by these observations, chelation is of no value in the treatment of manganese intoxication.

Exposure to manganese fumes produced in casting and arc burning of steel with greater than 10% manganese content has also been associated with parkinsonism.[19–21] It is not known if manganese fumes from conventional welding cause neurologic damage, but a comparison of patients and control subjects found that welding increased the risk of Parkinson's disease.[22]

The extrapyramidal syndromes differ somewhat between miners and industrial workers. The onset of disease in miners is marked by a period of psychosis before the extrapyramidal features emerge.[18] Dystonic features are often present[23] in addition to parkinsonian bradykinesia, rigidity, and impairment in postural reflexes. The psychotic phase is absent in foundry workers, and bradykinesia, rigidity, and impairment of balance are the prominent features with less dystonia.[12,13,15] Symptoms may progress after cessation of exposure.[24]

Cases of parkinsonism after chronic low exposure to manganese have been reported,[25] raising concern about manganese-containing pesticides increasing the risk of parkinsonism in rural areas.

The pathologic changes of manganese intoxication are most conspicuous in the globus pallidus and striatum, with only one report noting damage to the substantia nigra.[26] Positron emission tomography (PET) scans of four Taiwanese manganese smelters with mild parkinsonism have shown normal fluorodopa uptake in the striatum consistent with the notion that the clinical deficits are due to a postsynaptic lesion.[12,16,24] Magnetic resonance imaging (MRI) shows accumulation of manganese in the globus pallidus and striatum of experimentally intoxicated monkeys[27] and similar changes in an arc welder cutting steel.[21] This suggests that MRI may be a sensitive tool for detecting suspected manganese intoxication.

Some reports claim the parkinsonian features respond to levodopa (L-DOPA)[28] therapy while others report negative results.[15] Based on the pathologic and PET scan evidence, one would expect only a transient benefit at best because the postsynaptic site of action for dopamine in the striatum would be incapable of responding.

Carbon Monoxide

Carbon monoxide intoxication is rarely encountered as an occupational hazard. It is usually the result of intentional exposure as part of a suicide attempt or accidental exposure due to faulty furnaces or inadvisable burning of coal or gas in poorly ventilated spaces.[29] The few cases that are work related have usually occurred in utility workers.[30] In the vast majority of cases, signs of diffuse neurologic dysfunction overshadow the parkinsonian symptoms.[30] Parkinsonian features usually appear as delayed sequelae.[29] Treatment with hyperbaric oxygen has prevented both the acute and delayed sequelae.[31] Autopsied cases show ischemic necrosis of cortex and cerebellum, while pallidal necrosis accounts for the parkinsonian features.[32] Only a handful of patients with a pure parkinsonian syndrome have been reported. One such patient, a survivor of a suicide attempt, showed hypodense bilateral pallidal lesions on CT scan and, as expected, did not respond to L-DOPA therapy.[33]

Permanent neurologic sequelae occur only when the exposure is sufficient to render the individual comatose, and they do not result from chronic low-level exposure to operating machines in the workplace. One possible exception was the case of a man who was rendered unconscious on at least two occasions while operating a gas engine concrete saw before parkinsonism developed.[32] However, because of a good response to L-DOPA he may have had an unrelated IP. Cases of persistent subtle neuropsychological deficits following moderate exposure in workplace accidents have been reported.[34] Firefighters, an example of individuals at high risk for carbon monoxide exposure, were surveyed by questionnaire and found to have an increased incidence of Parkinson's disease.[35] An ascertainment bias in favor of a greater proportion of ill people responding leaves open the question of whether chronic low exposure to carbon monoxide may be a cause of parkinsonism.

1-Methyl-4-Phenyl-1,2,3,6-Tetrahydropyridine

In separate incidents, young-onset parkinsonism developed in two chemists who used MPTP as a starting material for the synthesis of other chemicals, raising the possibility of intoxication from cutaneous absorption or vapor inhalation.[36,37] With this in mind, Barbeau and colleagues[38] examined a group of pharmaceutical company employees variously exposed to MPTP and found a parallel in the incidence of extrapyramidal signs and the level of exposure. A comprehensive study of chemists synthesizing or using MPTP has not been done, but it has not emerged as an important occupational hazard.

Paraquat and diquat are chemically related to MPTP and are used as herbicides, providing a possible environmental cause of parkinsonism in farm workers. However, only rare case reports have associated use of these chemicals with Parkinson's disease.[39] It must be noted, however, that a large number of farm workers exposed to pesticides are migratory, with historically poor health care and documentation. Although epidemiologic studies show an increased incidence of young-onset Parkinson's disease in persons living in rural North America, no association with a specific herbicide or pesticide has been found.[40]

The major importance of MPTP is the question it raises about the possibility of an MPTP-like or other environmental agent that may be responsible for IP and its use as an experimental model for the study of IP and other neurotoxins specific for a particular neuronal system.

IS THERE AN ENVIRONMENTAL CAUSE FOR IDIOPATHIC PARKINSONISM? THE EXAMPLES OF MPTP AND THE PARKINSON'S DISEASE–AMYOTROPHIC LATERAL SCLEROSIS DEMENTIA COMPLEX OF GUAM

MPTP

Two developments on either side of the Pacific Ocean have intrigued medical scientists and renewed interest in environmental factors as etiologically important in IP and perhaps other neurodegenerative diseases of unknown cause. In 1983, Langston and colleagues[41] reported the appearance of acute parkinsonism in four heroin addicts who had injected "synthetic heroin" obtained from a chemist who clandestinely attempted to make a meperidine (Demerol) analogue, MPPP. The toxic chemical was identified as MPTP, a reaction product of the intended MPPP. A similar case had already been reported in a student who had been attempting to make the same meperidine analogue for his own use and committed suicide after severe parkinsonism developed.[42] Subsequently, four more cases have been added to the list,[43] including a man who "snorted" the drug.[44]

The reasons for the intense interest generated by this episode are severalfold. MPTP is the first neurotoxin that causes such selective damage to result in signs and symptoms virtually indistinguishable from those of the idiopathic disease. It produces the clinical and pathologic equivalent of the human condition in monkeys,[1,45,46] which provides an experimental model for study of the disease. It is a relatively simple compound related to other industrial and "natural" chemicals (e.g., the herbicide paraquat and pyridines present in cigarette smoke), raising the possibility that exposure to an MPTP-like molecule in our environment may be critical for the development of IP.

In experimental animals MPTP neurotoxicity can be prevented by pretreatment with a monoamine oxidase inhibitor to prevent its oxidation to the actual toxic molecule, MPP^+.[47] This has raised the possibility of a "protective" therapy to prevent the formation of a neurotoxin from an exogenous or endogenous protoxin. This idea was given impetus by a retrospective uncontrolled study claiming slower progression of disease in patients treated with the monoamine oxidase inhibitor deprenyl.[48] Two placebo-controlled, double-blind prospective trials were then organized to test the hypothesis that treatment of early IP with deprenyl could slow the progression of the disease. Both studies, a smaller single center study[49] and a larger multicenter trial,[50] clearly demonstrated that the use of deprenyl delayed the onset of disability in early untreated IP, possibly because it slows the progression of the disease. If deprenyl truly slows the progression of early IP, a potentially momentous discovery leading to a new therapeutic strategy for neurodegenerative diseases will have occurred. The immediate implications for IP are clear, including a practical economic benefit. It has been estimated that for every extra week that parkinsonian patients can work, $10 million are saved in taxes and disability payments in the United States.[51]

In the seven addicts with MPTP-induced parkinsonism, moderate to severe signs developed over a short period, as one might anticipate from a poisoning. If MPTP is to serve as a model for IP, there should be examples of an insidious onset and slower progression like the idiopathic disease. Twenty-two addicts who injected smaller amounts of the same drug from the illicit California laboratory have now developed mild parkinsonism.[52] Two addicts without parkinsonism have had PET scans showing diminished uptake of fluorodopa intermediate between normal and symptomatic addicts and Parkinson's disease patients.[53] This "presymptomatic" group also will be watched for the development of overt parkinsonism,[54] which would support the theory that a subclinical toxic injury could be followed by a latent asymptomatic interval until the superimposed effects of aging would reduce the remaining neurons to a critically low level; at this time the symptoms of the disease would become manifest.[55,56]

The Parkinson's Disease–Amyotrophic Lateral Sclerosis Dementia Complex of Guam

Meanwhile, a story that is taking longer to unfold is taking place across the Pacific Ocean on Guam, where a high incidence of amyotrophic lateral sclerosis (ALS), Parkinson's disease, and dementia in various combinations or in a relatively pure form occurs in the native Chamorro population. Recent reviews summarize the clinical, pathologic, and epidemiologic evidence, which has excluded genetic and infectious causes and favors an environmental etiology.[57,58]

Historical accounts indicate that Lytico-bodig (the Chamorron name for the PD-ALS-dementia complex) had been present for many decades before World War II, but the incidence increased in the first two decades after the war and then was followed by a subsequent steady decline as the diet has become westernized.[59] One hypothesis favors a link between the ingestion of an indigenous food and these disorders. Spencer and associates[60] have summarized the evidence that increased use of the seed of the false sago palm *Cycas circinalis* as a foodstuff during the Japanese occupation during World War II would account for the increase in incidence following the war with a subsequent decline as the diet has become westernized.

Two components of the cycad nut with neurotoxic properties are being studied. A metabolite of cycasin, the major toxin in cycads, is receiving the most attention after studies of b-*N*-methylamino-ʟ-alanine (BMAA) have suggested that it is less likely to be the toxic ingredient.[61]

The Epidemiology of Idiopathic Parkinsonism

It has been suggested that IP is a disease of the age of industrialization because it was not described until 1817 by Parkinson and less than 80 years later was considered by Gowers and Charcot to be among the most common neurologic diseases encountered in their clinics.[62] The discovery of MPTP as a specific neurotoxin and the likelihood of a dietary factor as a cause of Guamanian PD-ALS-dementia have given impetus to new epidemiologic studies looking for evidence of environmental factors as a sole or contributing cause for Parkinson's disease.

Wherever investigated, IP has been found in all ethnic groups.[63–67] In a door-to-door community survey, the most reliable of epidemiologic survey methods, the prevalence of IP in blacks and whites in Mississippi was found to be equal (103 and 159/100,000).[68] However, geographic differences in prevalence rates were noted.[63,69,70] In other door-to-door surveys in China (49/100,000)[65] and Nigeria (67/100,000),[71] the lower prevalence rate in these relatively nonindustrialized countries has been cited as support of the idea that environmental factors associated with industrialization might predispose to the development of PD. A possible exception to this is a recent report of a door-to-door survey of the Parsi community in Bombay,[72] where the prevalence (328/100,000) is among the highest reported. In a follow-up case control study in China, where industrialization is relatively recent and exposures are easier to ascertain in this less mobile population, Tanner and colleagues[62] found that occupational or residential exposure to industrial chemical or printing plants and quarries was associated with an increased risk of developing PD while a decreased risk was associated with living in villages. However, a smaller case control study of the residents of homes for the elderly in Hong Kong[73] found an increased risk of IP associated with long residence in rural areas, with farming, with previous use of herbicides and pesticides, and with habitual consumption of raw vegetables. In North America an increased risk in young-onset PD was associated with living in a rural area and drinking well water.[40,69] However, this is not necessarily a contradiction to the industrialization hypothesis if herbicides and pesticides are among the offending agents.[74] Agricultural chemicals are used to a very limited extent in China, and exposure to them may be increased further in rural North America by drinking well water, which may act to concentrate the chemicals leached from overlying soil.[62] Well water has not been analyzed for agricultural chemicals; however, no particular agent, including paraquat, has been definitively associated with the increased risk.[40,75] Well water used by patients with young-onset IP patients did not differ from that used by control subjects in the content of 23 heavy metals.[40]

In a study of brains obtained from brain banks in the eastern United States, organochlorine pesticide residues were assayed in 20 IP, 7 Alzheimer's disease (AD), and 14 control brains.[76] Only two of the 16 pesticide residues screened were detected. One of them, a long-lasting residue of DDT, was found in the majority of brains from all three groups. Only deildrin was found in a disproportionate number of IP cases (6/20), in comparison to AD (1/20) and control brains (0/14). However, the levels were small, and it remains to be seen if chronic low-level exposure to this toxin is a factor in the development of IP in susceptible individuals.

Nonetheless, in Europe and North America at least, exposure to agricultural chemicals in particular and to wood pulp manufacturing has consistently emerged as a risk factor in epidemiologic studies. A case control study in Spain identified an increased risk for IP in those drinking well water for more than 40 years and those who had more than 5 years' exposure to pesticides.[77] In a similar study in Quebec, patients with IP were more likely to have had occupational or residential exposures to heavy metal industries, pesticides, well water, and cigarette smoke.[78] An earlier study in Quebec and a similar study in Sweden relying on pharmacy records of levodopa use to estimate the geographic variation in the prevalence of IP found the greatest prevalence in areas where vegetable farming[74] and wood pulp[67,74] and steel alloy[67] mills were the predominant industries.

Three recent case control studies using logistic regression analysis and mutivariate statistical methods to limit confounding variables have struck a similar theme. All three surveyed relatively rural regions of North America where agriculture and wood products were the dominant industries. One of the two Canadian studies found an increased risk for working in orchards and planar mills.[79] In the other, family history was the strongest predictor of risk followed by head trauma and herbicide use.[80] The U.S. study also found a significant association with family history. Insecticide exposure was a stronger predictor than herbicide use or rural residency at the time of diagnosis.[81]

However, it has been argued that the stability of the incidence rates over 40 years in Rochester, Minnesota, where the prevalence rate is among the highest recorded, is against an environmental cause,[82,83] especially those industrial or agricultural chemicals introduced since then.

PUGILISTIC ENCEPHALOPATHY

Also known as "dementia pugilistica" or "punch drunk syndrome," the more common features of pugilistic encephalopathy are dementia and a pseudobulbar, slow slurred speech accompanied by corticospinal signs of hyperreflexia, spasticity, and Babinski signs. Parkinsonian bradykinesia and masked facies are often present and occasionally a typical resting tremor is seen.[84,85] An interval of several years may elapse between the end of the boxing career and the onset of symptoms.[85,86] The reason for the latent interval is unknown. As has been hypothesized for Parkinson's disease and Alzheimer's disease, it has been proposed that subclinical damage (in this case from trauma) becomes clinically manifest decades later as a consequence of age-related neuronal attrition.[55,86] Postmortem examinations have shown cerebral atrophy, ventricular enlargement, and atrophy of cerebellar folia. Microscopically there are neurofibrillary tangles and degeneration of the substantia nigra.[87]

Only one epidemiologic study has been done to assess the prevalence of clinical neurologic abnormalities.[88] Former professional boxers were randomly selected for study from the national register in Great Britain. Of 224 examined, 17% were found to have the punch drunk syndrome. The prevalence rose to 28% in former boxers over the age of 50. The prevalence also increased with increased exposure (number of bouts). An even higher percentage of active amateur[89] and former boxers without history of neurologic or psychiatric disease had evidence of brain damage on neuropsychological tests, electroencephalography (EEG) and computed tomographic (CT) brain scans.[90]

The Possible Role of Peripheral Trauma in Movement Disorders

The evidence is anecdotal and a causal association speculative, but there has been increasing interest in the possibility that peripheral trauma—that is, injury to a limb or the neck exclusive of head trauma—may play a role in triggering involuntary postures and movements, especially focal dystonia. Starting with the observations of the great French and English neurologists of the late nineteenth century, the association of hand cramps (writer's cramp, musician's cramp) with overuse from certain occupations has been noted. For a time this condition was known as "occupational neurosis," which conveyed the notion held by most physicians that this was primarily a psychiatric problem if not outright malingering. Although the pathophysiologic mechanism is still unknown, occupational cramp occurs with such regularity in certain pursuits, such as music (musician's cramp) that the association is no longer thought to be mere coincidence or a "neurosis." The growing acceptance of occupational cramp as an organic pathologic entity has given some support to the consideration that dystonia following trauma may be more than a coincidental association and may share a similar pathophysiologic mechanism. One report has noted an association of hand trauma and the development of focal dystonia in musicians.[91] Occupational cramp is discussed in more detail in Chapter 12, and the rest of this section is confined to the issue of dystonia and other involuntary movements following trauma.

Aside from the normal scientific caution in assigning any cause and effect relationship when the only evidence is anecdotal and our methods are insufficient to prove such an association, additional caution is advised because of the medicolegal implications. As we review the current literature we should be mindful of the following questions that require an answer before this matter can be elevated above the merely speculative. Why do dystonias or other disorders of movement occur so infrequently when minor trauma to limbs and neck is so common? Are there predisposing factors that make only a few susceptible? Only about 10% of patients with torticollis report a prior injury. Is this because the trauma may not be recalled by the others? How much time should be allowed between the episode of trauma and the onset of the movement disorder to consider it a causal association? The interval in reported cases varies from an immediate onset to 8 years. What mechanism can account for a perturbation in the periphery leading to dysfunction in central motor pathways, and how long would it take for the disordered physiology to develop? Finally, in an individual case one must decide if the abnormal movement or posture represents true neurologic dysfunction or is a contracture or a psychogenic disturbance.

DYSTONIA

Torsion dystonia is characterized by forceful and sustained muscle contractions or spasms that produce involuntary twisting movements or abnormal postures of the body or limbs or both. The speed and duration of the spasm may vary from myoclonic-like jerks ("myoclonic dystonia") or irregular tremor-like jerks (clonic) to continuous writhing (athetoid) movements or fixed posture (tonic). Characteristically it begins in one body part and the dystonic spasm occurs only when that part is voluntarily moved (action dystonia). During this early stage muscle tone may be entirely normal at rest. It may remain limited to one body part (focal dystonia) or gradually progress to involve another region (segmental dystonia) or become generalized. Generalized torsion dystonia is much more likely to begin in childhood, whereas segmental and focal dystonia most often have their onset in adulthood.[92,93]

Physiologically, dystonia is characterized by co-contraction of agonists and antagonists and overflow of the contraction to muscle groups inappropriately activated for the intended movement.[94] This inappropriate co-contraction appears to result from the lack of reciprocal inhibition of the antagonist muscles.[94–96] An abnormality of the suppression phase of certain brain stem reflexes in craniocervical dystonia (e.g., idiopathic blepharospasm, spasmodic torticollis) is consistent with defective control of inhibitory interneuronal networks.[97–99]

Dystonia can be classified according to the part of the body affected or to the etiology (idiopathic or symptomatic).[100] The most common symptomatic cause of generalized dystonia is static perinatal encephalopathy (cerebral palsy), which may be delayed in onset or undergo progression during adolescence.[101] Hemidystonia may be caused by a variety of lesions affecting the basal ganglia of one hemisphere, usually the putamen.[102,103] Most generalized and focal dystonia is idiopathic. Known or suspected occupational causes are listed in Table 7.1.

Sheehy and Marsden[104] speculated that trauma might be a specific trigger in some cases of idiopathic torticollis based on a review of the literature in which preceding neck trauma was recorded in 9% of 414 cases. A similar 12% of individuals in a recent series of patients receiving botulinum injections recalled an incident of trauma preceding the onset of their torticollis.[105] However, the interval between the incident of trauma and the onset of the torticollis was quite lengthy in some cases, and if the interval was limited to 3 months or less only 5% of the cases qualified. The onset of torticollis immediately (within 24 hours) after a neck injury has been described ("posttraumatic torticollis").[106,107] However, the reported cases differed in several respects from idiopathic torticollis. A marked reduction in neck movement and a fixity of posture unusual for idiopathic torticollis were seen. The abnormal posture did not go away with sleep or respond to sensory tricks. Muscle hypertrophy was prominent in some patients, similar to two patients with trapezius hypertrophy reported by Mattle and colleagues.[108] One of their patients had an accessory nerve transected during a lymph node biopsy. This phenomenon of neurogenic hypertrophy in response to nerve trauma instead of the expected atrophy is most commonly seen in the calf following S1 root lesions. The authors have seen a similar case of marked hypertrophy of trapezius and other cervical muscles following a C6 radiculopathy secondary to an acute herniated disk relieved by surgery. However, only two of the 11 patients with posttraumatic torticollis had evidence of a radiculopathy.

A variety of injuries, usually minor, have been associated with focal dystonia. In the reported cases the injury is to the body part later affected by the dystonia, and the interval between the presumed precipitating injury has varied from hours to 8 years. A typical history is a sprain or direct blow to a limb followed weeks to months later by the abnormal movement. In some cases of limb dystonia, evidence of a nerve entrapment or root compression is seen rather than a direct injury.[109,110] In a subset of the injured patients, a reflex sympathetic dystrophy also develops.[111,112] Oromandibular dystonia and spasmodic dysphonia have been reported following facial trauma or oral or laryngeal surgery.[112,113] Axial dystonia or hemidystonia has been reported in association with whiplash, back strain, or a fall onto the buttocks or back.[109,114]

PAINFUL LEGS AND MOVING TOES SYNDROME

Under the apt title, "Painful legs and moving toes," Spillane and colleagues[115] described a distinctive syndrome of rhythmic undulating movements of the toes (usually of one foot, although bilateral cases have occurred) with a severe pain that usually precedes the onset of the movements in the affected foot and leg. No cause or effective treatment has been found, but a common story is a history of sciatica and lumbar disk disease.[115–117] Other root and peripheral nerve lesions have been described, including herpes zoster, a traumatic injury of the cauda equina, a sacral root cyst, and a musculocutaneous neuropathy.[115,116] A similar syndrome in the arm and fingers has been reported in a woman with a radiation brachial plexopathy.[118] Trauma to the leg was implicated in five cases, but in two of them the interval between the event and the first symptoms was 2 and 10 years.[119] Because of the frequency of associated root or peripheral nerve lesions it has been suggested that the movements are caused by posterior root fibers firing spontaneously and that this input to the spinal cord induces the firing of the related motor neurons and interneurons.[116]

OTHER MUSCLE SPASMS

Other involuntary movements, sometimes described as muscle spasms but otherwise unclassifiable as dystonia, chorea, or myoclonus, have occurred following trauma or in association with root or peripheral nerve lesions (Table 7.3). They may be short-lived and cramp-like or very prolonged, producing a fixed posture. Some of the cases of posttraumatic torticollis may belong in this category (see the section on dystonia). A frequent accompaniment is reflex sympathetic dystrophy. Brief spasms of hand muscles have been described in patients with radiculopathy secondary to cervical spondylosis.[120] The author has seen two similar cases, one in a patient who had a prior cervical fracture-dislocation without apparent neurologic sequelae.

SEGMENTAL MYOCLONUS

Myoclonus is an involuntary, brief, shock-like muscle contraction that cannot be voluntarily suppressed. It can be caused by lesions at many levels of the central nervous system, including cerebral cortex, brainstem, and spinal cord. Segmental myoclonus refers to spontaneous discharges of neurons in brain stem or one or several contiguous segments of the spinal cord that produce rhythmic or arrhythmic contractions in muscle groups innervated by those neurons. It is included here because not only might it be a sequela of spinal cord injury but it has been reported after lesions of spinal roots or peripheral nerve.[111,114,121,122] Excluding doubtful cases in which an accompanying central lesion could have been responsible, five of 37 cases reported by Jankovic and Pardo[122] had a peripheral lesion as the only presumptive cause, with a latency varying from immediate onset to 30 days.

Another reason for including segmental myoclonus is a suggestion that one form, hemifacial spasm, may serve as a useful model for understanding how a peripheral lesion could lead to involuntary movements that appear to require the participation of central motor mechanisms in brain stem and

TABLE 7.3
Movement Disorders Possibly Associated with
Peripheral Trauma, Overuse, and Other Local Factors

Movement Disorder	*Associated Factors*
Dystonia	
Segmental/hemidystonia	Whiplash, back strain, fall[109,114]
Focal dystonia	
Musician's cramp	Overuse, trauma (?), nerve entrapment[172]
Writer's cramp	Hand trauma, nerve entrapment (?)[173]
Torticollis	Trauma (usually neck)[104,106,107]
Oromandibular	Facial trauma, oral surgery[112,113]
Spasmodic dysphonia	Vocal cord surgery[113]
Limb	Minor trauma to limb[170]
	With nerve injury[109,110]
	Reflex sympathetic dystrophy[111,112]
"Painful legs and moving toes"	Root compression, trauma[115,119]
Unclassifiable muscle spasms	Reflex sympathetic dystrophy[111]
	Root compression[120]
	Plexus, peripheral nerve lesions[110,118]
Segmental myoclonus	Neck trauma, spinal trauma and surgery, radiculopathy, reflex sympathetic dystrophy[111,122]

spinal cord.[123] Hemifacial spasm is associated with a focal compression of the facial nerve that may be the result of a tumor or ectatic basilar artery, or, in the more common idiopathic form, of abnormal blood vessels that, when removed, result in a cure in a high percentage of cases.[124] One hypothesis to explain the spontaneous discharges of the nerve is ephaptic transmission ("cross-talk" with adjacent fibers carrying afferent impulses) at the site of the irritation. There is some electrophysiologic support for this,[125] but other physiologic recordings obtained during surgical decompression of the nerve were compatible with participation of the facial nucleus motor neurons themselves in the abnormal discharges and against ephaptic transmission alone as the sole mechanism.[126] Thus, it is tenable to suggest that the local compression of the nerve causes ectopic excitation and ephaptic transmission, producing antidromic as well as orthodromic traffic that results in a reorganization of the neuronal apparatus and hyperexcitability of the motor neurons.[123] This may serve as an example of how a peripheral nerve injury can, in some instances, induce a change in the excitability of central motor neurons.

It is not difficult to conceive that such a mechanism may be operative at spinal and brain stem levels, which explains some cases of segmental myoclonus, painful legs and moving toes, and muscle spasms with reflex sympathetic dystrophy, but this does not explain how peripheral trauma can produce reorganization of neuronal networks across several synapses in the basal ganglia to produce dystonia. Based on cases of symptomatic dystonia due to lesions in basal ganglia, it has been proposed that idiopathic dystonia results from a disturbance in striatopallidal-thalamic input to the supplementary motor area (SMA), whereas in posttraumatic focal dystonia, the disturbance is in the SMA itself as a result of altered sensory information from a painful limb or neck, disturbing sensorimotor integration and motor commands from the SMA.[127] However, because peripheral trauma rarely causes dystonia and only 5–10% of focal dystonias are associated with trauma, trauma alone is unlikely to be the primary cause. Trauma may be a nonspecific trigger for the appearance of the symptoms in those predisposed to development of dystonia because of genetic or other factors. With this in mind, Jankovic and Van Der Linden[112] identified 23 patients with presumptive trauma-induced dystonia or tremor that satisfied their criteria of an obvious topographic and temporal relationship between the trauma and the movement disorder with a latency of no longer than a year. Of the 23, 15 had possible predisposing factors, including a family history of dystonia or essential tremor, prior exposure to neuroleptics (including one who had a dystonic reaction), and possible perinatal static encephalopathy.

Movement Disorders of Brain Stem-Cerebellar Origin

This section discusses abnormalities of movement (tremor, ataxia, intention myoclonus, opsoclonus) that often occur together in the same patient, reflecting a common pathophysiology in a derangement of cerebellar motor pathways and associated neuronal systems in brain stem and diencephalon. Occupational causes of these movement disorders (see Table 7.1) seldom result in an isolated symptom or sign—for example, ataxia—but are part of a broader picture of neurologic injury in which the movement disorder may be a prominent or disabling feature. Because tremor is often more readily observed and is a sign of several occupationally related movement disorders, it is featured separately (Table 7.4). The relative prominence of the motor abnormality usually depends on the severity and duration of exposure. For example, in acrylamide intoxication ataxia is prominent in acute or subacute high exposure, whereas a peripheral neuropathy may be the only neurologic abnormality in less severe chronic intoxication.[128]

INDUSTRIAL TOXINS
Mercury

Organic mercurials are still responsible for poisoning epidemics, but inorganic elemental mercury intoxication, which causes a characteristic tremor and intention myoclonus, has seldom been seen since it was discovered to be responsible for the "mad hatter's" syndrome.[129] Sporadic cases of acute exposure are still reported,[130] but the major con-

TABLE 7.4
Occupational Causes of Tremor

Cause	Type of Tremor	Associated Features
Mercury	I,P	Intention myoclonus
Chlordecone	I,P	Gait ataxia, opsoclonus
Methyl bromide	I,P	Ataxia, intention myoclonus
Dioxin	I,P	Dystonia
HPNS	I,P,R	Myoclonus, fasciculations
Carbon disulfide	I,P,R	Parkinsonism, ataxia
Manganese	R	Parkinsonism, dystonia
MPTP	R	Parkinsonism
Pugilistic encephalopathy	R,P	Parkinsonism, dementia, spasticity

I = intention; P = postural; R = resting; HPNS = high-pressure neurologic syndrome; MPTP = 1-methyl-4-phenyl-1,2,3,6-tetrahydropyridine.

cern has shifted to chronic low-level exposure—for example, in dentists.[131] Polyneuropathy has been the only consistent finding, but in a careful case control study of workers from a single plant exposed to elemental mercury over 20 years earlier, a significant correlation between exposure and declining neurologic function, especially tremor and coordination, was noted.[132]

Tremometers have been used in some studies to look for evidence of neurologic deficits that are not clinically or functionally apparent in workers exposed to concentrations of elemental mercury vapors considered to be safe. Subtle differences from control subjects in tremor frequency and amplitude[133,134] were found that confirmed other uncontrolled studies.[135,136] The degree of change roughly correlated with the level of urinary mercury, and the effects were reversible on reduction of mercury exposure. Because of the wide variability in test results among individuals, it is doubtful that tremorographic recordings have any advantage over monitoring of urine mercury as a practical means for identifying workers with increased exposure.[135] Also, the changes in tremor noted are of dubious functional significance.

Chlordecone (Kepone)

Chlordecone is an organochlorine pesticide that is no longer manufactured after multiorgan toxicity was discovered in 23 workers in a Virginia chemical plant.[137] Symptoms and signs of central nervous system involvement were prominent and included postural and intention tremor, mental changes, gait difficulty, and headache in nine, three of whom had benign intracranial hypertension.[138] Of special note was the presence of opsoclonus, an unusual disorder of eye movements usually secondary to viral encephalitides[139] or a paraneoplastic manifestation of a neoplasm.[140] At the time it was first described as a manifestation of chlordecone intoxication, it was the first example of a toxic cause.[138] Subsequently, opsoclonus has also been seen in amitriptyline overdose,[141] thallium and organophosphate poisoning,[142] intoxication with lithium and haloperidol,[143] and intoxication with toluene[144] (see the following section). A follow-up evaluation of 16 of the 23 revealed a persistent neurologic abnormality, a coarse tremor in only one of the workers.[145]

Toluene

Definite neurologic impairment has occurred only in subjects addicted to solvent vapor inhalation.[144] Persistent neurologic dysfunction has been noted after chronic toluene abuse. The most prominent disability was cognitive impairment, with cerebellar ataxia the next most significant clinical disability. In contrast, a case control study of rotogravure printers with long-term toluene exposure failed to find any difference from control subjects on a series of clinical, neurophysiologic, and neuropsychological tests.[146]

Acrylamide

The most common neurologic manifestation of acrylamide intoxication from industrial exposure is a peripheral neuropathy.[128] Only with more severe acute or subacute intoxication have central nervous system symptoms appeared, consisting of a diffuse encephalopathy and an ataxia that appears before evidence of a polyneuropathy and is likely to reflect cerebellar damage.

Methyl Bromide

Methyl bromide intoxication causes widespread neurologic dysfunction, but in some cases ataxia, dysarthria, intention tremor, and myoclonus have been the most prominent features.[147] A permanent severe intention myoclonus has been described after accidental exposure during fumigation of a house, but a posthypoxic intention myoclonus secondary to a status epilepticus could not be excluded.[148]

HIGH-PRESSURE NEUROLOGIC SYNDROME

When divers are exposed to pressures exceeding 20 atm, a series of neurologic symptoms known as the high-pressure neurologic syndrome occur.[149] The neurologic dysfunction is a direct result of the high pressure and not a consequence of the "bends." The major features are a mild, generalized slowing of electroencephalographic activity and a tremor that may occur at rest and combine features of a postural and intention tremor. Associated features may include muscular fasciculations, myoclonus, incoordination, dizziness, and sleep disturbance.

Impact of Movement Disorders on the Workplace

Specific occupational exposures that may be responsible for movement disorders have been reviewed, but these account for the minority of cases encountered in the workplace. An equally important problem for occupational medicine is the accommodation of the patient and the workplace to meet each other's needs. The effort to keep a person with a physical disability gainfully employed is often of mutual advantage to the employer and the employee. For the employer the effort to keep an experienced employee on the job may be less expensive than placing the worker on disability and training a replacement. In addition, many employers are obligated under state and federal law to reasonably accommodate employees with disability in the workplace. For the employee there are direct benefits—economically, physically, and emotionally—to being gainfully employed.[150,151]

Legally, the Americans with Disabilities Act (ADA) entitles all qualified persons the right to a job, regardless of disability. As far as employment is concerned, the two most important provisions of the ADA are that it prohibits discrimination against employees or potential employees who have a disability, and it requires reasonable accommodation in the workplace for persons with disabilities.[152] Therefore, it benefits employee, employer, and society to rehabilitate employees with medical problems. This requires commitment and education of the employer and the employee.

The most common movement disorder is parkinsonism, which is used in this chapter as a prototype for all movement disorders under discussion. Although typically a disease found in people over age 55, the incidence of IP in the 20- to 40-year-old age group is thought to be more common than currently reported.[153] This consideration and the fact that other movement disorders are found in the young as well as the old constitute issues for the workplace. Employment-related problems have not been formally studied for persons with movement disorders. Nonetheless, studies on the impact of other chronic illnesses in the workplace would suggest that specific problems can be identified and extrapolated to the population of individuals with movement disorders.

Two categories of problems in the workplace specific to movement disorders are discussed in this chapter: (1) those related to the patient's disease or treatment, and (2) those related to the attitudes and actions of the employer, coworkers, and employee.

IDIOPATHIC PARKINSONISM

IP is a chronic progressive disease with individual variation in symptoms, and, generally, a slow rate of progression. Work limitations change over time, and accommodation to these changes is a dynamic process.

In early-stage IP (Hoehn and Yahr stage I and II), the most common presenting symptom is involuntary resting tremor; this is the symptom most obvious to the patient and others. Underlying the tremor may be bradykinesia and rigidity, which are noticed when the patient attempts to use the affected extremity. In stage I symptoms are unilateral, and they become bilateral in stage II. In stage II there is more generalized slowness, some masked facies, and slight stooping of posture. Drugs are administered according to severity of symptoms and perceived interference with work and daily activities.

In stages III and IV patients begin to experience more difficulty with gait and balance in spite of drug therapy. The stride may be shorter, with occasional shuffling and difficulty in initiating movement. Turns may be less stable, and problems with balance may result in a tendency to fall forward or backward. At this stage of the disease, many patients have been on drug therapy for some time and may start to experience long-term side effects seen with chronic use of antiparkinsonian drugs. The two most troubling side effects are the fluctuating motor response and dyskinesias. In the fluctuating motor response patients may go from being extremely mobile to being quite parkinsonian many times throughout the day. Dyskinesias are choreiform, writhing, involuntary movements that are thought to be a result of dopaminergic overstimulation. Both of these problems may be helped by dosage adjustment but not completely eradicated.

Impact of Physical Symptoms on the Workplace

The significance of physical limitations imposed by parkinsonism, therapy, or both is dictated by job requirements. As an example, job performance may be more compromised in work requiring a lot of walking than in work that involves mostly sitting at a desk. Tremor does not usually interfere with motor activity because it is present only at rest. Nonetheless, it becomes a psychological impediment because it is distracting and can be misinterpreted as anxiety. It also becomes more pronounced with stress. If an employee is in a visible position with the public, it is best to directly acknowledge that the tremor is not a sign of nervousness to prevent misunderstanding and subsequent lack of confidence.

The bradykinesia and rigidity of upper extremities may result in difficulty with writing and activities requiring fine motor movement. Adaptations to word processing or dictation can be extremely helpful in maintaining productivity. Occupational therapists should visit the work site and make recommendations about adaptations of the work environment.[154]

Slowness of gait and impaired balance are usually later stages of the disease but do not necessarily prevent employment. Careful evaluation and necessary adaptations of the physical work environment should be made if the job necessitates physical labor or climbing. Referral to a physical therapist can be helpful with gait retraining and/or ambulation aids.

Although not as common, speech can be affected, producing rapid speech, motor dysarthria, and hypophonia. These symptoms may fluctuate with the medication and should be evaluated in regard to jobs that require a significant amount of telephone contact. Day-to-day communication on the job may be facilitated by speech therapy. Hypophonia may be helped by referral for speech amplification devices.

Other symptoms include cognitive decline and fatigue. Although estimates of prevalence are difficult due to lack of uniform criteria, dementia is thought to occur in approximately 35–45% of people with IP and at later stages of disease.[155] Typically, there is loss of recent and retrograde memory, diminished concentration and attention, and perceptual and visuospatial deficits. Disorders of cognition can be accentuated by stress. Neurologic evaluation can be very helpful in determining cognitive limitations and provides a basis for job reassignment or retirement. Early recognition and intervention can prevent an insidious process of job failure and loss of self-esteem.

Fatigue is a common symptom in Parkinson's disease. The exact cause is unknown but is probably the synergistic effect of several mechanisms. These include altered sleep patterns, sedation from medications, depression, deconditioning from immobility, decreased ventilatory capacity, and the disease itself. Reduced work hours and/or education in techniques for energy conservation can prevent premature departure from the workforce.[154,156]

Impact of Drug Therapy on the Workplace

Side effects seen with antiparkinsonian therapy can have implications for the workplace. Anticholinergics are used to control tremor. Centrally acting anticholinergics such as trihexyphenidyl and benztropine can impair memory and cause blurred vision. If these side effects occur, they should be evaluated in relationship to job requirements and, if possible, other drugs should be prescribed.

Dopaminergics, levodopa, and dopamine agonists are used to treat the other symptoms of parkinsonism. Long-term side effects, dyskinesias, and the fluctuating motor response can directly impact the work environment.

Although dyskinesias are extremely visible, most people with these disorders do not find them disabling and associate the extra movements with good mobility. The problem is usually with coworkers or clients who do not understand and find the continuous movement disconcerting. This is best handled by education and open discussion among employees, coworkers, and clients in the workplace. Like tremor, dyskinesia is made worse with excitement or stress.

On the other hand, the fluctuating response can be extremely disabling. These fluctuations are not always predictable. It can be very disconcerting to be completely normal one moment and then quite parkinsonian (slow and tremulous) the next. This uncertainty can produce fear and anxiety for an employee. Coworkers may interpret this pattern as lack of motivation because the employee may be capable one moment and unable to function the next. Although some of these fluctuations in response to drugs may be alleviated by dose adjustment, education for employee and coworker is critical to cope with this variability.[154,157,158]

Impact of Psychological Factors on the Workplace

The attitude of the employer, coworker, and employee is more difficult to define and is, perhaps, a leading factor in early retirement or request for disability status.[157–159]

Example: Mr. J.

> Mr. J. is a 47-year-old senior escrow officer with a 3-year history of IP, which is manifested by tremor and left-sided bradykinesia. Although his symptoms were not completely eradicated with antiparkinsonian medication, he had no functional limitations. His employer and coworkers were told about his diagnosis and potential limitations.
>
> Mr. J. had been a very successful businessman and had handled increasing responsibility easily. After the diagnosis of parkinsonism, he noted that increased pressure, stress, and longer hours all resulted in more visible symptoms and excessive fatigue. Although he was able to sustain his productivity, he became increasingly self-conscious and anxious. He worried that his coworkers and clients were losing their confidence in him because of his tremor and other parkinsonian signs. In addition, he began to doubt his own ability, and because of his fear of failure, he quit his job prematurely.

This example illustrates that lack of education and proper counseling for employee, employer, and coworkers can result in unnecessary termination. A more active role from health care providers in educating employers and the public about the disease may be helpful in facilitating adaptation in the workplace.[157–160] For Mr. J., counseling regarding reassignment to another department, which had less public visibility and more flexible hours, might have prevented loss of a valued employee. Employers, understandably, have difficulty recognizing the individual variability that exists within Parkinson's disease in terms of physical symptoms and prognosis and need ongoing education from health care professionals. Employee assistance programs that provide access to ongoing counseling and evaluation, education programs, and supervisor training are potential ways to change negative attitudes in the work setting.[157–162]

The patient's attitude and psychological state represent a major factor in continued employment. The changes resulting from chronic illness threaten self-confidence and self-esteem.[163] In a study to identify the problems of cancer patients returning to work, it was found that of 379 cancer patients, aged 30–59 with no evidence of active cancer, only 64% described themselves as fully employable.[164] Although the reasons for this percep-

TABLE 7.5
National Organizations for Parkinson's Disease*

United Parkinson Foundation (International)
360 West Superior Street
Chicago, IL 60610

The American Parkinson Disease Association, Inc.
116 John Street
New York, NY 10034

The Parkinson Disease Foundation
William Black Medical Research Building
640 West 168th Street
New York, NY 10032

National Parkinson Foundation, Inc.
1501 Ninth Avenue N.W.
Miami, FL 33136

---

*These organizations can direct people to local support groups.

tion were not delineated, changes in body image and self-esteem secondary to chronic illness have been shown to affect perceptions of work success.[154,157–159,163–165] The health care provider has the responsibility to instigate counseling, referral to local support groups (Table 7.5), and vocational rehabilitation rather than to immediately consider disability.[161,162]

In summary, the problems of the patient with Parkinson's disease in the workplace can be easily extrapolated to movement disorders in general. Most have visible signs, varying physical limitations, and slow progression of disease symptoms. Dysfunction in the work setting may be a product of the physical limitations imposed by the movement disorder or by the perceptions of coworkers, the public, and employees of the motor signs of the disorder. Problems in the workplace need to be addressed by the employer, coworkers, and the patient and his or her health care providers. These interventions require objective evaluation to determine the degree of physical and potential cognitive disability and the necessity for job reassignment, education, and assistance programs, as well as to carefully monitor the physical and psychological condition of the patient.

References

1. Forno LS, Langston JW, DeLanney LE, Irwin I, Ricaurte GA. Locus ceruleus lesions and eosinophilic inclusions in MPTP-treated monkeys. Ann Neurol 1986;20:449–455.

2. Megro F. Les syndromes Parkinsoniens par intoxication sulfo-carbonee. Rev Neurol 1930;49:518–518.
3. Gordy ST, Trumper M. Carbon disulfide poisoning: Report of 21 cases. Ind Med 1940;9:231–234.
4. Lewy FH. Neurological, medical and biochemical signs and symptoms indicating chronic industrial carbon disulfide absorption. Ann Intern Med 1941;15:869–883.
5. Peters HA, Levine RL, Matthews CG, Sauter SL, Rankin JH. Carbon disulfide-induced neuropsychiatric changes in grain storage workers. Am J Ind Med 1982;3:373–391.
6. Peters HA, Levine RL, Matthews CG, Sauter S, Chapman L. Synergistic neurotoxicity of carbon tetrachloride/carbon disulfice (80/20 fumigants) and other pesticides in grain storage workers. Acta Pharmacol Toxicol 1986;59(Suppl 7):535–546.
7. Peters HA, Levine RL, Matthews CG, Chapman LJ. Extrapyramidal and other neurologic manifestations associated with carbon disulfide fumigant exposure. Arch Neurol 1988;45:537–540.
8. Chapman LJ, Sauter SL, Henning RA, Levine RL, Matthews CG, Peters HA. Finger tremor after carbon disulfide based pesticide exposures. Arch Neurol 1991;48:866–870.
9. Richter R. Degeneration of the basal ganglia in monkeys from chronic carbon disulfide poisoning. J Neuropathol Exp Neurol 1945;4:324–353.
10. Gottfried MR, Graham DG, Morgan M, Casey HW, Bus JS. The morphology of carbon disulfide neurotoxicity. Neurotoxicology 1985;6:89–96.
11. Mena I. The role of manganese in human disease. Ann Clin Lab Sci 1974;4:487–491.
12. Huang CC, Chu NS, Lu CS et al. Chronic manganese intoxication. Arch Neurol 1989;46:1104–1106.
13. Wang JD, Huang CC, Huang YH, Chiang JR, Lin JM, Chen JS. Manganese induced parkinsonism: an outbreak due to an unrepaired ventilation control system in a ferromanganese smelter. Br J Ind Med 1989;46:856–859.
14. Cook DG, Fahn S, Brait KA. Chronic manganese intoxication. Arch Neurol 1974;30:59–64.
15. Greenhouse AH. Manganese intoxication in the United States. Trans Am Neurol Assoc 1971;96:248–249.
16. Wolters EC, Huang C–C, Clark C et al. Positron emission tomography in manganese intoxication. Ann Neurol 1989;26:647–651.
17. Cotzias GC. Manganese in health and disease. Physiol Rev 1958;38:503–532.
18. Mena I, Marin O, Fuenzalida S, Cotzias GC. Chronic manganese poisoning—clinical picture and manganese turnover. Neurology 1967;17:128–136.
19. Whitlock CM,Jr., Amuso SJ, Bittenbender JB. Chronic neurological disease in two manganese steel workers. Am Ind Hyg Assoc J 1966;27(5):454–459.
20. Tanaka S, Lieben J. Manganese poisoning and exposure in Pennsylvania. Arch Environ Health 1969;19:674–684.
21. Nelson K, Golnick J, Korn T, Angie C. Manganese encephalopathy: utility of early magnetic resonance imaging. Br J Ind Med 1993;50(6):510–513.
22. Siemers E, Robbins B, Hui S. Environmental Agents Associated with Parkinson's Disease (3rd ed). Philadelphia: Annual Symposium on the Etiology and Pathogenesis of Parkinson's Disease, 1989.

23. Barbeau A. Manganese and extrapyramidal disorders. Neurotoxicology 1984;5:5–27.

24. Huang CC, Lu CS, Chu NS et al. Progression after chronic manganese exposure. Neurology 1993;43:1479–1482.

25. Ferraz HB, Bertolucci PHF, Pereira JS, Lima JGC, Andrade LAF. Chronic exposure to the fungicide maneb may produce symptoms and signs of CNS manganese intoxication. Neurology 1988;38:550–553.

26. Bernheimer H, Birkmayer W, Hornykiewicz O, Jellinger K, Seitelberger F. Brain dopamine and the syndromes of Parkinson and Huntington—clinical, morphological and neurochemical correlations. J Neurol Sci 1973;20:415–425.

27. Eriksson H, Tedroff J, Thomas KA et al. Manganese induced brain lesions in Macaca fascicularis as revealed by positron emission tomography and magnetic resonance imaging. Arch Toxicol 1992;66(6):403–407.

28. Cotzias GC, Papavasiliou PS, Ginos J, Steck A, Duby S. Metabolic modification of Parkinson's disease and of chronic manganese poisoning. Annu Rev Med 1971;22:305–326.

29. Choi IS. Delayed neurologic sequelae in carbon monoxide intoxication. Arch Neurol 1983;40:433–435.

30. Garland H, Pearce J. Neurological complications of carbon monoxide poisoning. Q J Med 1967;36:445–455.

31. Myers RA, Snyder SK, Emhoff TA. Subacute sequelae of carbon monoxide poisoning. Ann Emerg Med 1985;14:1163–1167.

32. Ringel SP, Klawans HL. Carbon monoxide-induced Parkinsonism. J Neurol Sci 1972;16:245–251.

33. Klawans HL, Stein RW, Tanner CM, Goetz CG. A pure parkinsonian syndrome following acute carbon monoxide intoxication. Arch Neurol 1982;39:302–304.

34. Fennell EB, Booth MP, Moberg PJ, Gallagher TJ. Neuropsychological evaluation of 13 cases of acute simultaneous exposure to moderate levels of carbon monoxide [abstract]. Neurology 1991;41(Suppl 1):237.

35. Minerbo GM, Jankovic J. Prevalence of Parkinson's disease among firefighters [abstract]. Neurology 1990;40(Suppl 1):348.

36. Langston JW, Ballard PA Jr. Parkinson's disease in a chemist working with 1-methyl-4-phenyl-1,2,5,6-tetrahydropyridine. N Engl J Med 1983;309:310.

37. Burns RS, LeWitt PA, Ebert MH, Pakkenberg H, Kopin IJ. The clinical syndrome of striatal dopamine deficiency. Parkinsonism induced by 1-methyl-4-phenyl-1,2,3,6-tetrahydropyridine. N Engl J Med 1985;312:1418–1421.

38. Barbeau A, Roy M, Langston JW. Neurological consequence of industrial exposure to 1-methyl-4-phenyl-1,2,3,6-tetrahydropyridine. Lancet 1985;1:747.

39. Sechi GP, Agnetti V, Piredda M et al. Acute and persistent parkinsonism after use of diquat. Neurology 1992;42:261–264.

40. Rajput AH, Uitti RJ, Stern W et al. Geography, drinking water chemistry, pesticides and herbicides and the etiology of Parkinson's disease. Can J Neurol Sci 1987;14(Suppl 3):414–418.

41. Langston JW, Ballard P, Tetrud JW, Irwin I. Chronic parkinsonism in humans due to a product of meperidine-analog synthesis. Science 1983;219:979–980.

42. Davis GC, Williams AC, Markey SP. Chronic parkinsonism secondary to intravenous injection of meperidine analogues. Psychiatry Res 1979;1:249–254.

43. Ballard PA, Tetrud JW, Langston JW. Permanent human parkinsonism due to 1-methyl-4-phenyl-1,2,3,6-tetrahydropyridine (MPTP): seven cases. Neurology 1985;35:949–956.
44. Wright JJ, Wall RA, Perry TL, Paty DW. Chronic parkinsonism secondary to intranasal administration of product of meperidine-analogue synthesis. N Engl J Med 1984;310:325–325.
45. Burns RS, Chiueh CC, Markey SP, Ebert MH, Jacobowitz DM, Kopin IJ. A primate model of parkinsonism: selective destruction of dopaminergic neurons in the pars compacta of the substantia nigra by 1-methyl-4-phenyl-1,2,3,6-tetrahydropyridine. Proc Natl Acad Sci USA 1983;80:4546–4550.
46. Crossman AR, Clarke CE, Boyce S, Robertson RG, Sambrook MA. MPTP-induced Parkinsonism in the monkey: neurochemical pathology, complications of treatment and pathophysiological mechanisms. Can J Neurol Sci 1987;14:428–435.
47. Langston JW. MPTP: insights into the etiology of Parkinson's disease. Eur Neurol 1987;26(Suppl 1):2–10.
48. Birkmayer W, Knoll J, Riederer P, Youdim MBH, Hars V, Marton J. Increased life expectancy resulting from addition of L-deprenyl to Madopar treatment in Parkinson's disease: a long-term study. J Neural Transm 1985;64:113–127.
49. Tetrud JW, Langston JW. The effect of Deprenyl (Selegiline) on the natural history of Parkinson's disease. Science 1989;245:519–522.
50. Parkinson Study Group. Effects of tocopherol and deprenyl on the progression of disability in early Parkinson's disease. N Engl J Med 1993;328:176–183.
51. Lewin R. Big first scored with nerve diseases. Science 1989;245:467–468.
52. Tetrud JW, Langston JW, Garbe PL, Ruttenber AJ. Mild parkinsonism in persons exposed to 1-methyl-4-phenyl-1,2,3, 6-tetrahydropyridine (MPTP). Neurology 1989;39:1483–1487.
53. Calne DB, Langston JW, Martin WRW et al. Positron emission tomography after MPTP: observations relating to the cause of Parkinson's disease. Nature 1985;317:246–248.
54. Langston JW. The Discovery of MPTP: How Far Will It Take Us? In P Jenner (ed), Neurotoxins and Their Pharmacological Implications. New York: Raven, 1987;153–161.
55. Calne DB, McGeer E, Eisen A, Spencer PS. Alzheimer's disease, Parkinson's disease, and motoneurone disease: abiotropic interaction between ageing and environment? Lancet 1986;2:1067–1070.
56. Calne DB, Langston JW. Aetiology of Parkinson's disease. Lancet 1983;2:1457–1459.
57. Spencer PS. Guam ALS. Parkinsonism-dementia: a long-latency neurotoxic disorder caused by slow toxin(s) in food? Can J Neurol Sci 1987;14(Suppl 3):347–357.
58. Garruto RM, Yase Y. Neurodegenerative disorders of the Western Pacific: the search for mechanisms of pathogenesis. TINS 1986;9:368–374.
59. Garruto RM, Yanagihara R, Gajdusek DC. Disappearance of high-incidence amyotrophic lateral sclerosis and parkinsonism-dementia on Guam. Neurology 1985;35:193–198.
60. Spencer PS, Nunn PB, Hugon J et al. Guam Amyotrophic lateral sclerosis-parkinsonism-dementia linked to a plant excitant neurotoxin. Science 1987;237:517–522.

61. Kisby GE, Ellison M, Spencer PS. Content of the neurotoxins cycasin (methylazoxymethanol B-D-glucoside) and BMAA (B-N-methylamino-L-alanine) in cycad flour prepared by Guam Chamorros. Neurology 1992;42:1336–1340.
62. Tanner CM, Chen B, Wang W et al. Environmental factors and Parkinson's disease: a case-control study in China. Neurology 1989;39:660–664.
63. Schoenberg BS. Environmental risk factors for Parkinson's disease: the epidemiologic evidence. Can J Neurol Sci 1987;14(Suppl 3):407–413.
64. Rajput AH, Offord KP, Beard CM, Kurland LT. Epidemiology of parkinsonism: incidence, classification and mortality. Ann Neurol 1984;16:278–282.
65. Li S, Schoenberg BS, Wang C et al. A prevalence survey of Parkinson's disease and other movement disorders in the People's Republic of China. Arch Neurol 1985;42:655–657.
66. Cosnett JE, Bill PLA. Parkinson's disease in blacks: observations on epidemiology in Natal. S Afr Med J 1988;73:281–283.
67. Aquilonius SM, Hartvig P. A Swedish county with unexpectedly high utilization of anti-parkinsonian drugs. Acta Neurol Scand 1986;74:379–381.
68. Schoenberg BS, Anderson DW, Haerer AF. Prevalence of Parkinson's disease in the biracial population of Copiah County, Mississippi. Neurology 1985;35:841–845.
69. Tanner CM, Chen B, Wang WZ et al. Environmental factors in the etiology of Parkinson's disease. Can J Neurol Sci 1987;14(Suppl 3):419–423.
70. Lux WE, Kurtzke JF. Is Parkinson's disease acquired? Evidence from a geographic comparison with multiple sclerosis. Neurology 1987;37:467–471.
71. Schoenberg BS, Osuntokun BO, Adeuja AOG. Comparison of the prevalence of Parkinson's disease in black populations in the rural US and in rural Nigeria: door-to-door community studies. Neurology 1988;38:645–646.
72. Bharucha NE, Bharucha EP, Bharucha AE, Bhise AV, Schoenberg BS. Prevalence of Parkinson's disease in the Parsi community in Bombay, India. Arch Neurol 1988;45:1321–1324.
73. Ho SC, Woo J, Lee CM. Epidemiologic study of Parkinson's disease in Hong Kong. Neurology 1989;39:1314–1318.
74. Barbeau A, Roy M. Uneven prevalence of Parkinson's disease in the province of Quebec [abstract]. Can J Neurol Sci 1985;12:169–170.
75. Rajput AH, Uitti RJ. Paraquat and Parkinson's disease. Neurology 1987;37:1820–1821.
76. Fleming L, Mann JB, Bean J, Briggle T, Sanchez-Ramos JR. Parkinson's disease and brain levels of organochlorine pesticides. Ann Neurol 1994;36(1):100–103.
77. Jimenez–Jimenez FJ, Gonzales DM, Gimenez-Roldan S. Exposure to well water drinking and pesticides in Parkinson's disease: a case-control study from the southeast area of Madrid [abstract]. Proceedings of the Ninth International Symposium on Parkinson's Disease. Mississauga, Ontario: Medical Education Services, 1988;118.
78. Campanella G, Roy M, Masson H. A case-control study of Parkinson's disease in southern Quebec: exposure to metals and pesticides [abstract]. Proceedings of the Ninth International Symposium on Parkinson's disease. Mississauga, Ontario: Medical Education Services, 1988;118.
79. Hertzman C, Wiens M, Bowering D, Snow B, Calne DB. Parkinson's disease: a case-control study of occupational and environmental risk factors. Am J Ind Med 1990;17:349–355.

80. Semchuk KM, Love EJ, Lee RG. Parkinson's disease: a test of the multifactorial etiologic hypothesis. Neurology 1993;43:1173–1180.
81. Butterfield PG, Valanis BG, Spencer PS, Lindeman CA, Nutt JG. Environmental antecedents of young-onset Parkinson's disease. Neurology 1934;43:1150–1158.
82. Duvoisin RC. On the Cause of Parkinson's disease. In CD Marsden, S Fahn (eds), Movement Disorders. London: Butterworth, 1982.
83. Eldridge R, Rocca WA, Ince SE. Parkinson's Disease: Evidence Against Toxic Etiology and for an Alternative Theory. In SP Markey, N Castagnoli, AJ Trevor, IJ Kopin (eds), MPTP: A Neurotoxin Producing a Parkinsonian Syndrome. New York: Academic, 1986;355–367.
84. Critchley M. Medical aspects of boxing, particularly from a neurological standpoint. Br Med J 1957;1:357–362.
85. Mawdsley C, Ferguson FR. Neurological disease in boxers. Lancet 1963;2:795–801.
86. Friedman JH. Progressive parkinsonism in boxers. South Med J 1989;82(5):543–546.
87. Corsellis JAN, Bruton CJ, Freeman–Browne D. The aftermath of boxing. Psychol Med 1973;3:270–283.
88. Roberts AH. Brain Damage in Boxers. London: Pitman, 1969.
89. McLatchie G, Brooks N, Galbraith S et al. Clinical neurological examination, neuropsychology, electroencephalography and computed tomographic head scanning in active amateur boxers. J Neurol Neurosurg Psychiatry 1987;50:96–99.
90. Casson IR, Siegel O, Sham R, Campbell EA, Tarlau M, DiDomenico A. Brain damage in modern boxers. JAMA 1984;251(20):2663–2667.
91. Charness ME. The relationship between local injury and focal dystonia in performing artists [abstract]. Neurology 1989;39(Suppl 1):246–247.
92. Marsden CD. The problem of adult-onset idiopathic torsion dystonia and other isolated dyskinesias in adult life (including blepharospasm, oromandibular dystonia, dystonic writer's cramp, torticollis and axial dystonia). Adv Neurol 1976;14:259–276.
93. Marsden CD, Harrison MJG. Idiopathic torsion dystonia (dystonia musculorum deformans): a review of 42 patients. Brain 1974;97:793–810.
94. Marsden CD, Rothwell JC. The physiology of idiopathic dystonia. Can J Neurol Sci 1987;14:521–527.
95. Panizza ME, Hallett M, Nilsson J. Reciprocal inhibition in patients with hand cramps. Neurology 1989;39:85–89.
96. Panizza M, Lelli S, Nilsson J, Hallett M. H-reflex recovery curve and reciprocal inhibition of H-reflex in different kinds of dystonia. Neurology 1990;40:824–828.
97. Nakashima K, Rothwell JC, Thompson PD et al. The blink reflex in patients with idiopathic torsion dystonia. Arch Neurol 1990;47:413–416.
98. Nakashima K, Thompson PD, Rothwell JC, Day BL, Stell R, Marsden CD. An exteroceptive reflex in the sternocleidomastoid muscle produced by electrical stimulation of the supraorbital nerve in normal subjects and patients with spasmodic torticollis. Neurology 1989;39:1354–1358.
99. Tolosa E, Montserrat L, Bayes A. Blink reflex studies in focal dystonias: enhanced excitability of brainstem interneurons in cranial dystonia and spasmodic torticollis. Move Disord 1988;3(1):61–69.

100. Fahn S, Marsden CD, Calne DB. Classification and Investigation of Dystonia. In CD Marsden, S Fahn (eds), Movement Disorders 2. London: Butterworth, 1987:332–358.

101. Burke RE, Fahn S, Gold AP. Delayed-onset dystonia in patients with "static" encephalopathy. J Neurol Neurosurg Psychiatry 1980;43:789–797.

102. Brett EM, Hoare RD, Sheehy MP, Marsden CD. Progressive hemi-dystonia due to focal basal ganglia lesion after mild head trauma. J Neurol Neurosurg Psychiatry 1981;44:460.

103. Marsden CD, Obeso JA, Zarranz JJ, Lang AE. The anatomical basis of symptomatic hemidystonia. Brain 1985;108:463–483.

104. Sheehy MP, Marsden CD. Trauma and pain in spasmodic torticollis. Lancet 1980;1:777–778.

105. Tsui J. Personal communication, 1989.

106. Truong DD, Dubinsky R, Hermanowicz N, Olson WL, Silverman B, Koller WC. Posttraumatic torticollis. Arch Neurol 1991;48:221–223.

107. Goldman S, Ahlskog JE. Posttraumatic cervical dystonia. Mayo Clin Proc 1993;68:443–448.

108. Mattle HP, Hess CW, Ludin HP, Mumenthaler M. Isolated muscle hypertrophy as a sign of radicular or peripheral nerve injury. J Neurol Neurosurg Psychiatry 1991;54:325–329.

109. Schott GD. The relationship of peripheral trauma and pain to dystonia. J Neurol Neurosurg Psychiatry 1985;48:698–701.

110. Scherokman B, Husain F, Cuetter A, Jabbari B, Maniglia E. Peripheral dystonia. Arch Neurol 1986;43:830–832.

111. Marsden CD, Obeso JA, Traub MM, Rothwell JC, Kranz H, La Cruz F. Muscle spasms associated with Sudeck's atrophy after injury. Br Med J 1984;288:173–176.

112. Jankovic J, Van Der Linden C. Dystonia and tremor induced by peripheral trauma: predisposing factors. J Neurol Neurosurg Psychiatry 1988;51:1512–1519.

113. Brin MF, Fahn S, Bressman SB, Burke RE. Dystonia precipitated by peripheral trauma. Neurology 1986;36(Suppl 1):119.

114. Schott GD. Induction of involuntary movements by peripheral trauma: An analogy with causalgia. Lancet 1986;2:712–716.

115. Spillane JD, Nathan PW, Kelly RE, Marsden CD. Painful legs and moving toes. Brain 1971;94:541–556.

116. Nathan PW. Painful legs and moving toes: evidence on the site of the lesion. J Neurol Neurosurg Psychiatry 1978;41:934–939.

117. Schoenen J, Gonce M, Delwaide PJ. Painful legs and moving toes: a syndrome with different physiopathologic mechanisms. Neurology 1984;34:1108–1112.

118. Verhagen W, Horstink M, Notermans S. Painful and moving fingers. J Neurol Neurosurg Psychiatry 1985;48:384–389.

119. Schott GD. "Painful legs and moving toes": the role of trauma. J Neurol Neurosurg Psychiatry 1981;44:344–346.

120. Satoyoshi E, Doi Y, Kinoshita M. Pseudomyotonia in cervical root lesions with myelopathy. Arch Neurol 1972;27:307–313.

121. Banks G, Nielsen VK, Short MP, Kowal CD. Brachial plexus myoclonus. J Neurol Neurosurg Psychiatry 1985;48:582–584.

122. Jankovic J, Pardo R. Segmental myoclonus. Arch Neurol 1986;43:1025–1031.

123. Marsden CD. Peripheral movement disorders [abstract]. Annual course on Movement Disorders. American Academy of Neurology 1989;51–58.
124. Jannetta PJ, Abbasy M, Maroon JC, Ramos FM, Abir MS. Aetiology and definitive microsurgical treatment of hemifacial spasms. J Neurosurg 1977;47:321–328.
125. Nielsen VK. Pathophysiology of hemifacial spasm. Neurology 1984;34:418–426.
126. Moller AR, Jannetta PJ. Hemifacial spasm: results of electrophysiologic recording during microvascular decompression operations. Neurology 1985;35:969–974.
127. Katz RT, Williams C. Focal dystonia following soft tissue injury: three case reports with long-term outcome. Arch Phys Med Rehabil 1990;71:345–348.
128. LeQuesne PM. Clinical and morphological findings in acrylamide toxicity. Neurotoxicology 1985;6:17–24.
129. Neal PA, Jones RR. Chronic mercurialism in the hatter's fur-cutting industry. JAMA 1938;110:337–343.
130. Roullet E, Nizou R, Jedynak P, Lhermitte F. Myoclonies d'intention et d'action revelatrices d'une intoxication professionnelle par le mercure. Rev Neurol 1984;140:55–58.
131. Shapiro IM, Cornbluth DR, Sumner AJ. Neurophysiological and neuropsychological functions in mercury-exposed dentists. Lancet 1982;2:1147–1150.
132. Albers JW, Kallenbach LR, Fine LJ et al. Neurological abnormalities associated with remote occupational elemental mercury exposure. Ann Neurol 1988;24:651–659.
133. Roels H, Gennart JP, Lauwerys R, Buchet JP, Malchaire J, Bernard A. Surveillance of workers exposed to mercury vapour: Validation of a previously proposed biological threshold limit value for mercury concentration in urine. Am J Ind Med 1985;7:45–71.
134. Chapman LJ, Sauter SL, Henning RA, Dodson VN, Reddan WG, Matthews CG. Differences in frequency of finger tremor in otherwise asymptomatic mercury workers. Br J Ind Med 1990;47:838–843.
135. Langolf GD, Chaffin DB, Henderson R, Whittle HP. Evaluation of workers exposed to elemental mercury using quantitative tests of tremor and neuromuscular functions. Am Ind Hyg Assoc J 1978;39:976–984.
136. Verberk MM, Salle HJA, Kemper CH. Tremor in workers with low exposure to metallic mercury. Am Ind Hyg Assoc J 1986;47(8):559–562.
137. Cannon SB, Veazey JM, Jackson RS et al. Epidemic kepone poisoning in chemical workers. Am J Epidemiol 1978;107:529–537.
138. Taylor JR, Selhorst JB, Houff SA, Martinez AJ. Chlordecone intoxication in man. I. Clinical observations. Neurology 1978;28:626–630.
139. Baringer JR, Sweeney VP, Winkler GF. An acute syndrome of ocular oscillations and truncal myoclonus. Brain 1968;91:473–480.
140. Dropcho E, Payne R. Paraneoplastic opsoclonus-myoclonus: association with medullary thyroid carcinoma and review of the literature. Arch Neurol 1986;43:410–415.
141. Au WJ, Keltner JL. Opsoclonus with amitriptylene overdose. Ann Neurol 1979;6:87.
142. Pullicino P, Aquilina J. Opsoclonus in organophosphate poisoning. Arch Neurol 1989;46:704–705.

143. Cohen WJ, Cohen NH. Lithium carbonate, haloperidol and irreversible brain damage. JAMA 1974;230:1283–1287.
144. Hormes JT, Filley CM, Rosenberg NL. Neurologic sequelae of chronic solvent vapor abuse. Neurology 1986;36:698–702.
145. Taylor JR. Neurological manifestations in humans exposed to chlordecone: follow-up results. Neurotoxicology 1985;6:231–236.
146. Juntunen J, Matikainen E, Antti-Poika M, Suoranta H, Valle M. Nervous system effects of long-term occupational exposure to toluene. Acta Neurol Scand 1985;72:512–517.
147. Moses H, Klawans HL. Bromide Intoxication. In PJ Vinken, GW Bruyn (eds), Intoxications of the Nervous System, Part I. Vol. 36: Handbook of Clinical Neurology. Amsterdam: North Holland, 1979;291–318.
148. Prockop LD, Smith AO. Seizures and action myoclonus after occupational exposure to methyl bromide. J Fla Med Assoc 1986;73:690–692.
149. Halsey MJ. Effects of high pressure on the central nervous system. Physiol Rev 1982;62:1341–1377.
150. Layton C. Employment, unemployment, and response to the general health questionnaire. Psychol Rep 1986;58:807–810.
151. Stagner S. The role of education in the employability of persons with a history of cancer. American Cancer Society: Proceedings of the Workshop on Employment, Insurance and the Patient with Cancer. New Orleans: American Cancer Society, 1987;58–61.
152. Hoffman B. Taking Care of Business: Employment, Insurance and Money Matters. In F Mullan, B Hoffman (eds), Charting the Journey: An Almanac of Practical Resources for Cancer Survivors. Mount Vernon, NY: Consumers Union of the United States, 1990:97–113.
153. Gershanik O. Parkinsonism of Early Onset. In J Jankovic, E Tolosa (eds), Parkinson's Disease and Movement Disorders. Munich: Urban & Schwarzenberg, 1988:191–204.
154. Berry DL, Catanzaro M. Persons with cancer and their return to the workplace. Cancer Nursing 1992;15(1):40–46.
155. Mayeaux R. Mental Status. In WC Koller (ed), Handbook of Parkinson's Disease. New York: Marcel Dekker, 1987:127–139.
156. Piper BF, Lindsey AM, Dodd MJ. Fatigue mechanisms in cancer patients: developing nursing theory. Oncol Nurs Forum 1987;14(6):17–23.
157. Crothers HM. Employment problems of cancer survivors: local problems and local solutions. American Cancer Society: Proceedings of the Workshop on Employment, Insurance and the Patient with Cancer. New Orleans: American Cancer Society, 1987;51–57.
158. Dudas S, Carlson CE. Cancer rehabilitation. Oncol Nurs Forum 1988;15(2):183–188.
159. Feldman FL. The return to work: the question of workability. American Cancer Society: Proceedings of the Workshop on Employment, Insurance and the Patient with Cancer. New Orleans: American Cancer Society, 1987;27–35.
160. Leeds B. The concept of worksite counseling. American Cancer Society: Proceedings of the Workshop on Employment, Insurance and the Patient with Cancer. New Orleans: American Cancer Society, 1987;45–47.
161. Mor–Barak ME. Social support and coping with stress: implications for the workplace. Occupational Medicine: State of the Art Reviews 1988;3:663–675.

162. Sheppard CA. Cancer rehabilitation and vocational rehabilitation: conflict, compromise and cooperation. American Cancer Society: Proceedings of the Workshop on Employment, Insurance and the Patient with Cancer. New Orleans: American Cancer Society, 1987;36–40.
163. Lambert C, Lambert V. Psychosocial impacts created by chronic illness. Nurs Clin North Am 1987;22:527–533.
164. Mellette S. The cancer patient at work. Cancer J Clinicians 1985;35:360–373.
165. Holland J. Special problems of cancer patients returning to work. Trans Assoc Life Insur Med Dir Am 1985;69:87–94.
166. Ley CO, Gali FG. Parkinsonian syndrome after methanol intoxication. Eur Neurol 1983;22:405–409.
167. Melamed E, Lavy S. Parkinsonism associated with chronic inhalation of carbon tetrachloride. Lancet 1977;1(8019):1015.
168. Rosenberg NL, Myers JA, Martin WRW. Cyanide-induced parkinsonism: clinical, MRI, and 6–fluorodopa PET studies. Neurology 1989;39:142–144.
169. Nayernouri T. Posttraumatic parkinsonism. Surg Neurol 1985;24:263–264.
170. Koller WC, Wong GF, Lang A. Posttraumatic movement disorders: a review. Move Disord 1989;4:20–36.
171. Klawans HL. Dystonia and tremor following exposure to 2,3,7,8-tetrachlorodibenzo-p-dioxin. Move Disord 1987;2:255–261.
172. Lederman RJ. Occupational cramp in instrumental musicians. Med Probl Perform Art 1988;3:45–51.
173. Sheehy MP, Marsden CD. Writer's cramp—a focal dystonia. Brain 1982;105:461–480.

CHAPTER 8

Chemically Induced Toxic Neuropathy

James W. Albers, M.D., Ph.D.
Mark B. Bromberg, M.D., Ph.D.

Patients with chemically induced toxic neuropathy are uncommon compared to those with hereditary, metabolic, or inflammatory etiologies. Physicians evaluating patients with neuromuscular disorders must be alert for potential occupational, recreational, or pharmaceutical exposures, as well as for new epidemics with new or old chemicals, because improvement typically follows removal from exposure. Although drug-related neuropathies are among the most common toxic neuropathies,[1] they are not included in this chapter but are reviewed elsewhere.[2,3] The number of chemicals with neurotoxic potential is increasing in the workplace and environment. Many chemicals have well-established peripheral neurotoxicity, while others are implicated only by isolated case reports or by epidemiologic group comparisons demonstrating minor statistically significant differences of uncertain clinical importance between exposed and unexposed workers. Chemically induced toxic neuropathies play an important role as experimental probes in studying the mechanism of other acquired or hereditary neuropathies. Identification of a chemically induced neuropathy depends on thorough clinical, electrodiagnostic, and laboratory evaluations designed to establish the presence and etiology of neuropathy. This chapter includes a discussion of methods for evaluating patients with suspected peripheral neurotoxic disorders and descriptions of neuropathies associated with specific industrial and agricultural chemicals, including several for which neurotoxicity remains controversial.

Evaluation of Suspected Peripheral Neuropathy

The evaluation of patients with suspected chemically induced peripheral neuropathy is identical to the evaluation of any patient with a suspect neuropathy, regardless of cause. It includes a thorough history and physical examination. On the basis of identified symptoms and signs, the physician attempts to localize the disorder within the nervous system. Additional laboratory studies, including electrophysiologic evaluations, may be required to establish the underlying pathophysiology or identify underlying or concurrent conditions.

CLINICAL EXAMINATION

The clinical examination represents the most fundamental level of testing in the evaluation of suspected neuropathy. It consists of a history, a physical examination, and laboratory studies. The history is an important component of the examination. In brief, it includes a review of chief complaints; a description of the present illness; a review of systems seeking other symptoms; and social, industrial, exposure, family, and past medical histories.

For patients with suspected neuropathy, the description of sensory and motor symptoms is important, as are the distribution and temporal profile of individual complaints. Patients complaining of "numbness" must further characterize their complaint to determine if they mean tingling, loss of sensation, or even weakness. The presence of hyperesthesia or hyperpathia is important. Small-fiber involvement produces complaints reflecting postural hypotension, palpitations, bladder or bowel impairments, sexual dysfunction, or abnormal sweating. Most patients with chemically induced neuropathy have symmetric involvement with a distal predilection.

The neurologic examination constitutes an important component of the physical examination, but it is not performed in isolation and should not ignore other aspects of the general physical examination. Table 8.1 lists findings commonly associated with large-fiber peripheral neuropathy. Patients with neuropathy do not demonstrate abnormalities of mental status unless a component of a toxic encephalopathy is also present. Cranial nerve function is usually normal, with the exception of mild facial weakness or hypesthesia. Peripheral motor dysfunction may be present, consisting of decreased muscle tone and weakness. Weakness typically is symmetric, involving distal extremity muscles, most pronounced in the lower extremities. When present, weakness most commonly involves toe extensors (extensor digitorum brevis), foot dorsiflexors (anterior tibialis), and intrinsic hand muscles (e.g., first dorsal interossei or hypothenar). Unilateral abnormalities usually reflect isolated lesions associated with focal or cumulative nerve trauma. Reflexes are either

TABLE 8.1
Findings Commonly Associated with Peripheral Neuropathy*

	Predominant fiber size involvement		
Sign	Large fiber: Axonal	Demyelinating	Small fiber: Axonal
Weakness	Prominent, early distal > proximal	Prominent if conduction block, distal and proximal	Mild distal
Atrophy	Prominent	Proportional to disuse	Minimal
Sensory loss:			
Vibration	Prominent	Prominent	Minimal
Touch pressure	Prominent	Prominent	Minimal
Joint position (JP)	If severe	If severe	Normal
Pain-temperature	Minimal loss	Minimal loss	Prominent (dissociated loss)
Sensory level trunk	No	No	No
Abnormal station	Proportional to JP loss	Proportional to JP loss	Normal
Reflexes	Early impairment	Early impairment	May be preserved

*Overall distribution of signs: symmetric, distal greater than proximal, lower greater than upper extremity.

absent or hypoactive, and the Achilles reflexes are usually absent in any clinically significant large-fiber neuropathy. Pathologic reflexes should not be present, and there should be no abnormalities of coordination, rapid alternating movements, station, or gait disproportionate to weakness or sensory loss. A postural tremor sometimes is present in association with large-fiber sensory loss.

Clinically apparent sensory abnormalities are common. The typical stocking-glove distal distribution of sensory loss characteristic of a distal axonopathy or neuropathy is shown in Figure 8.1. In a large-fiber neuropathy, abnormal vibratory sensation is a frequent finding, most apparent in the distal lower extremities (e.g., at the great toe). However, absent vibratory sensation proximally at the iliac crest should suggest spinal cord involvement and not a severe neuropathy. Joint position sensation may be abnormal in the toes but usually is normal more proximally. Abnormalities of fine touch and touch-pressure sensations are more difficult to quantify but usually are detectable in large-fiber disease. With small-fiber involvement, pin-pain sensation is impaired in a stocking-glove distribution, as is perception of temperature (hot or cold). Abnormalities of

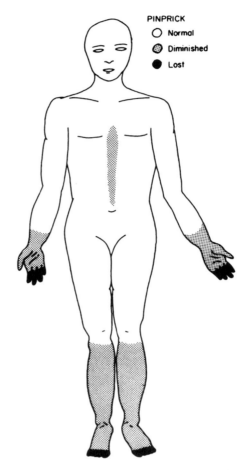

FIGURE 8.1   Schematic of the stocking-glove distal distribution of sensory loss characteristic of a distal axonopathy or neuropathy. The diminished sensation over the midthorax reflects involvement of the distal intercostal nerves. (Reprinted with permission from HH Schaumburg, PS Spencer, PK Thomas [eds]. Disorders of Peripheral Nerves. Philadelphia: Davis, 1983;10.)

discriminatory sensation such as stereognosis, dual simultaneous stimulation, or two-point discrimination should not be selectively impaired or abnormal disproportionate to primary modality sensory loss.

The neurologic examination is efficient, reliable, and reproducible, with demonstrated clinical validity and sensitivity. Clinical abnormalities are often present in asymptomatic individuals, and the examination can establish the magnitude of neurologic impairment. The full clinical examination allows recognition of patterns of abnormalities potentially related to toxic exposure or other causes. Identification of such patterns is important in establishing etiology. Standard laboratory evaluations of blood, urine, hair, nails, and cerebrospinal fluid may be used as part of the medical evaluation. Laboratory data are interpreted in the context of the complete examination, and minor deviations from normal may or may not have clinical relevance, depending on other findings. Histologic examination of nerve or muscle tissue also may be important in establishing a diagnosis. The neurologist uses additional tests to evaluate specific components of the nervous system, including the electrophysiologic measures described below.

ELECTRODIAGNOSTIC EXAMINATION

A variety of electrodiagnostic tests are available for evaluating subclinical or clinically evident neuropathy. These tests have widespread clinical application and are reliable and reproducible. Nerve conduction studies and needle electromyography (EMG) are sensitive measures, able to detect subclinical abnormalities.[4] They also are objective and largely independent of patient effort or cooperation. They can be used to identify the distribution and severity of a peripheral disorder and frequently can identify the underlying pathophysiology.[5] The term *electromyography* technically refers to the needle examination but often is used in reference to both nerve conduction and needle EMG examinations. Both are important in evaluating patients with neuropathy but evaluate components of the peripheral nervous system from different perspectives. Based on the results of these studies, the electromyographer must determine whether there is predominant involvement of sensory or motor fibers and determine whether the findings reflect axonal degeneration, primary or secondary demyelination, or a combination of each.[6]

Nerve conduction studies consist of recordings of the amplitude and conduction velocity of the sensory nerve action potential (SNAP) or compound muscle action potential (CMAP) following percutaneous nerve stimulation.[6] Amplitude measures are sometimes overlooked but reflect in part the size and number of nerve or muscle fibers.[7] This permits assessment of whether a neuropathy is of primarily axonal or demyelinating type.[8] Examples of ulnar SNAPs and CMAPs recorded following supramaximal percutaneous stimulation at several sites along the nerve are shown in Figures 8.2 and 8.3, allowing calculation of the sensory or motor conduction velocity.

The most frequent peripheral manifestation of a neurotoxic exposure is axonal neuropathy or a symmetric "dying-back" pattern (Figure 8.4). Because the largest fibers often are preferentially involved, reduced amplitude or absent SNAPs are common. Reduced CMAP amplitude, particularly in distal lower-extremity muscles, results from any axonal neuropathy involving motor fibers. The amplitude reduction related to axonal loss is demonstrated schematically in Figures 8.5 and 8.6 using a computerized

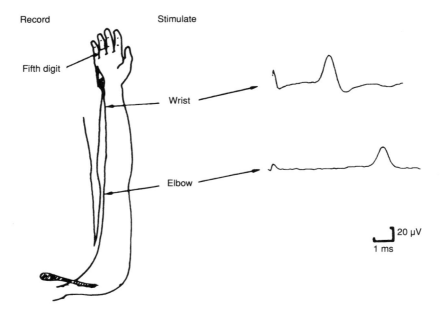

FIGURE 8.2   Sensory nerve action potentials (SNAPs) recorded from digit 5 using ring electrodes following percutaneous stimulation of the ulnar nerve at the wrist and the elbow. Calibration bars represent 1 ms and 20 µV.

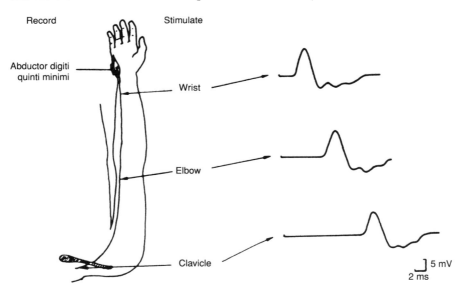

FIGURE 8.3   Ulnar compound muscle action potentials (CMAPs) recorded from the hypothenar muscle using surface electrodes following percutaneous stimulation of the ulnar nerve at the wrist, elbow, and clavicle. Calibration bars represent 2 ms and 5 mV.

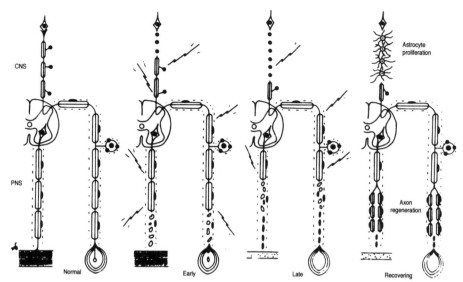

FIGURE 8.4   Schematic diagram of the features characteristic of a toxic distal axonopathy or neuropathy. With progressive involvement, axonal degeneration advances proximally (dying-back) by the late stage. CNS=central nervous system; PNS=peripheral nervous system. (Reprinted with permission from HH Schaumburg, PS Spencer, PK Thomas [eds]. Disorders of Peripheral Nerves. Philadelphia: Davis, 1983;10.)

model of the motor nerve, before and after loss of 75% of axons. Amplitude also reflects the distribution of conduction velocities within the nerve. When the distribution increases, the duration of the response also increases and the amplitude decreases. With short distances between stimulation and recording sites, amplitudes are larger than those recorded with long distances because of normal temporal dispersion of the responses. This difference is accentuated when the conduction velocity distribution is abnormally increased, and the presence of abnormal temporal dispersion can be important in differentiating acquired from hereditary neuropathies. Other physiologic abnormalities such as segmental demyelination may result in conduction block, further reducing evoked response amplitude. Technical factors such as limb temperature also affect recorded amplitudes (Figure 8.7). When these factors are controlled, amplitude measures reflect an important component of peripheral nerve function.[7]

Conduction velocity measures reflect transmission time for the largest myelinated nerve fibers. It is expressed as a velocity in meters per second between two points along the nerve or as a latency (milliseconds) along a fixed length of nerve. For motor studies, the distal latency also includes a neuromuscular transmission time. Conduction velocity reflects nerve size, amount of myelin, nodal and internodal lengths, axonal resistance, and nerve temperature.[6,7] Borderline-low conduction velocity may

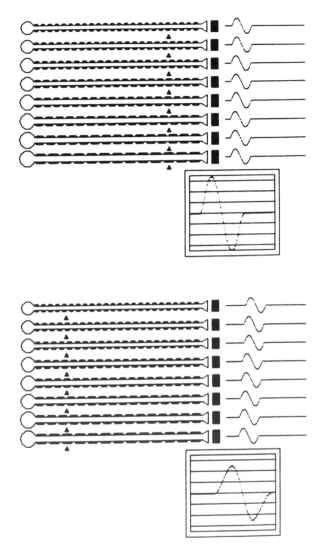

FIGURE 8.5   Computer model of peripheral motor nerve, demonstrating summation of eight individual muscle fiber action potentials to produce the compound muscle action potential (CMAP) shown below each nerve in the schematic screen. Individual axons are of slightly different sizes and therefore conduct at different velocities. Muscle fibers are denoted by solid bars to the right of each axon. Arrows represent stimulation sites. Upper recording: resultant CMAP following distal nerve stimulation. Lower recording: resultant CMAP following proximal nerve stimulation. (Reprinted from JW Albers. Inflammatory Demyelinating Polyradiculoneuropathy. In WF Brown, CF Bolton [eds], Clinical Electromyography. Boston: Butterworths, 1987;209–244. With permission of Butterworths Publishers, copyright 1987.)

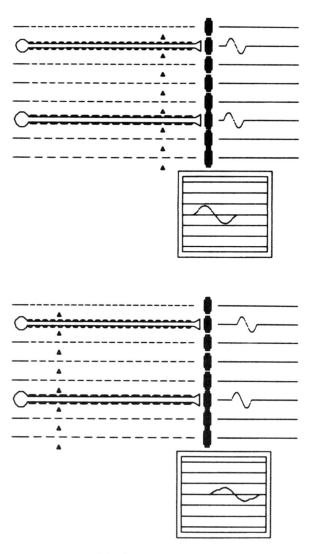

FIGURE 8.6 Computer model of axonal degeneration in peripheral motor nerve described in Fig. 5, following random loss of 75% of axons. Resultant CMAP after distal (upper screen) and proximal (lower screen) stimulation. Note that the amplitude is reduced with distal and proximal stimulation, but the distal latency and conduction velocity are essentially normal. (Reprinted from JW Albers. Inflammatory Demyelinating Polyradiculopathy. In WF Brown, CF Bolton [eds], Clinical Electromyography. Boston: Butterworths, 1987. Pp. 209–244. With permission of Butterworths Publishers, copyright 1987.)

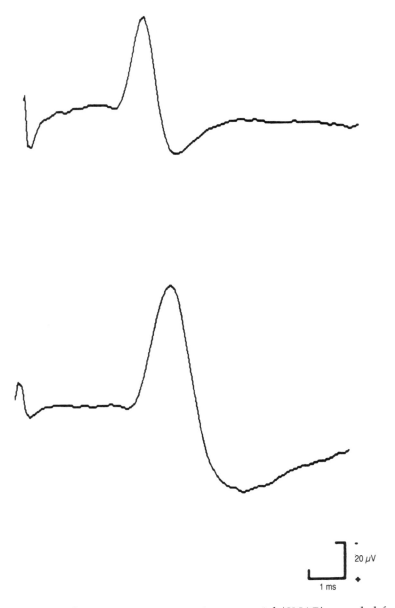

FIGURE 8.7   Median sensory nerve action potential (SNAP) recorded from the index finger following supramaximal percutaneous stimulation at the wrist. Top tracing: study performed with mid-palm temperature of 33.0°C. Lower tracing: repeat study after limb cooling with mid-palm temperature of 28.3°C. The SNAP amplitude increased by 42% and the distal latency (peak) increased by 30% over initial values. The distal latency increase corresponded to approximately 0.2 ms per degrees Centigrade.

result from axonal loss associated with neurotoxic exposures or following selective loss of large fibers, whereas lesions of the myelin sheath more commonly result in dramatic reduction of conduction velocity. In addition to primary axonal loss and demyelination, there also may be metabolic abnormalities associated with reduced conduction velocity.[4] The range of conduction velocities in a given nerve can be determined, although these measures have had limited utility in toxic neuropathy evaluations.[9]

Conduction times over the entire motor nerve can be approximated by F-wave latency measures. The F-wave results from antidromic motor nerve stimulation, with activation of some anterior horn cells and transmission of an orthodromic response along the same axon. The response can be recorded from muscle and the latency from stimulation to response onset can be determined. Diffuse conduction abnormalities are accentuated by the long conduction distances. H-wave studies also can be used to measure conduction over long nerve segments but are used infrequently in the evaluation of toxic neuropathy because of lack of specificity.[10] Sensory and motor conduction studies are sensitive only to dysfunction of large myelinated nerve fibers. Skin potential responses (sympathetic skin potentials) are one measure of smaller unmyelinated nerve fibers.[11] These potentials are recorded between areas of high and low sweat gland density, occurring spontaneously or in response to a variety of stimuli. Because few toxins have been associated with selective loss of small nerve fibers, this technique has had limited application to toxic neuropathy.

Neuromuscular transmission can be evaluated by several techniques, including repetitive motor nerve stimulation to demonstrate abnormal fatigue. An abnormal response consists of a decrease in the CMAP amplitude (decremental response). This is seen in conditions with defective neuromuscular transmission, such as myasthenia gravis or anticholinesterase intoxication. These studies also have limited application to the evaluation of toxic neuropathy but are an important component of the evaluation of any patient who complains of abnormal fatigability.

Nerve conduction studies and measurement of neuromuscular transmission must be rigorous, using standardized laboratory techniques.[7] Complete nerve conduction studies including amplitude, distal latency, and conduction velocity should be performed and reported, along with normal values. Population normal values usually are reported as three standard deviations from the mean when the data are normally distributed, or as a normal range when the distribution is not symmetric. Different values exist for different age groups and some measures vary according to patient size (height, finger circumference, limb length).[12] Minor abnormalities such as slightly prolonged distal latencies or equivocally reduced conduction velocities usually are clinically insignificant and must be interpreted in the context of the complete electrodiagnostic and clinical examinations. Patients with clinically evident neuropathy typically have substantial electrodiagnostic abnormalities in appropriate nerves, with findings well beyond the range of normal. The distribution of abnormality should be consistent with the clinical examination, and appropriate for neuropathy. Confusing or contradictory findings should result in the evaluation of additional nerves to clarify the evaluation or identify any isolated abnormalities.

Electromyography is a very sensitive indicator of ongoing or prior axonal degeneration. The subjective evaluation of fibrillation potentials or positive waves at rest is easily performed and reproducible. When factors unrelated to neuropathy (other localized disease, local trauma, end-plate recordings) are excluded, distal lower-extremity abnormalities usually represent the earliest findings in subclinical axonal neuropathy.[13] The needle examination is used in several ways. As a sensitive indicator of axonal degeneration, it may demonstrate the only abnormality in an early axonal neuropathy.[14] It also can be used to identify the chronicity of a given finding, differentiating acute, subacute, and chronic peripheral disorders. This may be useful in identifying evidence of residual abnormalities, independent from toxic neuropathy. EMG also can be used to identify focal disorders such as radiculopathy in distributions not easily evaluated by nerve conduction studies.

A standard evaluation can be outlined (Table 8.2), although the strategy differs depending on the severity of the disorder.[6,15] The electrodiagnostic examination establishes the presence or absence of neuropathy with a high degree of accuracy. A complete electrodiagnostic examination requires motor and sensory conduction studies on multiple nerves in upper and lower extremities. Bilateral studies usually are performed on several nerves to evaluate symmetry, recognizing that isolated mononeuropathies superimposed on a generalized neuropathy are common. When symptoms or signs are minimal, evaluation is directed toward the most sensitive or susceptible nerves. Conversely, absent lower-extremity responses provide no information about possible demyelination and cannot be used to document progression, making it important to study less involved nerves. Careful attention must be given to measuring evoked response amplitudes. When combined with the clinical examination, the results may suggest a specific diagnosis.

Using appropriately defined normal data, individual patients or groups of patients exposed to a common neurotoxin may be compared to population normal values. Individual patients may be considered abnormal only when their findings exceed the normal laboratory values and only when normal variations such as anomalous innervation have been excluded. Findings explained by local trauma or focal nerve or root damage cannot be used as evidence of a diffuse process. Only after the entire electrodiagnostic and clinical examinations have been considered can it be determined whether abnormal findings are related to the presence of a toxic neuropathy. Small abnormalities in the mean values for a specific measure in a population of patients may be statistically apparent when compared to population normal values even when individual differences are not outside the normal range.[7] However, these statistically significant differences may or may not have clinical significance for individual patients.

TABLE 8.2
Representative Electrodiagnostic Protocol for
Evaluating Suspected Peripheral Neuropathy

Conduction studies[a]
1. Test most involved site if mild or moderate, least involved site if severe.
2. Evaluate peroneal motor nerve (extensor digitorum brevis); stimulate ankle and below fibular head. Measure F-wave latency.[b]
3. If abnormal, evaluate tibial motor nerve (abductor hallucis); stimulate ankle and knee. Measure F-wave latency.
4. If no responses, evaluate
   a. Peroneal motor nerve (anterior tibialis); stimulate below fibular head and knee.
   b. Ulnar motor nerve (hypothenar); stimulate wrist and below elbow. Measure F-wave latency.
   c. Median motor nerve (thenar); stimulate wrist and elbow. Measure F-wave latency.
5. Evaluate sural nerve (ankle); stimulate calf.
6. Evaluate median sensory nerve (index finger); stimulate wrist and elbow. If response is absent or focal entrapment is suspected, record from wrist and stimulate midpalm; evaluate ulnar sensory nerve (fifth digit); stimulate wrist.
7. Additional nerves can be evaluated if findings are equivocal. Definite abnormalities should result in
   a. Evaluation of contralateral extremity.
   b. Evaluation of specific suspected abnormality.
Needle examination
1. Examine anterior tibialis, medial gastrocnemius, vastus lateralis, biceps brachii, first dorsal interosseous (hand), and lumbar paraspinal muscles.
2. Any abnormality should be confirmed by examination of at least one contralateral muscle looking for symmetry.

---

[a]Muscles in parentheses indicate recording site for conduction studies.
[b]All F-wave latency measurements are for distal stimulation sites. Record as absent if no response after 10–15 stimulations.
Source: Modifed from JW Albers, PD Donofrio, TK McGonagle. Sequential electrodiagnostic abnormalities in acute inflammatory demyelinating polyradiculoneuropathy. Muscle Nerve 1985;8:528–539.

Selected Examples of Peripheral Neurotoxins

An encyclopedic summary of all chemicals found in the workplace and environment and known to cause peripheral nervous system damage in humans or experimental animals is beyond the scope of this chapter. A selection of several established peripheral neurotoxins (excluding medications) are discussed in this section, along with several chemicals whose peripheral toxicity is controversial. The more common industrial or agricultural uses of each chemical are described, and the port of entry, metabolism, and excretion are noted. Whenever possible, well-established neurotoxic mechanisms are described, along with the neurologic, electrodiagnostic, and pathologic consequences of exposure. Central nervous system involvement, when it occurs in association with peripheral abnormalities, is also described. Findings and studies important in establishing the diagnosis are presented, as are known treatments. The classification system used is not exclusive and is used for convenience.

ORGANIC SOLVENTS AND RELATED ORGANIC COMPOUNDS

Carbon Disulfide

Carbon disulfide has had widespread industrial application since 1851, initially as a phosphorus solvent used to make matches. It is now used commonly in the production of viscose rayon fiber, cellophane, plywood, and pesticides.[16,17] It is a colorless liquid that evaporates at room temperature and can be absorbed by inhalation or skin contact.[16] The mechanism of neurotoxic action is unknown but is associated with giant axonal swellings, which are also seen in several other toxic neuropathies.[18] The majority of inhaled or absorbed carbon disulfide is biotransformed; the metabolites are eliminated in the urine and can be measured to document exposure.[17]

As with many organic compounds, neurologic consequences of carbon disulfide exposure involve the central and peripheral nervous systems. High-level industrial exposures in the late nineteenth century reportedly resulted in evidence of encephalopathy and signs of extrapyramidal dysfunction and peripheral neuropathy.[16,19]

Acute, fulminate manifestations are now rare, and the majority of carbon disulfide–associated neurotoxicity currently results from years or decades of chronic low-level industrial exposure.[16] With chronic exposures, symptoms and signs of neuropathy predominate, often in association with extrapyramidal symptoms and nonspecific neurasthenia.[17,20–22] The latter symptoms occasionally are referred to as myasthenic conditions, but the implication is in reference to neurotic or psycho-asthenic states, not weakness or abnormal fatigue associated with defective neuromuscular transmission such as myasthenia gravis.[17] Neuropathic symptoms include numbness and weakness of the lower extremities to a greater extent than in the upper extremities, in association with distal weakness, absent lower-extremity muscle stretch reflexes, and impaired perception of pin, touch, and vibration sensations.[18] Examination of 16 workers with at least 10 years of exposure to carbon disulfide in a rayon plant demonstrated clinical and electrodiagnostic evidence of neuropathy in ten.[23] In seven workers, the neuropathy was believed to be caused by carbon disulfide exposure alone, whereas in three others, competing causes of neuropathy were identified.

Evaluations of workers with carbon disulfide exposures generally below 20 parts per million (ppm) are reported by Putz-Anderson and associates.[24] Although abnormalities at these levels were previously described, only marginal effects were found and no significant behavioral changes. Furthermore, symptom prevalence was not consistently related to exposure levels. At higher exposures (levels ≤40 ppm), Seppalainen and Tolonen[25] report motor conduction slowing in the lower limbs suggestive of a subclinical neuropathy. Johnson and associates[26] also demonstrated electrodiagnostic differences in ulnar motor, peroneal motor, and sural sensory conduction studies between carbon disulfide–exposed and unexposed workers. These differences occurred without an increase of symptoms in the exposed workers, indicating that clinically asymptomatic workers had physiologically detectable differences. Small (<5%) but significantly (p<.05) reduced conduction velocities were found in the exposed versus comparison groups for the sural and peroneal nerves. These small differences are of questionable clinical significance but are supported by a dose-response relationship between peroneal conduction velocity and cumulative carbon disulfide exposure. A reduction in the ratio of the proximal to distal peroneal CMAP amplitudes was also found in exposed workers, perhaps reflecting abnormal temporal dispersion from an increase in the range of conduction velocities.

Similar findings are reported by Corsi and associates.[27] The prevalence of neuropathy appears to be related to the degree of exposure, with slight reductions in maximum and slow motor conduction velocities. Reexamination of 12 subjects with neuropathy 4 years later demonstrated no improvement. They conclude that the findings are consistent with a permanent axonal neuropathy, although this interpretation is suspect because conduction velocity measures are a poor reflection of the magnitude of axonal degeneration or regeneration.[27] Nevertheless, recovery is slow and sometimes incomplete, suggesting that spinal cord involvement may occur as well.[18] Needle EMG demonstrates fibrillation potentials, consistent with axonal degeneration.[18]

Taken together, the clinical and electrodiagnostic findings are consistent with a mild, distal sensorimotor neuropathy of the axonal type, characteristic of many toxic neuropathies as reported by Schaumburg and Spencer.[18] In laboratory animals, carbon disulfide exposure induces neuropathy; peripheral nerve abnormalities as reported by Gottfried and associates[28] are characterized by paranodal and internodal swellings and ongoing axonal degeneration. The swellings appear to represent neurofilament accumulations. Peripheral myelin is decreased and thin, and the number of microtubules is decreased. Schwann cell processes intrude into the axoplasm, and Schwann cells have increased cytoplasmic content with proliferation around demyelinated axons. The morphologic findings in carbon disulfide neuropathy are similar to those associated with hexacarbons and acrylamide.[28] Treatment consists of removal from exposure.

Cyanide

Cyanide is one of the most potent and rapid-acting poisons known. Hydrogen cyanide, a gas, and cyanide salts, such as potassium cyanide, are readily absorbed from the lungs and the gastrointestinal tract. Acute ingestion of as little as 300 mg may be lethal. Chronic industrial exposure is rare and usually results from the use of cyanide salts in electroplating in the metallurgic industry or from exposure to pesticides containing cyanide. Chronic exposure also occurs with consumption of certain stone fruit seeds (apricots, peaches, wild cherries, and bitter almonds) or the cassava plant.[29,30] Clinical features as described by Osuntokun[29] include painful paresthesias that are initially noted in the feet and later occur in the hands. These sensory symptoms are followed by distal weakness. On examination, proprioceptive loss and weakness are associated with a broad-based, ataxic gait. Other neurologic features include optic atrophy, cochlear-type hearing loss, and occasional signs of cortical tract involvement. Symptomatic individuals have elevated plasma levels of thiocyanate. Motor nerve conduction studies indicate normal or mildly slow conduction velocity. Needle EMG demonstrates the variable presence of denervation.[29]

Acute cyanide toxicity is due to reaction with trivalent iron in the cytochrome oxidase system throughout the body, preventing cellular respiration.[31] Treatment is based on competitive binding of cyanide from cytochrome oxidase to trivalent iron of methemoglobin. Nitrate is administered to produce methemoglobin, and thiosulfate then is given to form thiocyanate from cyanomethemoglobin. Thiocyanate is rapidly excreted in urine.[31]

Peterson and associates[32] describe patients with sickle cell disease who were treated with sodium cyanate and developed clinical neuropathy with electrodiagnostic evidence of low-amplitude or absent motor and sensory evoked responses, as well as some slowing of nerve conduction velocities in lower extremities. In the upper extremities, mild slowing of motor and sensory conduction velocities occurred. Needle EMG demonstrated evidence of denervation with increased spontaneous activity and mild neurogenic motor unit changes. A portion of asymptomatic patients showed similar but less severe changes. Sural nerve biopsy provided supportive evidence of primary axonal degeneration with secondary demyelination. Clinical and electrical improvement occurred with cessation of exposure.

Ethyl Alcohol

Ethyl alcohol has been associated with several neurologic disorders potentially related to direct neurotoxic effects of alcohol or its metabolites, nutritional disorders, genetic factors, or combinations of these.[33] The role of ethyl alcohol in the pathogenesis of neuropathy has been controversial because most individuals who consume large amounts of alcohol forgo other foods and may become nutritionally compromised.[34] Peripheral neuropathies with clinical similarities to those seen with high alcohol consumption are common in vitamin-deficient states, especially deficiency of thiamine in beriberi, and alcoholic neuropathy is generally thought to result from deficiency of thiamine and other B vitamins.[34] Support for a nutritional cause includes evidence suggesting that neuropathy is not induced by excessive alcohol in individuals receiving nutritional supplementation.[34] However, other studies indicate that alcohol impairs axonal transport,[35] and Behse and Buchthal[36] report that a typical alcohol neuropathy can occur in the setting of normal nutrition.

Setting aside the nutritional controversy, the incidence of neuropathy in alcoholic patients is high.[33,34] The neuropathy may be subclinical, with electrodiagnostic abnormalities only.[34] When symptomatic, the findings described by Victor and associates[34] and Charness and colleagues[33] include paresthesias and painful distal dysesthesias with foot pain and muscle cramps as common early symptoms. The neuropathy is gradually progressive, and symmetric distal weakness appears, along with gait ataxia. Involvement may become severe, with distal paralysis and proximal weakness. Sensory loss is prominent, with distal defects of fine touch, pin-pain, and vibratory sensations. There may be evidence of dysautonomia. Muscle stretch reflexes are absent distally and reduced proximally. Progression may be slow, stepwise, or rapid over months.

Nerve conduction abnormalities reported by Behse and Buchthal[36] include low-amplitude sensory nerve action potentials, most abnormal in patients with greatest involvement. Sensory nerve conduction velocity may be mildly slowed. Compound muscle action potential amplitudes may be markedly reduced, especially when recorded from weak distal muscles. Although occasional descriptions emphasize a predominantly demyelinating neuropathology,[33,34] motor conduction velocity is only mildly slowed, more consistent with an axonal neuropathy.[36] The presence of axonal involvement is supported by needle EMG, which shows evidence for denervation and reinnervation even in asymptomatic individuals, but most prominently in weak muscles.[36] Rarely, the electrodiagnostic evaluation provides evidence suggestive of a proximal myopathy, although this almost always coexists with a generalized neuropathy.[33] The pathologic changes in peripheral nerve initially were described as showing prominent demyelination, but more recent studies document primary axonal damage and mild secondary demyelination.[36] Treatment consists of removal from exposure and nutritional supplementation.

Ethylene Oxide

Ethylene oxide is used extensively in the biomedical industry as a gas sterilant for heat-sensitive materials and is manufactured in great quantities as a precursor for industrial chemicals.[37,38] Ethylene oxide is readily absorbed following inhalation. It is water soluble and reacts in water to form ethylene glycol. The neurotoxic mechanisms of cell damage are unknown, but it is thought that some molecule produced in the cell body and transported to the nerve axon is involved.[38] It is a highly reactive epoxide and is a direct alkylating agent, making it mutagenic, although the relationship to human cancer is controversial.[39]

Ethylene oxide neurotoxicity has been demonstrated to produce central and peripheral nervous system damage in animals and humans.[38,40] Reports exist of human toxicity following subacute (weeks) and chronic (months) exposure in industrial settings, associated with and without demonstrable gas leaks.[37,41] Although acute encephalopathy is associated with ethylene oxide exposure, the most common neurologic consequence of exposure is peripheral neuropathy. Neuropathy occurs at low-level exposure, when damage to other tissues is not apparent.[38] In two patients reported by Gross and associates,[37] distal extremity numbness and weakness developed associated with clinical evidence of distal sensory loss and areflexia. Three patients reported by Finelli and associates[41] had similar symptoms and findings, plus distal lower-extremity weakness. Removal from exposure resulted in progressive improvement. Within a 4- to 6-month follow-up period, the most severely involved patients described by Finelli and associates demonstrated normal examinations except for absent Achilles muscle stretch reflexes (one patient) and difficulty in heel walking (one patient). Windebank and Blexrud[38] demonstrated ethylene oxide neurotoxicity in vitro and suggest that residual ethylene oxide in dialyzers after sterilization may contribute to progressive neuropathy in patients receiving chronic hemodialysis.

Electrodiagnostic studies of ethylene oxide–associated neuropathy are consistent with a distal axonopathy characterized by primary axonal degeneration and secondary demyelination, preferentially involving the distal portion of axons.[41] Findings include mild motor conduction velocity slowing (none slower than 80% of the lower limit of normal), low-amplitude responses, and needle EMG evidence of positive waves and fibrillation potentials with polyphasic motor units, all most prominent in the distal lower extremities. In follow-up evaluations, denervation potentials disappeared and motor unit action potential amplitude increased, consistent with ongoing reinnervation. In another patient, conduction studies demonstrated improvement and there was evidence of reinnervation, although active denervation potentials persisted. The patient with the least severe clinical involvement had normal conduction studies, including sural sensory responses.[41]

Finelli and associates[41] suggest a difference in individual vulnerability to ethylene oxide, similar to that associated with several other toxic exposures, because only some exposed workers show involvement of the peripheral nervous system. Nevertheless, the clinical symptoms and signs and the electrodiagnostic abnormalities are very similar among the reported patients, and the variable involvement may reflect differential exposures as opposed to differences in vulnerability. Finelli and associates[41] also suggest that identification of symptomatic individuals should result in clinical and electrodiagnostic evaluation of coworkers to detect asymptomatic neuropathy.

Trichloroethylene

Trichloroethylene (TCE) is a chlorinated hydrocarbon with extensive industrial and household use as a cleaner, solvent, and degreasing agent. It has been used medically as an anesthetic and as an analgesic agent.[42] TCE is a colorless, highly volatile liquid. Its most important route of entry is by inhalation, but also can be absorbed orally and through the skin. As an analgesic agent, TCE was used in the treatment of trigeminal neuralgia, as a self-administered drug during obstetric procedures, and during dental extractions and other short operative procedures.[42] It was estimated that as many as 60,000 patients a year received TCE as an anesthetic agent, and the National Institute of Occupational Safety and Health (NIOSH) reports that the total number of individuals occupationally exposed to TCE may have been in excess of 3.6 million in 1974.[43,44] Metabolism is via microsomal mixed-function oxidases in the liver. Biotransformation produces chlorohydrate, which is rapidly metabolized to trichloroethanol and trichloroacetic acid, more water-soluble products that are excreted in the urine.[45] Exposure can be monitored by urinary excretion of the TCE metabolites.[46]

Neurotoxicity primarily involves the central nervous system, and acute exposure results in headache, nausea, and incoordination, although there are many contradictory statements regarding its neurotoxic effects.[42] Chronic TCE exposure is associated with dizziness, light-headedness, headache, fatigue, nausea, vomiting, and alcohol intolerance, and symptom prevalence is increased in exposed compared to unexposed workers.[46,47] In the study by DeFalque,[47] neurologic signs do not demonstrate a significant relation to exposure intensity.

Acute TCE exposure is associated with trigeminal nerve dysfunction, involving both motor and sensory components.[48] Feldman and associates[49] describe a TCE-intoxicated patient with lethargy, confusion, constricted visual fields, unilateral paresis of accommodation, bilateral trigeminal anesthesia, and masseter muscle weakness. Impaired extraocular eye movement and asymmetric ptosis, facial weakness, reduced taste perception of the anterior two-thirds of the tongue, and hoarse voice were also seen. Muscle stretch reflexes and extremity sensation were intact. Over an 18-month period, facial anesthesia improved, as did other symptoms and signs. This picture of multiple cranial mononeuropathies has been reported by others.[50,51] Two of four TCE-exposed workers reported by Buxton and Hayward,[51] including one in whom severe multiple cranial mononeuropathies developed, had ptosis, reduced eye movements, facial and bulbar muscle weakness, and findings referable to trigeminal nerve dysfunction. In the most severely involved patient, muscle stretch reflexes were difficult to elicit but they were normal in the other patients. No evidence of a diffuse neuropathy was seen, and the depressed muscle stretch reflexes could reflect brain stem involvement. Trichloroethylene also has been associated with multiple cranial mononeuropathies after general anesthesia, presumably related to a breakdown product (dichloracetylene) resulting from reaction between TCE and soda lime.[52] When contact with soda lime was avoided, TCE was regarded as a safe anesthetic agent,[53] although the effects on the trigeminal nerve of exposure to impure TCE were so predictable that it was used in the treatment of trigeminal neuralgia.[30]

Although the term *neuropathy* often is used in association with TCE, evidence of peripheral nerve involvement is sparse and "multiple cranial mononeuropathies" may be a more appropriate description. In general, the trigeminal nerve is relatively spared by most toxins that affect other peripheral nerves.[52] When facial and extremity sensation are equally impaired, the likely lesion is a neuronopathy affecting dorsal root and trigeminal ganglia, as seen in pyridoxine overdose producing virtually total large-fiber sensory loss.[54]

Electrodiagnostic evaluations demonstrate prolonged facial nerve latencies that may reflect involvement of cranial nuclei.[48] The patient reported by Feldman and associates[49] demonstrated substantially prolonged facial latencies (needle electrode recordings) that progressively improved and were recorded as normal 120 weeks after exposure. They also found a reduced ulnar sensory nerve distal conduction velocity (finger to wrist) 2 weeks after exposure. However, the wrist-to-elbow conduction velocity was faster at this time than in subsequent recordings, suggesting a potential measurement discrepancy or other technical difficulty. Conduction velocity returned toward normal but remained borderline-reduced 34 weeks after exposure in this patient, with no signs or symptoms referable to the ulnar nerve. Other abnormalities included the presence of H waves recorded following ulnar nerve stimulation, with a latency identical to the F-wave latency (the H-wave latency should be shortened). The significance of this is unclear, although the presence of an H-wave recorded in intrinsic hand muscles is not necessarily abnormal. Based on these findings, Feldman et al. believe that the reversibly slowed nerve conduction velocity most likely reflected demyelination and remyelination, perhaps from the lipid solvent effect of TCE, which alters large and small fibers in proportion to the amount of myelin. Feldman and associates[55] also report that blink reflex latencies were prolonged for individual workers with direct TCE exposure, and average latencies for a group of individuals exposed to TCE through the public drinking water were significantly longer than laboratory control latencies. Blink reflex studies are technically difficult compared to conventional nerve conduction studies and demonstrate greater response variability. Nevertheless, normal values have been established using standardized procedure, and these studies provide a potential means of evaluating facial and trigeminal reflex pathways following toxic exposure.[56] Long-term exposure at about the threshold limit value demonstrated an equivocal reduction in the mean sural conduction velocity in 31 printing workers compared to 28 age-matched control subjects, but no abnormality of motor nerves or blink reflexes.[57] While these findings can be explained by slight abnormality of the trigeminal and sural nerves, they are of limited clinical significance.

The underlying pathology of TCE-associated dysfunction remains unclear, particularly with reference to any potential peripheral effect. Necropsy examination of the patient reported by Buxton and Hayward[51] revealed abnormalities involving the brainstem nuclei and tracts, the trigeminal nerve, and sensory roots. These findings are consistent with extensive axonal degeneration and demyelination in a distribution consistent with the clinical findings. Cavanagh and Buxton[58] suggest that the trigeminal neuropathy associated with TCE exposure reflects a chemically induced reactivation of latent orofacial herpes simplex virus, not a direct neurotoxic effect.

Hexacarbons

Hexacarbon compounds are used as industrial solvents and are implicated in neuropathies in industrial settings and following solvent inhalant abuse. They consist of a six-member carbon chain with different substitution groups. N-hexane, the unsubstituted molecule, is found in industrial and household glues and is associated with neuropathy in factory workers and following volitional inhalation of vapors.[59,60] Methyl-n-butyl ketone (MBK) is a commonly used substituted hexacarbon. Chronic high-dose exposure to this compound may occur in the workplace.[61,62] Both compounds gain access to the body across the skin and respiratory membranes. Oxidative metabolism takes place in the liver, and both compounds ultimately form 2,5-hexanedione, which is believed to be the neurotoxic agent.[63] Another similar substituted hexacarbon, methyl ethyl ketone (MEK), is not neurotoxic but may promote neuropathy due to other hexacarbons with which it is frequently mixed.[64]

Occupational exposure to n-hexane is associated with a sensorimotor polyneuropathy of the dying-back type, characterized by stocking-glove sensory loss to all modalities, distal weakness, and absent ankle reflexes.[65–69] High doses of n-hexane produce a subacute and severe neuropathy with substantial distal weakness and sensory loss,[59] and examples of pure motor neuropathy associated with occupational hexacarbon exposure are unusual.[68,70] Eight children and adolescents reported by Lalloo and associates[70] did have a predominately motor neuropathy attributable by the authors to abuse of n-hexane. This contrasts to the description by Herskowitz and associates[59] of three adult cabinet finishers with prolonged and intense exposure to n-hexane in whom distal symmetric weakness, sensory loss to all modalities, and distal areflexia occurred. Identification of a pure motor neuropathy also is inconsistent with the known abnormalities on sural nerve biopsy, described below.

Improvement follows removal from exposure, but those most acutely and severely affected experience incomplete recovery. An important observation is continued progression of the neuropathy for several months after cessation of exposure, before improvement commences.[18] Some reports of patients with neuropathy following voluntary inhalation of glue or thinner containing n-hexane emphasize the prominence of motor compared to sensory findings, whereas others document distal sensory impairments.[70–73] The neuropathy associated with MBK exposure initially results in slowly progressive sensory impairment characterized by acral and pedal numbness with mild loss of touch, pin, and vibratory sensations, as reported by Allen and associates.[61] Reflexes are relatively preserved, although ankle reflexes are usually reduced or absent. With further progression, weakness and atrophy of intrinsic hand and foot muscles occur. An associated constitutional sign is weight loss.[61]

Nerve conduction studies in hexacarbon-exposed but asymptomatic individuals may be normal or may suggest the existence of a subclinical neuropathy in the form of mildly slowed motor conduction velocities.[62] In symptomatic individuals exposed to *n*-hexane, motor and sensory evoked amplitudes are reduced and conduction velocities are slowed.[65,67,73,74] Lalloo and coworkers[70] describe nerve conduction abnormalities for two patients exposed to *n*-hexane, as an impurity in the benzine (not benzene) they were inhaling. Nerve amplitudes were not reported, but conduction velocities were in the range of 35–40% of the lower limit of normal. Chang and colleagues[67] describe evaluations of 56 printers exposed to *n*-hexane. In 20 of the 56 exposed workers, symptomatic sensorimotor neuropathy developed, supported by electrophysiologic and clinical abnormalities. Initial findings consisted of reduced sensory amplitudes, followed by reduced motor amplitudes and reduced conduction velocities consistent with primary axonal degeneration with secondary demyelination. All motor conduction velocities for the cabinet finishers described above were moderately slowed.[59] Urinary excretion of 2,5-hexanedione has been correlated with the degree of conduction slowing.[75]

Substantial reductions in conduction velocity frequently are interpreted as evidence of primary demyelination, a finding atypical of most toxic neuropathies. However, hexacarbon neuropathy may be an exception to this concept.[76] Sumner and others attribute conduction slowing to the secondary myelin sheath damage (described below) that occurs in relationship to the multifocal giant axonal swellings.[60,76] Kuwabara and associates[72] report transient multifocal conduction block in a patient with *n*-hexane neuropathy. Changes in nerve conduction velocity or partial conduction block may be explained by secondary or passive changes to myelin caused in part by the axonal swelling. Distribution of conduction velocity measurements in *n*-hexane neuropathy suggests initial involvement of the faster fibers, but involvement of all fibers at higher exposure levels.[77] Slowing along central nervous system fiber tracts producing prolonged visual and somatosensory evoked potentials also is reported.[74,78] Electromyographic examination demonstrates positive waves and fibrillation potentials, with large motor units and decreased recruitment.[61] In general, clinical and electrodiagnostic improvement follows removal from exposure, although conduction slowing and unobtainable responses may persist in the lower extremities of the most severely involved patients; denervation activity disappears and is replaced by large-amplitude motor unit action potentials.[79]

Pathology studies of exposed humans and exposed experimental animals demonstrate axonal swellings at both peripheral and central ends of nerve fibers, with changes ranging from disturbance of the myelin with preserved axons to multifocal axonal distention with paranodal swelling and neurofilamentous masses.[65,67,72,76,77,80] The varied pathologic changes may be due to the presence of other hydrocarbons or to the severity of the neuropathy. The axonal swellings consist of neurofilament aggregates, which may accumulate because of abnormalities of fast and slow axonal transport mechanisms.[60,81,82] Couri and Milks[83] suggest that covalent interaction with lysyl residues causes cross-linking of axonal neurofilaments and disruption of axonal flow. 2,5-Hexanedione shares a similar configuration of carbonyl groups with other neurotoxic carbon compounds such as 2,5-heptanedione and 3,6-octanedione, but the neurotoxicity of each is likely related to metabolism to 2,5-hexanedione.[84] Specific treatment is not known other than reduction or elimination of exposure.

Methyl Bromide

Methyl bromide is a colorless, faintly odored gas that has been used as a fumigant, fire extinguisher, refrigerant, and insecticide.[31] It is absorbed by the lungs following inhalation. Acute intoxication results in symptoms and signs, including nausea, anorexia, vomiting, headache, slurred speech, unsteady gait, and difficulty concentrating, that are typical of most organic vapors.[85] Following mild exposure, recovery is complete; severe exposures may be fatal, with widespread systemic involvement of the lungs, kidneys, and nervous system including delirium and seizures.[31] Chronic toxicity has been associated with involvement of the central and peripheral nervous systems, resulting in findings consistent with pyramidal, cerebellar, and peripheral nerve involvement.[31,85] A sensorimotor neuropathy associated with daily methyl bromide exposure over 3 months is reported by Kantarjian and Shaheen.[85] In the eight patients described, distal paresthesias developed, followed by objective superficial distal sensory loss to all modalities, distal weakness, and unsteady gait. Achilles reflexes were absent (four patients) or hypoactive. None demonstrated symptoms of systemic illness. Electrodiagnostic evaluations were not performed, but a clinical diagnosis of neuropathy was established. Within 6–8 months of removal from exposure, no neurologic abnormalities were detectable.

Methylhexane

Butylazo-hydroxy-methylhexane (BHMH) is a methylhexane that was used briefly as an industrial agent in the manufacture of reinforced plastic bathtubs. An outbreak of encephalopathy and peripheral neuropathy is reported by Horan and coworkers.[86] In seven of 18 workers subacute central and peripheral nervous system dysfunction developed, characterized by dizziness, paresthesias, muscle weakness, incontinence, memory loss, and visual loss. The symptoms characteristic of a sensorimotor neuropathy began distally and were associated with prolonged sensory latency, fibrillation potentials, and decreased motor unit recruitment. Slow improvement occurred following removal from exposure. Demonstration of this outbreak resulted in withdrawal of BHMH from distribution. The product was subsequently shown to be a potent neurotoxin in rats, causing loss of axons in the peripheral nerves and spinal cord, and degeneration of optic nerve tracts. BHMH was described as a prototype for a new family of neurotoxic aliphatic hydrocarbon compounds.[86]

Styrene

Styrene is a colorless, volatile organic solvent that has been associated with central nervous system behavioral effects, as well as with a possible peripheral neuropathy.[87–90] It has widespread application in the plastics industry, particularly in the polyester resin boat industry.[91] Styrene is readily absorbed following inhalation.[31] Behavioral effects have been described, but peripheral nervous system effects are less clear.

Rosen and associates[91] identified seven of 33 individuals with paresthesias in fingers and toes following chronic styrene exposure. In this pilot study, designed to compare the effects of different levels of styrene exposure, neurologic examinations did not identify peripheral or central nervous system abnormalities. Nevertheless, electrodiagnostic evaluations demonstrated the following mild findings, which were consistent with a sensory neuropathy. Motor conduction studies were normal. Sensory conduction studies demonstrated slightly reduced amplitudes and conduction velocities compatible with axonal loss. Sensory nerve action potential duration also was increased. Statistically significant abnormalities existed for only one of the exposure groups described by Rosen and coworkers.[91] When the ten workers with possible sensory neuropathy were compared to remaining subjects, they were found to be significantly older (54.9 versus 39.7 years). The investigators felt that significant electrodiagnostic differences existed between the two groups of workers even after compensation for age. There also were significant exposure differences, with the older workers having greatest exposure. The authors conclude that the older workers were more prone to development of styrene-induced neurotoxicity than were the younger workers.[91]

Cherry and Gautrin[90] evaluated 70 workers exposed to styrene. They found mild sensory nerve conduction deficits in 23% of workers exposed to less than 50 ppm and in 71% of workers exposed to more than 100 ppm, but no conduction slowing in a small group of five men exposed to more than 100 ppm for less than 4 weeks. A lower risk of sensory conduction deficit was associated with wearing a mask and current consumption of alcohol, but there was no indication that neurotoxicity was related to individual differences in the capacity to metabolize styrene. Others have reported sensory but not motor conduction slowing in a small sample of 11 styrene-exposed workers compared to control subjects.[89] They also found increased R-R interval variability on electrocardiography and concluded that styrene may affect peripheral sensory fibers, as well as autonomic nervous activity.

These results of styrene-induced neurotoxicity have not been confirmed in animal models. Seppalainen[88] evaluated and compared sensory conduction velocities in styrene-exposed animals and control animals. No difference was detected after 11 weeks of exposure. Failure to identify a clear dose-response relationship in human subjects further reduces the clinical significance of the reported work, although a possible peripheral neurotoxic effect cannot be excluded.

Toluene

Toluene (methyl benzene) is used as a solvent and thinner in many industrial settings. Exposure is mostly through the respiratory tract and less so across skin. Toluene is eliminated through the lungs or converted to hippuric acid and excreted in urine.[92] Individuals at risk are those working with toluene-containing lacquers and thinners, glues, and cleaning liquids, and individuals addicted to sniffing toluene. The neurotoxic effects of toluene appear to be confined to the central nervous system in the form of dose-related neurobehavioral abnormalities, such as drowsiness, headache, impaired coordination, cerebellar dystaxia, eye movement abnormalities, anosmia, and hearing changes.[93–95] White-matter changes on magnetic resonance imaging (MRI) strongly correlate with identified neuropsychological impairments.[96] Despite high levels and prolonged exposure following volitional inhalation of toluene almost continuously for 5 years, no abnormalities on nerve conduction studies or needle EMG are noted.[93] Reports of neuropathy due to toluene in glue sniffing can be explained by the presence of *n*-hexane in the glue.[97] To date, there is little convincing evidence that pure toluene or other aromatic hydrocarbons cause peripheral neuropathy.[98]

Mixtures of Organic Solvents

Exposure to organic solvents commonly occurs in the form of mixtures, and it is often difficult or impossible to relate effects to a specific solvent, or to study workers in an environment where exposure is limited to a single solvent. Furthermore, it is theoretically possible that combined solvents may potentiate the effects of an individual solvent in the same dose. The neurotoxic potential of organic solvent mixtures is controversial.[58,99–102] In occupational settings, this is complicated further because the use of individual solvents may vary over time, and exposure estimations are difficult.[103] Organic solvents are volatile and readily absorbed through the lungs, but they also can be absorbed through the skin. Because they are lipid-soluble, they distribute to both the central and peripheral nervous systems.[104] Organic solvents are metabolized mainly in the liver and excreted primarily through exhalation of unchanged solvent or in the urine as unchanged solvent or solvent metabolites.[105]

Acute exposure to organic solvent vapors causes narcosis. Chronic exposure has been associated with central and peripheral nervous system impairment, although reservations have been expressed regarding the diagnosis of chronic organic solvent intoxication because of difficulty in differentiating solvent intoxication from other neurologic disorders or normal individual variation.[106]

Peripheral manifestations of organic solvent exposure, excluding aliphatic hydrocarbons such as *n*-hexane, are uncommon.[98,100] In an evaluation of 42 workers exposed to organic solvent mixtures, Fagius and Gronqvist[107] identified only one plausible and two suspected cases of neuropathy. Comparison of the exposed and control workers demonstrated no significant differences. Grouping according to exposure levels demonstrated a longer mean median distal latency for the control subjects compared to exposed workers. This was attributed to random variation, although other observed abnormalities were attributed to organic solvent exposure. Cherry and associates[100] evaluated 96 solvent-exposed workers. Although they demonstrated excess symptoms in the exposed group, they found no evidence of abnormal nerve conduction studies suggestive of a peripheral disorder.

In an evaluation of 34 workers exposed primarily to mixtures of organic solvents, Matikainen and Jantunen[103] found nine workers with diminished reflexes or sensory findings, or both, suggestive of peripheral neuropathy. However, clinical and neurophysiologic findings tended to be more prominent in the older workers and control subjects were younger than the exposed workers. The most prominent findings involved workers whose exposure included carbon disulfide, although carbon disulfide was not believed to be responsible for the overall findings. Furthermore, symptoms and signs of peripheral neuropathy have been found in exposed workers whose solvent mixture exposures do not include substantial amounts of either hexacarbons or carbon disulfide.[108–111]

Elofsson and coworkers[112] evaluated 80 industrial spray painters with long-term exposure to mixtures of organic solvents. Compared to control workers, symptoms consistent with peripheral neuropathy such as paresthesias were significantly increased in the exposed workers, as were other symptoms not necessarily related to peripheral neuropathy. Quantified neurologic examination of peripheral function did not reveal any significant group differences, although exposed workers had a significantly higher vibration threshold than the reference group. The increased threshold was not necessarily associated with sensory symptoms. Electrodiagnostic evaluation of median, peroneal, and sural nerves demonstrated significant group differences for sural nerve measurements. The differences consisted of reduced amplitude and conduction velocity for exposed compared to control workers. There also were small (less than 3%) but statistically significant reductions in motor and sensory conduction velocities for exposed compared to control workers consistent with a mild axonal neuropathy.

Juntunen and coworkers[113] report similar findings in a retrospective study of 37 patients exposed to organic solvents, although a clear-cut exposure-effect relationship could not be established. Halonen et al.[114] identified abnormal vibration perception thresholds in four of 90 shipyard workers exposed to organic solvents. Seven additional workers also had increased upper-extremity perception thresholds, although a significant correlation between vibratory perception thresholds and duration of solvent exposure could not be demonstrated. Gregersen and coworkers[115] report that symptoms and signs of peripheral neuropathy are not significantly increased in workers exposed to organic solvents compared to unexposed control subjects. Nevertheless, solvent exposure and neurotoxic signs were weakly correlated, suggesting the possibility of a dose-effect relationship.

Floden and associates[116] report that workers fulfilling their criteria for organic solvent-associated psycho-organic syndrome also have an increased frequency of neuropathy in comparison with workers without any evidence of psycho-organic syndrome, although these investigators do not include conventional clinical examination criteria or criteria that would necessarily be considered diagnostic of a sensorimotor neuropathy. They conclude that it is reasonable that patients with psycho-organic syndrome also have an increased frequency of neuropathy; nevertheless, the clinical and electrodiagnostic findings are inconclusive.

Hormes and associates[98] identified neurologic abnormalities in 13 of 20 chronic abusers of solvent vapors. All abnormalities were referrable to the central nervous system, and they found no evidence of peripheral neuropathy. Maizlish and associates[117] found evidence of mild neuropathy in 16% of 240 workers, some of whom were exposed to mixtures of organic solvents; no neuropathy was clinically significant. Comparisons of exposed and nonexposed workers showed a slightly higher frequency of symptoms in exposed workers, but this difference was not related to solvent level, making the finding of questionable importance. The highest level of symptoms was found for workers with exposures of 5–24 ppm, while workers with exposures of 25–124 ppm demonstrated fewer symptoms than any other exposure group. Segregation of symptoms into those related to sleep disturbances, neurasthenia, intoxication, or peripheral symptoms demonstrated no significant differences between exposed and nonexposed groups. Exposed workers had slightly but significantly reduced vibratory sensation at the foot and diminished ankle reflexes compared to unexposed workers. However, after controlling for age, sex, alcohol intake, and examiner, the only significant relationship between solvent concentration and neurologic function was diminished two-point discrimination at the foot. No firm evidence was found for a dose-response relationship between neurologic function and low-level organic solvent mixture exposures in this study. Grasso and coworkers[118] were unable to demonstrate that long-term industrial exposure to solvents other than carbon disulfide results in a functional neurologic impairment. They comment that the uniformity with which nerve conduction changes are reported following solvent exposure suggests that a relationship is possible, although they emphasize that inattention to limb temperature and to accuracy in reproducibility of recording techniques may account for some of the findings.

In summary, prolonged exposure to mixed solvents has been associated with mild nonprogressive encephalopathy with or without evidence of neuropathy, although Spencer and Schaumburg[119] point out that supportive neuropathologic or experimental animal studies are lacking. The combined findings suggestive of a chronic solvent-induced encephalopathy were described as "chronic painter's syndrome" by Arlien-Soborg and associates.[104] Others failed to find a convincing dose-response effect to solvent exposure, casting doubt on the presence of a distinct or typical painter's syndrome.[99,102,120,121] Comparison of groups of workers receiving disability pensions for work-related abnormalities demonstrated no differences on neuropsychological testing between construction workers (unexposed to solvents) and painters (exposed).[121] Such evaluations provide no evidence to support a typical solvent syndrome. Finally, reanalysis of the neuropsychological test data from a group of workers originally diagnosed with solvent induced toxic encephalopathy (painter's syndrome) found that previously reported impairments could not be confirmed when the influence of age, education, and intelligence was considered.[122]

Few organic solvents unequivocally induce chronic, long-lasting nervous system changes; the extent of reversibility is related to the specific chemical, the dose, and the duration of exposure.[119] The best examples of organic solvent mixtures producing neuropathy contain *n*-hexane or methyl-*n*-butyl ketone.[119] When these are excluded, the findings are less clear. Because evaluation of the peripheral nervous system is less complicated than evaluation of the central nervous system, the picture of neuropathy is usually clear; it would therefore seem that the presence of neuropathy following exposure to mixtures of organic solvents would not be so controversial. In the many reports of exposure to solvent mixtures, disparate findings are often combined and statistical techniques used to identify small differences of uncertain clinical significance between exposed and control groups.[119] While there is sufficient evidence to justify further evaluations, compelling data supporting a causal relationship are unavailable.[119]

Acrylamide

Acrylamide is a water-soluble crystal with many industrial uses, including mining processes, disposal of industrial wastes, as a grouting agent, and as a strengthener in paper and cardboard.[123] It is rapidly absorbed following all routes of administration, and its neurotoxicity is independent of route. Because of its rapid distribution throughout body water, it quickly disappears from the serum with a half-life of less than 2 hours; only small amounts persist in nervous tissue for more than 14 days.[124] Acrylamide is metabolized in the liver and excreted primarily in the urine. Neurotoxicity is associated with distal axonal degeneration of long axons, although the precise mechanism is unknown. Current evidence suggests that acrylamide interferes with the fast axonal transport systems, particularly in the distal axon.[125,126] In addition, Gold and associates[125] established an association between neurofilament content and fiber caliper, suggesting a direct toxic effect of acrylamide on slow axonal transport.

Acrylamide administration induces a sensorimotor neuropathy involving primarily the distal limbs. The peripheral abnormalities are characteristic of those associated with a variety of other metabolic and toxic neuropathies.[127] The earliest manifestations include distal numbness and an unsteady gait. There may be excessive sweating and evidence of an exfoliative dermatitis.[18] Additional clinical features summarized by Schaumburg and Spencer[18] include distal weakness, unsteady gait, diffuse loss of reflexes, and diminished perception of vibratory sensation. Paresthesias are uncommon. Diffuse loss of reflexes is atypical of most mild toxic neuropathies that demonstrate selective loss of the Achilles reflexes. This diffuse loss is more characteristic of the neuropathy associated with vincristine, which is thought to selectively involve muscle spindles. Similarly, the ataxia and hyporeflexia associated with acrylamide likely reflect muscle spindle degeneration.[80]

Electrodiagnostic evaluation usually reveals evidence of sensory and motor abnormalities. The most common findings are reduced or absent sensory evoked responses with minimal abnormality of conduction velocity. Some patients examined during recovery demonstrate marked dispersion of the compound muscle action potential, likely due to regeneration of distal axons.[123,128] The evidence of early muscle spindle involvement suggests that H-waves may be intact early in the course of illness, at a time when muscle stretch reflexes are absent. In describing three patients with acrylamide neuropathy, Fullerton[128] investigated whether pressure produced localized nerve damage, explaining the disproportionate distal slowing. The delay confined to the distal portion of nerves was found to be independent of whether the nerves traversed common compression sites.

Findings on sural nerve biopsy obtained during recovery from acrylamide neuropathy demonstrate evidence of axonal degeneration with regenerating fibers, and with predominant involvement of the large-diameter axons.[128] Electron microscopy examination of nerves obtained from acrylamide-intoxicated animals demonstrates neurofilament accumulation within axons.[125] Although degeneration occurs distally, neurofilaments initially accumulate in the paranodal region, suggesting that acrylamide may damage the axon directly.[129,130] Because central nervous system axons are also involved, Spencer and Schaumburg[130] describe the process as a central-peripheral distal axonopathy.

There is no known treatment for acrylamide neuropathy other than removal from exposure. As with most toxic neuropathies, individuals with mild impairment demonstrate complete recovery, usually over months, although they may have evidence of depressed muscle stretch reflexes or distal vibratory loss. Patients with severe neuropathy demonstrate continued improvement over months, but they may have residual distal weakness and atrophy, gait ataxia, and vibratory sensory loss.[18]

Dimethylaminopropionitrile

Dimethylaminopropionitrile (DMAPN) is structurally similar to acrylamide and also is produced from acrylonitrile. It is used as a catalyst in the manufacture of polyurethane foam and, in an acrylamide grouting compound, is used as a waterproofing agent in tunnels and sewer lines.[131] DMAPN is readily absorbed following oral, respiratory, or dermal contact. From industrial exposure, DMAPN has been associated with urinary hesitancy and distal paresthesias. Pestronk and associates[132] report that the paresthesias and numbness first appear in the distal lower extremities, spread more proximally in the legs, and then appear in the hands. Sexual function also is impaired. Examination demonstrates impaired pin-pain, temperature, and light-touch sensations symmetric in the distal limbs and in the lower sacral dermatomes. Distal weakness is present and muscle stretch reflexes are described as "sluggish" at the ankles.

Prominent urinary and sexual dysfunction are unusual components of most toxic neuropathies, although urologic involvement is described in some cases of acrylamide neuropathy.[132,133] Sacral dermatomal sensory loss also is unusual, and it is suggested that this pattern of loss is due to involvement of small nerve fibers, consistent with the early loss of temperature sensations with relative preservation of muscle stretch reflexes.[132] Involvement of the spinal cord or the cauda equina could cause similar symptoms and findings.[132] After removal from exposure, improvement has been documented, although some individuals continue to have evidence of peripheral nerve, sexual, bladder, and possible central nervous system dysfunction.[131]

Electrodiagnostic evaluations related to DMAPN demonstrate reduced sensory evoked responses with slightly prolonged distal latencies and low or borderline-low compound muscle action potential amplitudes. Conduction velocities are within normal limits or they may be mildly slowed in severely affected patients.[132] Pestronk and associates[132] report resolution of electrodiagnostic abnormalities 5 months after termination of exposure. Sural nerve biopsy shows evidence of axonal degeneration and axonal swelling with disordered neurofilaments, similar to the abnormalities associated with regenerating axons in acrylamide-intoxicated rats.[132] Iminodipropionitrile (IDPN), another neurotoxic nitrile initially studied in the search for a model of lathyrism, also is associated with defective axonal transport resulting in accumulation of neurofilaments in motor neurons and proximal axons.[134] Its application as a model for the axonopathies has been reviewed by Griffin and Price,[134] demonstrating the use of a neurotoxin in establishing pathogenic mechanisms with abnormalities in axonal structure and physiology.

ORGANOPHOSPHORUS COMPOUNDS

Organophosphorus (OP) compounds describe a large class of acetylcholinesterase inhibitors widely used as pesticides.[135–137] Accidental exposure occurs during manufacture and application, although OP poisoning as a result of accidental exposure is uncommon in the United States and serious examples are rarely seen.[137] Because these compounds are readily available, intentional overdosing is common in suicide attempts, particularly in India.[138] OP compounds gain entry through the lungs and gastrointestinal tract, and across the skin. Metabolism takes place in the liver and kidneys, and metabolites are excreted in the urine. Although acute toxicity is related to tight binding to acetylcholinesterase, enzymes involved in metabolism are not irreversibly bound.

Acute OP toxicity is related to slowly reversible or irreversible binding to and phosphorylation of acetylcholinesterase. Acetylcholinesterase inhibition alters the normal physiology of cholinergic synapses by allowing accumulation of acetylcholine.[137] Cholinergic overactivity at muscarinic synaptic junctions of the autonomic nervous system produce miosis, increased bronchial secretions, excessive sweating, gastric hyperactivity with abdominal cramps and diarrhea, and bradycardia.[139] Central muscarinic effects include anxiety, restlessness, headache, confusion, and convulsions. Overactivity at nicotinic neuromuscular junctions produces fasciculations and weakness. With sufficient dose, respiratory failure may result from weakness, airway obstruction, and depression of medullary respiratory centers.[139,140]

Laboratory findings associated with OP exposure include depression of serum cholinesterase activity and red blood cell (RBC) cholinesterase. Typically, serum cholinesterase is more labile than RBC cholinesterase and declines more rapidly with exposure. RBC cholinesterase activity closely reflects physiologic effects in the nervous system and is used to assess toxicity. Acute symptoms may develop after a 70% or greater decrease in baseline cholinesterase levels, but are not believed to occur with less marked levels of cholinesterase inhibition.[141] Acute muscarinic effects during the first 24 hours, including autonomic and medullary respiratory effects, are treated with atropine.[139] Reactivation of the phosphorylated cholinesterase can be hastened by several oxime compounds, of which pyridine-2-aldoxime methyl chloride (2-PAM, pralidoxime) is the most useful clinically. 2-PAM acts at the neuromuscular junction and reverses skeletal muscle weakness, but not at muscarinic sites.[136,142]

Several syndromes associated with OP intoxication have a delayed onset after acute exposure. A largely reversible weakness involving head and proximal muscles occurring 24–96 hours after acute intoxication during the initial recovery from the cholinergic phase has been described by Senanayake and Karalliedde[143] as an intermediate syndrome. The most interesting and well-studied late effect of OP intoxication is a rapidly progressive polyneuropathy occurring 2–4 weeks after acute exposure.[135] This OP-induced delayed neuropathy (OPIDN) as described by Senanayake and Johnson[144] is characterized by distal paresthesias, impaired reflexes, and progressive weakness. It is more likely to occur with subacute and chronic OP exposure than after a single large dose, and is often associated with subsequent appearance of a superimposed myelopathy.[137] Recovery follows, although it may be incomplete, and spasticity becomes a prominent late feature, consistent with corticospinal fiber involvement.[145] Intoxications of epidemic proportions occur after triorthocresyl phosphate (TOCP) ingestion. These include exposure to adulterated Jamaican ginger extract in the United States (jake leg paralysis) and contaminated cooking oil in Morocco.[145,146] The neuropathy as described by Aring[145] was heralded by dysesthesias, followed by progressive distal weakness.[146] Sensory testing was essentially normal, but subjective pain was common. Reflexes were reduced at the ankles, but were normal or brisk elsewhere. Recovery of strength was sometimes incomplete, and when a stable stage was reached after a year, spasticity was a prominent feature.[146,147]

Electrodiagnostic findings associated with OP intoxication depend on the timing of the evaluation. During acute intoxication, findings are similar to those associated with cholinesterase intoxication, which are sometimes observed in myasthenia gravis patients. Acetylcholinesterase inhibitors used to treat myasthenia gravis produce muscarinic and nicotinic effects identical to those seen in acute OP intoxication.[139] The response to high-dose exposure to medicinal and OP agents is a repetitive discharge of the motor nerve after a single depolarizing stimulus (Figure 8.8).[137,148,149] Such responses are the earliest and most sensitive alteration of acetylcholinesterase inhibition, regardless of the severity of intoxication.[137] The mechanism of repetitive discharges presumably involves recurrent depolarization of the postsynaptic end-plate by persistent acetylcholine, producing a prolonged end-plate potential.[150] In addition, excess acetylcholine may interact with receptors on the terminal axon just distal to the last myelinated node.[137] Activation of these receptors likely accounts for antidromic backfiring of the motor axon, producing spontaneous fasciculations, repetitive spontaneous discharges to a single action potential, and repetitive discharges to a single supramaximal stimulus.[137]

A decremental response occurs to repetitive supramaximal stimulation of the motor nerve in OP intoxication. The decreased CMAP ampli-

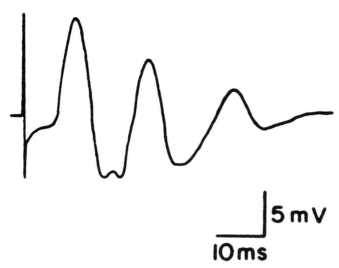

5mV

10ms

FIGURE 8.8   Repetitive discharges following the initial CMAP in response to a single supramaximal stimulation from a patient with acute OP intoxication. (From L Gutmann, R Besser. Organophosphate intoxication: pharmacologic, neurophysiologic, clinical, and therapeutic considerations. Semin Neurol 1990;10:46. With permission of Thieme Medical Publishers, Inc. [copyright 1990].).

tude is maximal with the second stimulus and is followed by a progressive increment in the response amplitude, similar to the decremental response to low rates of stimulation (e.g., 3 Hz) associated with myasthenia gravis. It differs from the response seen in myasthenia, however, in that the decrement response is most pronounced with higher stimulation rates and is dependent on CMAP duration; longer durations are associated with the appearance of decrement at lower stimulation rates.[151] CMAP recordings (20 Hz median nerve stimulation) obtained from a patient with OP intoxication are shown in Figure 8.9, demonstrating an initial severe depolarizing block (69 hours), a subsequent decremental response and repetitive discharges (day 4), and later improvement with a decrement-increment response (day 12). Similar decremental motor responses with normal nerve conduction studies and needle EMG, consistent with partial postsynaptic neuromuscular blockade and atypical of the decrement observed in myasthenia gravis or the myasthenic syndrome, have been reported for the "intermediate syndrome."[138,143,152]

CMAP recordings from workers with subclinical OP exposure have been reported by Jager et al.[149] to show abnormalities even after single exposures. However, interpretation of these data on subclinical exposure is unclear, given the absence of clinically evident weakness despite low-amplitude CMAPs and decrement to repetitive motor nerve stimulation. In addition, other studies of neuromuscular transmission by single fiber

20 Hz Stimulation

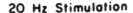

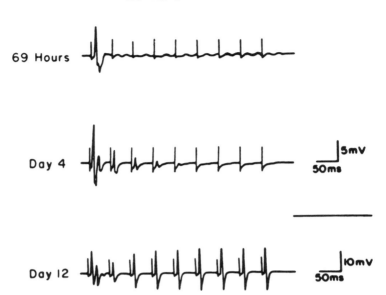

FIGURE 8.9   Decrement-increment response to 20 Hz supramaximal median stimulation (recording thenar muscles) and repetitive CMAP discharges recorded from a patient with OP intoxication, 3, 4, and 12 days after intoxication. (From L Gutmann, R Besser. Organophosphate intoxication: pharmacologic, neurophysiologic, clinical, and therapeutic considerations. Semin Neurol 1990;10:46. With permission of Thieme Medical Publishers, Inc. [copyright 1990].)

EMG techniques measuring jitter under similar conditions of OP exposure found no abnormalities referable to the neuromuscular junction.[153]

Electrodiagnostic findings in OPIDN include reduced SNAP and CMAP amplitudes, but normal nerve conduction velocities.[152,154] Needle EMG reveals signs of denervation with reduced recruitment consistent with the degree of weakness, and subsequent evidence of denervation and reinnervation.[144,152,154] Pathologic findings in OPIDN reported by Bischoff[155] and Cavanagh[156] include evidence of a central and peripheral distal axonopathy; in peripheral nerves there is axonal degeneration of motor and sensory fibers, and in the central nervous system there is loss of corticospinal tract fibers and sensory fibers in the dorsal column nuclei. Studies have demonstrated that axonal degeneration does not occur from isolated acetylcholinesterase inhibition. Rather, a neural protein with esteratic activity has been identified and named neurotoxic esterase (NTE).[157,158] NTE is distributed in the central and peripheral nervous systems and binds to neurotoxic organophosphorus compounds, although the steps leading to axonal degeneration are not established.[157–159] Inhibition of NTE (by phosphorylation) followed by loss of an alkyl group to produce a negatively charged phosphorylated NTE (aging) is an additional required step in the pathogenesis of OPIDN.[152] There is no known treatment for the delayed neuropathy.

Kaplan and associates[160] report eight patients in whom symptoms of a distal sensory neuropathy (axonopathy) developed after repeated respiratory and dermal chlorpyrifos exposure in enclosed, commercially fumigated sites. This reversible sensory neuropathy was associated with mild cognitive dysfunction in five of the patients, and evaluation demonstrated no other explanation for the neurologic disorder. This type of neuropathy has not been associated with OP compounds previously, and is distinct from OPIDN, described above.

METALS

Metals are used in many industrial applications and several have a history of medicinal application. Nevertheless, as a heterogeneous group they have neurotoxic effects, not only in the vicinity of the workplace but also in the general environment. Several of the most common neurotoxic metals are described below.

Arsenic

Arsenic is a toxic metalloid that has had both medicinal and homicidal applications.[31,161,162] Acute toxicity has been associated with numerous compounds containing arsenic, including pesticides, paints, wood preservatives, and mordants.[163] Chronic occupational exposure occurs in copper and lead smelting processes and in pesticide manufacturing.[48,163,164] Arsenic is readily absorbed from the gastrointestinal tract after ingestion, and a small portion is excreted in the feces. Following absorption, arsenic is rapidly excreted in the urine; the half-life of urinary excretion is approximately 3 weeks.[165] Even with low exposures, small amounts of arsenic accumulate in tissues; the magnitude of exposure is documented by the amount excreted in the urine or accumulated in hair or nails.[31] Transient increases in urinary excretion follow ingestion of certain seafoods containing organic arsenic.[164,166]

Arsenic-induced neuropathy is a common complication of arsenic intoxication. Like all metallic intoxications, arsenical neuropathy presents as one component of a systemic illness.[164] Following ingestion, symptoms suggest an acute gastrointestinal illness with nausea, vomiting, and diarrhea. Subsequently, symptoms and signs consistent with diffuse involvement appear, including dermatitis, encephalopathy, and cardiomyopathy in association with pancytopenia and abnormal liver function studies reflecting hepatitis.[164,167-169] Neuropathic features present subacutely 5–10 days after a single exposure and progress for weeks.[164,167-170] Initial neurologic complaints include symmetric distal numbness with painful paresthesias, unsteady gait, myalgia, and muscle cramping. Findings include ascending limb weakness, sensory loss affecting all modalities, and hypoactive or

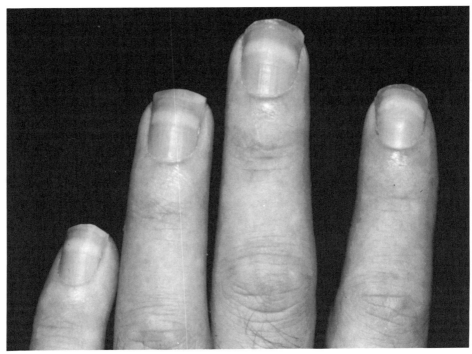

FIGURE 8.10   Mees' lines in the nails of a patient following arsenic intoxication resulting in severe sensorimotor neuropathy. (From JW Albers and MB Bromberg. Neuromuscular Emergencies. In GR Schwartz [ed], Principles and Practice of Emergency Medicine. Philadelphia: Lea & Febiger, 1992. With permission of Lea & Febiger [copyright 1990].)

absent reflexes. Severity depends on the magnitude of the arsenic load, varying from mild sensory loss with distal paresthesias to severe sensory loss with hyperpathia, dysautonomia, quadriplegia, and respiratory failure. Distinctive clinical features include hyperkeratosis, pigmented dermatitis, and Mees' lines.[167] Mees' lines appear 4–6 weeks after ingestion, growing out of the base of the nails (Figure 8.10), but are not pathognomonic for arsenic intoxication. Cerebrospinal fluid protein is frequently elevated, often between 150 and 300 mg/dl.[167] An aplastic anemia with pancytopenia and basophilic stippling develop with severe arsenic intoxication, and the diagnosis may be suggested by these findings.[167]

The neurologic presentation and early electrodiagnostic findings are suggestive of the Guillain-Barré syndrome.[167,171] Early electrodiagnostic findings include increased temporal dispersion and partial conduction block along motor nerves, slowed motor nerve conduction velocity, and low amplitude or absent sensory responses. Findings in motor nerves, shown in Figure 8.11, often fulfill criteria suggestive of acquired demyelination.[167,172] Serial studies, however, display features

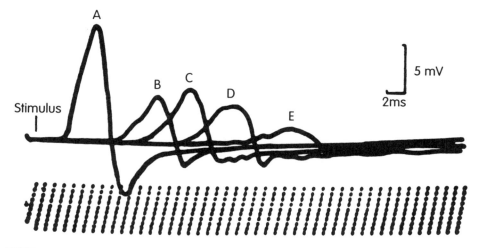

FIGURE 8.11   Surface recording of the CMAP recorded from the abductor digiti minimi muscle of a patient with acute arsenic intoxication, following percutaneous stimulation of the ulnar nerve at the wrist (A), below the elbow (B), above the elbow (C), at the axilla (D), and at Erb's point (E). Recording was performed 12 days after the onset of sensory complaints. Note the abnormal temporal dispersion and partial conduction block with stimulation at the elbow (B) and Erb's point (E). (From PD Donofrio et al. Acute arsenic intoxication presenting as Guillain-Barré–like syndrome. Muscle Nerve 1987;10:114. With permission of John Wiley & Sons, Inc. [copyright 1987].)

of a distal dying-back axonal neuropathy with progressive deterioration of evoked motor amplitudes and profuse fibrillation potentials.[167] Peripheral nerve histology demonstrates axonal (wallerian) degeneration involving larger-diameter fibers to a greater degree than the small fibers,[164] although reports suggesting primary segmental demyelination and remyelination exist.[170] Most likely the segmental demyelination is secondary to generalized axonal failure, appearing before there is clear evidence of axonal degeneration.

Chronic arsenic intoxication may result from occupational exposure in the smelting industry. The presence of a subclinical sensory neuropathy has been suggested using discriminate analysis of electrodiagnostic measures and arsenic load in a blinded evaluation of arsenic smelter workers.[48]

The laboratory diagnosis of arsenic intoxication is based on demonstration of increased urinary excretion. Blood levels are not usually helpful because of rapid clearance.[164] Intoxication also may be based on increased arsenic levels in hair and nails, because arsenic is bound to keratin in these growing tissues.[164]

Patients who survive the initial arsenic intoxication demonstrate partial or complete neurologic recovery over months to years, depending on the degree and extent of denervation. Patients with mild neuropathy recover completely, whereas patients with severe neuropathy may have residual distal sensory loss and weakness. Dimercaptopropanol (British antilewisite; BAL) interferes with binding of arsenic and increases its rate of urinary excretion.[164] Chelating agents such as penicillamine may increase tissue mobilization and the amount of arsenic excreted, but it is unclear whether dimercaptopropanol or penicillamine alters outcome.[164,165] Therapeutic plasma exchange has no apparent effect on outcome.[167]

Lead

The history of lead toxicity (plumbism) begins in antiquity and is intertwined with the development of industry in general and metallurgy in particular.[173] Lead is absorbed through the respiratory and gastrointestinal systems. Approximately 90% of the total body burden is in bone, and increased levels have occurred since the Industrial Revolution.[174] Diet is a major source of lead, especially among children who ingest lead pigment-based paint (pica). Paint chips may contain 6 mg lead per square centimeter.[175] Automobile exhaust contaminated by lead fuel additives is another source of exposure. An important nonoccupational source of lead is illicit whiskey made in lead-lined stills. Occupational exposures occur from lead smelting, reprocessing of lead-containing products (batteries, demolition of lead-painted structures), manufacturing of paint pigments, repairing of automobile radiators, and prolonged attendance in firearm shooting galleries.[174]

The effects of lead are widely distributed throughout the body and include hemopoietic, renal, hepatic, endocrinologic, cardiovascular, and reproductive systems. Acute toxic exposure causes gastrointestinal symptoms in the form of abdominal cramps, constipation, and anorexia. Chronic exposure may produce skin pallor, gingival lead line, weight loss, constipation, and signs and symptoms of anemia.[175] Acute and chronic exposures in children may cause encephalopathy and impaired cognition.[175,176] Neuropathy is rare but more common in adults than in children.[175] Lead neuropathy is primarily a motor neuropathy, reportedly involving upper before lower extremities.[177] Extensor muscles may be preferentially involved, causing a characteristic wrist and foot drop that may be asymmetric. Sensory loss is mild compared to weakness.[178]

Few individuals with symptomatic lead neuropathy have been studied using modern electrodiagnostic techniques. In a patient reported by Oh,[179] nerve conduction studies showed mild slowing of motor and sensory conduction velocities and reduced sensory amplitudes. Needle EMG showed abnormal spontaneous activity, reduced recruitment, and increased motor unit polyphasia, but the patient may have had a superimposed ethanol neuropathy. These findings are consistent with axonal involvement, as are sural nerve biopsy findings reported by Buchthal and Behse.[180] A lead-exposed worker with hand muscle atrophy but normal sensation had nerve conduction evidence of a focal ulnar mononeuropathy.[181] Resolution of nerve conduction abnormalities occurred over a few months in association with chelation, suggesting to the authors that subclinical entrapment may relate to increased nerve vulnerability in lead neuropathy.

The question of a subclinical lead neuropathy following chronic exposure is difficult to assess, particularly with regard to dose-response relationships and threshold serum lead levels associated with nerve conduction abnormalities.[173,182,183] Support for a subclinical neuropathy is in the form of nerve conduction abnormalities in exposed subjects (documented by work histories and measures of serum lead levels) compared to unexposed control populations. Specific findings include abnormal temporal dispersion or partial conduction block of peroneal motor nerve conduction,[184] slowing of motor or sensory conduction velocities,[175,185] and preferential reduction of the slower conducting components of motor nerves.[186,187] Needle EMG findings supportive of an axonal neuropathy include abnormal spontaneous activity and mild abnormalities of motor unit action potentials.[187,188] Attempts have been made to define a threshold by correlating the magnitude of changes with the serum lead level. Serum levels of 30 mg/dl are associated by Schwartz and associates[189] with slow conduction in motor nerves. In adults, serum levels of 50 mg /dl,[190] 70 mg /dl,[188] and 80 mg/dl[185] are associated with slow conduction velocity.

Arguments that a subclinical neuropathy has not been convincingly demonstrated in subjects with serum lead levels below 60 mg/dl include studies showing no significant changes in conduction velocity at this level when compared to unexposed control populations,[191] significant changes in isolated nerves but all conduction velocities within the normal population range,[192] no significant change in conduction velocity in a prospective study of exposed workers,[190] and slowed sural nerve conduction without underlying histologic abnormalities.[180] From the statistical standpoint, there is concern for making multiple statistical comparisons and broad inferences from statistically significant but isolated differences. From the methodologic standpoint, many studies have design flaws.[182] Evaluation of 95 workers occupationally exposed to lead for more than 9 years whose blood lead concentrations were below or slightly above 70 mg/100 ml (the hygienic border value) failed to identify clinical evidence of neuropathy in any of the workers.[193] Furthermore, quantitative sensory and electrodiagnostic evaluations were normal when compared to those of age-matched controls subjects, suggesting that peripheral lead neuropathy is unusual when blood lead levels are kept within an acceptable range.

Pathologic studies of nerves from asymptomatic subjects using modern techniques also are limited. Buchthal and Behse[180] report a reduction in the number of myelinated fibers in the sural nerve, although they were within the normal range, and mild changes in myelin. The changes were insufficient to account for the slowed conduction described above. Data from experimental animals exposed to lead may not be helpful because of marked species differences in response to lead.[194] Lead neuropathy in rats and guinea pigs demonstrates primary demyelination, but few consistent changes are noted in nerves of nonhuman primates.[194] This raises the further question of whether the parameter of nerve conduction velocity is the appropriate one to measure in humans. If lead causes axonal loss, the amplitude of the sensory evoked response would be expected to be a more sensitive measure. Yet, in studies in which amplitude has been measured, it has been higher in exposed subjects.[180] In summary, the electrophysiologic and pathologic data from subjects with serum levels below 60 mg/dl have not convincingly demonstrated a subclinical peripheral neuropathy. Abnormalities that have been reported are mild and are present as averaged differences in the sample population. Thus, it is questionable whether small changes in conduction velocity, which are within the normal range, can be used to suggest a subclinical lead neuropathy in an asymptomatic individual.

Lead levels reflecting recent exposure can be measured in blood and urine. Body stores can be measured indirectly in urine as mobilized lead after chelation by calcium disodium (calcium disodium versenate).[195] There are various measures of the effect of lead on heme synthesis. An elevation of free erythroporphyrin is thought to reflect altered iron incorporation in heme at the mitochondrial level. The resultant reduction in heme synthesis causes an anemia of the microcytic and hypochromic type, and basophilic stippling of red cells.[196] There are similarities in the metabolic alterations of heme synthesis occurring from acute intermittent porphyria and lead toxicity, although lead intoxication appears to interrupt later stages of metabolism.[197] With lead intoxication, there may be pronounced urinary excretion of delta-aminolevulinic acid and coproporphyrinogen, in part as a consequence of aminolevulinic acid dehydrase inhibition.[198] In porphyria, there also is an increase in urinary porphobilinogen, which is less evident in lead poisoning.[173,198]

Symptomatic patients with high lead levels, especially following acute toxicity, have been treated primarily with calcium disodium ethylenediaminetetraacetic acid (CaNa$_2$EDTA; Calcium Disodium Versenate),[199] and with penicillamine.[200] CaNa$_2$EDTA chelates with lead by displacing calcium, drawing primarily from bone stores of lead. It is poorly absorbed from the gastrointestinal tract and after intravenous administration is excreted almost entirely in urine.[201] Renal toxicity is of concern and is usually reversible, but may be fatal.[199] Penicillamine may be used alone or with CaNa$_2$EDTA.[201] In chronic exposures resulting in peripheral neuropathy, halting exposure and use of chelation therapy have been reported by Feldman and associates,[175] with improvement over several months to years.

Similarities between the primary motor neuropathy caused by lead and motor neuron disease (amyotrophic lateral sclerosis [ALS]) have been noted, and a relationship between occult plumbism and motor neuron disease has been questioned.[202] Several trials have been undertaken to administer chelation therapy to patients with motor neuron disease but without known lead exposure. The results demonstrated no improvement or change in rate of progression, and there were a number of side effects, some of which may have hastened death.[174,203]

Mercury

Mercury and its compounds have been used for centuries and once were among the most widely prescribed medications. The neurotoxicity of mercury is well established, particularly in reference to occupational exposures. Mercury has many uses. In metal form, it is an excellent electrical conductor and is used in switches and other electrical apparatus. It is used as an antiseptic, as a wood preservative, in tanning and felt treatments, in the chloralkali industry, in paint manufacturing, in thermometers, in amalgam in dental fillings, and in the production of nuclear weapons.[204–206] Mercury is absorbed by the lungs or through the skin following direct contact. After ingestion, it is partially absorbed by the gastrointestinal tract, depending on its form, with elemental mercury being absorbed very poorly. Absorbed mercury is transformed in blood and tissues and excreted in the bile and urine.[205] The mechanism of mercury intoxication is not known, but it is thought to combine and interfere with sulfhydryl groups in enzymes or structural proteins.[164]

The diagnosis of mercury-associated neurotoxicity consists of demonstrating an appropriate neurologic syndrome in a setting of sufficient exposure with appropriate documentation of body burden.[164] Documentation of methyl mercury intoxication may be difficult because of the high affinity of the nervous system for methyl mercury and the lack of abnormal mercury excretion.[164] Inorganic or metallic mercury intoxication usually can be confirmed by abnormal urinary excretion, because excretion is slow with a half-life of approximately 60 days.[164] Urine measures reflect recent exposures and, to a lesser extent, body burden.[207] Blood levels of mercury can be measured but are poor indicators of body burden. Accumulation of mercury in tissues can be measured using hair levels or x-ray fluorescences of bone.[208]

The laboratory diagnosis of mercury intoxication is based on demonstration of increased urinary excretion in 24-hour urine collections or spot samples. Most studies have reported an increased likelihood of neurotoxic effects when urine mercury levels for individual patients exceed 500 µg per liter, and the number of peak levels exceeding 500 µg per liter following repeated exposures may be the best predictor of minimal neurologic impairments.[209,210]

Dimercaptopropanol has been used after acute mercury ingestion or inhalation, and dimercaptopropanol, dimercaptosuccinic acid, and penicillamine may increase tissue mobilization and excretion.[164,207,211] It is unclear whether the increased excretion is associated with mobilization of mercury from the nervous system,[164] although successful treatment of chronic inorganic mercury neurotoxicity using penicillamine has been reported by Markowitz and Schaumburg.[212] The efficacy of chelation, hemodialysis, and exchange transfusion in patients with organic mercury intoxication is not established.[213] Chelation should be used only in selected cases, depending on the exposure magnitude, the type of mercury exposure, and the clinical impairment.[207]

Elemental Mercury

Exposure to elemental mercury and its compounds produces symptoms and signs referable to the central and peripheral nervous systems, including behavioral manifestations, tremor, and neuropathy. The precise effects depend on the type of exposure, the dose, and the chemical state of the element.[164] In general, exposures are of three types: isolated inadvertent exposures, repeated single exposures, or chronic low-level exposures. Occupational exposure usually is monitored by urine excretion, and workers are removed from exposure when urine mercury levels exceed some threshold, such as 500 µg per liter. Differences between chronic low-level exposure and recurrent exposures are unclear, but recent evidence suggests that the magnitude of a single exposure or the number of repeated exposures may be a better indicator of peripheral neurotoxicity than overall duration of exposure.[204]

Acute high-level mercury vapor exposure produces erosive bronchitis and interstitial pneumonitis with pulmonary edema.[207] Respiratory symptoms may be combined with abdominal pain, nausea, vomiting, diarrhea, and renal insufficiency, as well as corrosive damage to other mucous membranes.[206] Neurologic symptoms appear approximately 24 hours later and include tremor, increased excitability, headache, perioral numbness, and slowed speech.[206,207] Findings related to isolated sublethal exposures are associated with spontaneous recovery.[211,214]

Chronic elemental mercury intoxication from repeated isolated or ongoing low-level exposures produces mental status changes called erethism and an abnormal static tremor of the outstretched hands. The term *erythism* was used in the late nineteenth century to describe a variety of features, including a tendency to blush, timidity, diffidence, shyness, loss of self-confidence, anxiety, a desire to remain unobtrusive, a pathologic fear of ridicule, an explosive loss of temper when criticized, insomnia, and hyperexcitability.[164,215–217] These nonspecific neuropsychological symptoms are generally interpreted as personality or behavioral changes, perhaps associated with memory and concentration impairments.[215] The behavioral changes develop in association with the most characteristic neurologic sign of mercury toxicity, postural tremor.[164,215] Abnormal tremor is an early manifestation of mercury toxicity (Hatter's shakes), demonstrating a dose-response effect in workers exposed to elemental mercury.[218,219] It is most apparent in the outstretched hands and differs from the coarse, low-frequency resting tremor characteristic of Parkinson's disease. Acrodynia is a rare and controversial syndrome of mercurialism that occurs in children, consisting of mental changes, abnormal sensation, photophobia, and peripheral vascular abnormalities with red swollen hands and cold, swollen feet with desquamation.[220,221] Mercury intoxication also produces a sensorimotor neuropathy.[164,181,204,222–224] Symptoms and signs include distal tingling and numbness, diminished vibration and position sensations, distal weakness, and reduced or absent reflexes.[222] There are reports of a syndrome resembling motor neuron disease,[225,226] although most descriptions include abnormal sensory nerve conduction studies.

A comparison of mercury-exposed workers at a thermometer factory with unexposed workers found that exposed workers reported more symptoms than referents, although the symptoms could not be associated with mercury exposure.[227] Static tremor, abnormal Romberg's sign, and difficulty with tandem gait were more prevalent among exposed workers, but evidence of neuropathy was not established.[227] Evidence of neuropathy among asymptomatic workers exposed to elemental mercury has been associated with elevated urinary mercury indexes.[223] In addition, comparison of previously exposed workers to workers with less exposure or no exposure demonstrates an increased prevalence of neuropathy and other findings consistent with central nervous system dysfunction.[204] Shapiro and associates[208] found that 30% of dentists with raised tissue levels of mercury had electrodiagnostic evidence of reduced mean sural and median motor conduction velocities compared to control subjects, findings consistent with subclinical neuropathy. Similar findings were reported by Richter and associates,[228] who reported distal EMG abnormalities in a group of asymptomatic thermometer factory workers. Mild slowing of average median motor conduction velocity was found in 16 workers chronically exposed to inorganic mercury compared to unexposed workers.[181] The reduced conduction velocity correlated with increased mercury levels in blood and urine and an increased number of neurologic symptoms, although sensory conduction abnormalities or group differences in these workers could not be demonstrated.

Electrodiagnostic evaluations of patients with established mercury neuropathy are limited. Barber reports two patients with mercuric oxide exposure, documented by needle EMG abnormalities, reduced sensory amplitudes, and reduced conduction velocities.[226] Vroom and Greer[229] report nine patients with mercury vapor exposure who had slightly reduced sensory and motor conduction velocities with prolonged distal latencies and neurogenic changes on needle EMG. Electrodiagnostic examination of a dentist intoxicated by mercury reported by Iyer and coworkers demonstrated borderline-low sensory amplitudes.[222] Comparison of mercury-exposed workers by Albers and coworkers[223] showed that workers with clinical evidence of mild neuropathy had reduced sensory evoked amplitudes, prolonged distal latencies, and increased likelihood of abnormalities on needle EMG compared to the remaining workers.

The combined clinical, electrodiagnostic, and epidemiologic descriptions suggest that elemental mercury exposure may be associated with a sensorimotor neuropathy of the axonal type. Neuropathy may be associated with central nervous system involvement or appear in isolation. Improvement following removal from exposure may be complete, except after years of exposure or particularly high-level exposure.[207]

Organic Mercury

The neurologic consequences of organic mercury compounds are generally more severe than those associated with inorganic compounds.[230] Organic mercury compounds are absorbed by inhalation of vapor, ingestion, or absorption through the skin. Organic mercury compounds such as methyl mercury are bound to plasma proteins and transported into cells by an unknown mechanism.[207] Organic mercury compounds may resist biologic degradation, and mercury is excreted slowly in the bile and the urine.[207] Inorganic mercury chloride discharged into Minamata Bay in Japan entered the food chain after conversion to methyl mercury.[35,231] Following ingestion of contaminated seafood, intoxicated patients developed ataxia, dysarthria, tremor, and mental impairment consistent with central involvement, as well as distal paresthesias suggestive of a sensory neuropathy.[164,231] Other reports of organic mercury poisoning include outbreaks in Iraq that followed ingestion of wheat seed treated with an organic mercurial fungicide.[149,213,232] Like the patients from Minamata, the Iraqi patients developed dysarthria, ataxia, constricted visual fields, evidence of encephalopathy, and prominent sensory symptoms thought to reflect peripheral involvement. Nevertheless, electrophysiologic evaluations reported by LeQuesne and colleagues[233] of 19 patients with organic mercury poisoning, including four severely involved patients, failed to demonstrate abnormalities, suggesting that the sensory disturbances reflected central nervous system dysfunction. Unremarkable electrodiagnostic evaluations of patients intoxicated with methyl mercury also are reported by Von Burg and Rustam.[230]

Thallium

Thallium is an element that resembles tin but is malleable like lead.[234] It is used industrially in glass and alloys. Historically, like mercury and arsenic, it has had therapeutic applications, including treatment of venereal diseases, tuberculosis, and ringworm.[164,234] It also has been used for rodent and insect control, and intoxications today involve accidental or homicidal poisoning. Thallium salts are water-soluble and are readily absorbed from the gastrointestinal and respiratory tracts and skin.[165] Thallium is distributed uniformly throughout the body and is eliminated via the gastrointestinal tract and kidneys.[234] The pathways of absorption and excretion follow those of potassium, and it enters cells through potassium channels.[165] The precise neurotoxic mechanism is unclear, although thallium is believed to interfere with oxidative phosphorylation.[165] It also may interfere with the sodium/potassium–adenosine triphosphatase (ATPase) system, and its biological effect may be related to binding of sulfhydryl groups.[164]

The neurotoxic effects of thallium have recently been summarized.[164,234] Following oral intoxication, nausea, vomiting, and diarrhea appear. Within days, pain and paresthesias develop in the distal extremities, followed by distal limb weakness and eventual atrophy.[164,165] As in acute arsenic intoxication, reflexes initially remain intact when sensory loss and weakness are clinically evident; this initial preservation of reflexes may be useful in differentiating thallium-induced neuropathy from an acute Guillain-Barré syndrome.[234] With increasing dose, central nervous system manifestations occur, including convulsions and coma.[164] Systemic manifestations include nephropathy, anemia, and hepatotoxicity. The hallmark of intoxication is alopecia.[164,234] Mees' lines, as seen in arsenic intoxication, may be apparent.[235] Alopecia develops several weeks after intoxication, and Mees' lines are not apparent for an even longer period of time, but neither are diagnostically helpful in the initial stages of clinical involvement.

Andersen[236] describes three cases of thallium neuropathy resulting from ingestion of thallium-contaminated milk. The most severely involved patient vomited repeatedly after drinking the milk and within hours experienced paresthesias in hands, feet, and tongue. Hyperalgesia and facial, bulbar, and lower-extremity weakness subsequently developed. Within 3 days the patient required intubation and subsequently became comatose and died. Botulism intoxication was suspected before demonstration of elevated serum thallium levels. The patient's husband experienced painful distal paresthesias, hypesthesia, distal weakness, urinary retention, obstipation, stomatitis, and anhidrosis. He became somnolent, and alopecia developed 2 weeks later. Recovery ensued over approximately 4 months. In a third exposed family member, only painful paresthesias and decreased vibration sensation developed.

The combination of abdominal pain, autonomic dysfunction, and progressive neuropathy is similar to abnormalities associated with acute porphyric neuropathy, although urinary excretion of porphobilinogen and delta-aminolevulinic acid is not increased in thallium neuropathy.[164,234] Chelation has not been reported as useful in the treatment of thallium poisoning.[164] Although potassium administration increases the excretion rate of thallium, this is of little practical benefit.[164] The degree of recovery depends on the severity of axonal degeneration and extent of regeneration and reinnervation.

There are few electrodiagnostic descriptions of thallium-induced neuropathy. Kalantri and associates[237] describe sequential evaluations of a victim of an apparent attempted homicidal poisoning. All findings were consistent with an axonal sensorimotor neuropathy. Pathologic evaluations reported by Cavanagh[165] demonstrated distal axonal degeneration with evidence of chromatolysis in dorsal root ganglion and anterior horn cells. All findings are consistent with a dying-back axonopathy involving sensory and motor axons. Whether this is related to a direct effect on the terminal axon or a primary effect on the cell body is not established.[164]

Tin

Organotins are used as stabilizers in plastic polymers and as catalysts in several processes including polyurethane formation and silicone and epoxy curing.[238] Trialkyl tin compounds are biocidal and have been used as repellents and wood product and textile preservatives.[239] They also are used agriculturally to treat fungal diseases and as disinfectants.[238] Of the large number of organotin compounds, the alkyl tins, triethyltin, and trimethyltin are known to be neurotoxic. They are absorbed through the skin and from the gastrointestinal tract. Their mechanism of action is unknown.

Besser and colleagues[240] associate acute trimethyltin exposure with a limbic-cerebellar syndrome consisting of disorientation, confabulation, amnesia, hyperphagia, seizures, nystagmus, ataxia, and a mild sensory neuropathy. Symptoms consistent with neuropathy consist of paresthesias in the legs. None of the symptomatic individuals exhibit reflex abnormalities or sensory loss, and electrodiagnostic studies were normal, except one individual who had a slightly reduced sural nerve conduction velocity but a normal amplitude. The clinical and electrodiagnostic evidence suggests that any peripheral component to trimethyltin exposure is minimal compared to the central nervous system manifestations.

Trimethyltin interferes with myelinogenesis in developing rats in the central nervous system but not in the sciatic nerve.[239] Rats chronically given triethyltin develop symmetric weakness in the hind legs and sensory loss in the tail, along with electrophysiologic and morphologic sciatic abnormalities.[241] The neuropathy was characterized by intramyelinic vacuole formation secondary to separation of myelin sheath lamellas. Axons contained increased numbers of neurofilaments and neurotubules. Acute triethyltin intoxication also is associated with central and peripheral nervous system edema.[238] Termination of exposure results in return of myelin sheath to normal without evidence of the myelin loss or axonal degeneration.[238]

Summary

Identification of chemically induced toxic neuropathy is an important but sometimes difficult task. In some respects, this task becomes easier as an increasing number of acquired and hereditary etiologies are identified. Over 40% of patients referred to neuromuscular centers for evaluation of undiagnosed neuropathy have inherited disorders, and over 33% are found to have a treatable or removable cause.[242] The task also is simplified by establishing reliable standards for identifying the presence and severity of neuropathy and establishing the underlying pathophysiology. Most toxic neuropathies are symmetric, with a prominent distal predilection for sensory and motor symptoms. Large fibers are commonly involved, and unequivocal distal vibratory sensation loss and diminished or absent muscle stretch reflexes are reliable early findings. Preservation of Achilles reflexes is incompatible with the diagnosis of clinically significant neuropathy, the only exceptions being rare forms of isolated small-fiber disease and some motor neuropathies early in their course.

The underlying pathophysiology is investigated using nerve conduction studies and needle EMG. Most chemically induced neuropathies are of the axonal type. Amplitude measurements are sensitive indicators of axonal loss, and the presence or absence of primary demyelination, rare in toxic neuropathy, is easily established using conduction measures.[243] Electromyographic evidence of partial distal denervation is characterized by symmetric fibrillation potentials. The needle EMG examination also is useful in establishing the duration of the disorder and identifying ongoing reinnervation. The most specific finding consistent with sensorimotor neuropathy is abnormal sensory evoked amplitudes; this localizes the lesion to the peripheral nervous system, at or distal to the dorsal root ganglia. There is no electrodiagnostic finding specifically diagnostic of a toxic etiology.

Clinical and electrodiagnostic findings of peripheral neuropathy should result in additional medical and laboratory investigations to identify systemic disorders associated with neuropathy or systemic findings associated with specific chemicals. Individual responses to neurotoxic exposure are important, although these usually reflect the magnitude of exposure necessary to produce involvement rather than a difference in the type of symptoms or neurologic findings. There may be different neurologic responses to increasing dosage, whereby low-level exposure results in symptoms and signs of mild neuropathy, and higher exposures produce superimposed evidence of encephalopathy, coma, and even death.

The most common industrial and agricultural chemicals associated with toxic neuropathy include some of the organic solvents and related compounds, neurotoxic nitriles, organophosphorus compounds, and metals. Simple association does not establish a toxic etiology and low-level exposure may produce transient, nonspecific complaints that are rarely helpful in establishing etiology. However, exposures sufficient to produce clinically evident neuropathy commonly are associated with other neurologic, systemic, and laboratory abnormalities. When present in appropriate combinations, such additional abnormalities help establish the diagnosis. Improvement over time after removal from exposure also is helpful in confirming the etiology; only rarely is the toxin so potent and the target so specific that irreversible peripheral damage ensues.

References

1. Sanenk Z. Toxic neuropathies. Semin Neurol 1987;7:9–17.
2. Goetz CG, Cohen MM. Neurotoxic Agents. In RT Joynt et al. (eds), Clinical Neurology. Philadelphia: Lippincott, 1990;1–83.
3. Albers JW, Bromberg MB. Neuromuscular Emergencies. In GR Schwartz (ed), Principles and Practice of Emergency Medicine. Philadelphia: Lea & Febiger, 1992;1544–1573.
4. Gregersen G. Diabetic neuropathy: influence of age, sex, metabolic control, and duration of diabetes on motor conduction velocity. Neurology 1967;17:972–980.
5. Behse F, Buchthal F, Carlsen F. Nerve biopsy and conduction studies in diabetic neuropathy. J Neurol Neurosurg Psychiatry 1977;40:1072–1082.
6. Albers JW. Clinical neurophysiology of generalized polyneuropathy. J Clin Neurophysiol 1993;10:149–166.
7. Daube JR. Electrophysiologic Testing in Diabetic Neuropathy. In PJ Dyck, PK Thomas, AK Asbury, AI Winegrad, D. Jr Porte (eds), Diabetic Neuropathy. Philadelphia: Saunders, 1987;162–176.
8. Donofrio PD, Albers JW. Polyneuropathy: classification by nerve conduction studies and electromyography. Muscle Nerve 1990;13:889–903.
9. Cummins KL, Dorfman LJ. Nerve fiber conduction velocity distributions: studies of normal and diabetic human nerves. Ann Neurol 1981;9:67–74.
10. Troni W, Carta Q, Cantello R. Peripheral nerve function and metabolic control in diabetes mellitus. Ann Neurol 1984;16:178–183.
11. Shahani BT, Halperin JJ, Bolu P et al. Sympathetic skin responses—a method of assessing unmyelinated axon dysfunction in peripheral neuropathies. J Neurol Neurosurg Psychiatry 1984;47:536–542.
12. Stetson DS, Albers JW, Silverstein BA et al. Effects of age, sex, and anthropometric factors on nerve conduction measures. Muscle Nerve 1992;15:1095–1104.
13. LaMontagne A, Buchthal F. Electrophysiological studies in diabetic neuropathy. J Neurol Neurosurg Psychiatry 1970;33:442–452.
14. Bastron JA, Thomas JE. Diabetic polyradiculopathy. Mayo Clin Proc 1981;56:725–732.
15. Albers JW. Common EMG Problems. In Course A: Fundamentals of EMG. Fifth Annual Continuing Education Course. Rochester, MN: American Association of Electromyography and Electrodiagnosis, 1982;59–67.
16. Allen N. Solvents and Other Industrial Organic Compounds. In PJ Vinken, GW Bruyn (eds), Handbook of Clinical Neurology. Amsterdam: Elsevier, 1979;361–389.
17. Seppalainen AM, Haltia M. Carbon Disulfide. In PS Spencer, HH Schaumburg (eds), Experimental and Clinical Neurotoxicology. Baltimore: Williams & Wilkins, 1980;356–373.
18. Schaumburg HH, Spencer PS. Human Toxic Neuropathy Due to Industrial Agents. In PJ Dyck, PK Thomas, EH Lambert, R Bunge (eds), Peripheral Neuropathy. Philadelphia: Saunders, 1984;2115–2132.
19. Lewey FH. Neurological, medical, and biochemical signs and symptoms indicating chronic industrial carbon disulfide absorption. Ann Intern Med 1941;15:869–883.

20. Vigliani EC. Carbon disulfide poisoning in viscose rayon factories. Br J Ind Med 1954;11:235–244.
21. Peters HA, Levine RL, Matthews CG et al. Carbon disulfide-induced neuropsychiatric changes in grain storage workers. Am J Ind Med 1982;3:373–391.
22. Peters HA, Levine RL, Matthews CG et al. Extrapyramidal and other neurologic manifestations associated with carbon disulfide fumigant exposure. Arch Neurol 1988;45:537–540.
23. Aaserud O, Hommeren OJ, Tvedt B et al. Carbon disulfide exposure and neurotoxic sequelae among viscose rayon workers. Am J Ind Med 1990;18:25–37.
24. Putz-Anderson V, Albright BE, Lee ST et al. A behavioral examination of workers exposed to carbon disulfide. Neurotoxicology 1983;4:67–78.
25. Seppalainen AM, Tolonen M. Neurotoxicity of long term exposure to carbon disulfide in the viscose rayon industry. A neurophysiological study. Work Environ Health 1974;11:145–153.
26. Johnson BL, Boyd J, Burg JR et al. Effects on the peripheral nervous system of workers' exposure to carbon disulfide. Neurotoxicology 1983;4:53–66.
27. Corsi G, Maestrelli GC, Picotti G et al. Chronic peripheral neuropathy in workers with previous exposure to carbon disulfide. Br J Ind Med 1983;40:209–211.
28. Gottfried MR, Graham DG, Morgan M et al. The morphology of carbon disulfide neurotoxicity. Neurotoxicology 1985;6:89–96.
29. Osuntokun BO. An ataxic neuropathy in Nigeria. A clinical, biochemical and electrophysiologic study. Brain 1968;91:215–248.
30. Schaumburg HH, Spencer PS, Thomas PK. Toxic Neuropathy: Occupational, Biological and Environmental Agents. In HH Schaumburg,PS Spencer, PK Thomas (eds), Disorders of Peripheral Nerves. Philadelphia: FA Davis, 1983;131–155.
31. Politis MJ, Schaumburg HH, Spencer PS. Neurotoxicity of Selected Chemicals. In PS Spencer, HH Schaumburg (eds), Experimental and Clinical Neurotoxicology. Baltimore: Williams & Wilkins, 1980;613–630.
32. Peterson CM, Tsairis P, Ohnishi A. Sodium cyanate induced polyneuropathy in patients with sickle-cell disease. Ann Intern Med 1974;81:152–158.
33. Charness ME, Simon RP, Greenberg DA. Medical progress: ethanol and the nervous system. N Engl J Med 1989;321:442–454.
34. Victor M, Adams RD,Collins GH. The Wernicke-Korsakoff Syndrome and Related Neurologic Disorders Due to Alcholism and Malnutrition. Contemporary Neurology Series, vol. 3. Philadelphia: F.A. Davis, 1989.
35. McLane JA. Decreased axonal transport in rat nerve following acute and chronic ethanol exposure. Alcohol 1987;4:385–389.
36. Behse F, Buchthal F. Alcoholic neuropathy: clinical, electrophysiological, and biopsy findings. Ann Neurol 1977;2:95–110.
37. Gross JA, Haas ML, Swift TR. Ethylene oxide neurotoxicity: report of four cases and review of the literature. Neurology 1979;29:978–983.
38. Windebank AJ, Blexrud MD. Residual ethylene oxide in hollow fiber hemodialysis units is neurotoxic in vitro. Ann Neurol 1989;26:63–68.
39. Steenland K, Stayner L, Greife A et al. Mortality among workers exposed to ethylene oxide. N Engl J Med 1991;324:1402–1407.
40. Hollingsworth RL, Rowe UK, Oyen F. Toxicity of ethylene oxide determined on experimental animals. Arch Ind Health 1956;13:217–210.

41. Finelli PF, Morgan TF, Yaar I et al. Ethylene oxide-induced polyneuropathy. A clinical and electrophysiological study. Arch Neurol 1983;40:419–421.
42. Waters EM, Gerstner HB, Huff JE. Trichloroethylene. I. An overview. J Toxicol Environ Health 1977;2:671–701.
43. Reactions grow to trichloroethylene alert. Chem Eng News 1975;19:41–43.
44. National Institute for Occupational Safety and Health. National Occupational Hazards Survey. Washington, DC: US DHEW 1974;1:74–127.
45. Wells JCD. Abuse of trichloroethylene by oral self-administration. Anesthesia 1982;37:440–441.
46. Jacobson JL, Jacobson SW, Humphrey HEB. Effects of in utero exposure to polychlorinated biphenyls and related contaminants on cognitive functioning in young children. J Pediatr 1990;116:38–45.
47. DeFalque RJ. The "specific" analgesic effect of trichlorethylene upon the trigeminal nerve. Anesthesiology 1961;22:379–384.
48. Feldman RG, Niles CA, Kelly Hayes M et al. Peripheral neuropathy in arsenic smelter workers. Neurology 1979;29:939–944.
49. Feldman RG, Mayer RM, Taub A. Evidence for peripheral neurotoxic effect of trichloroethylene. Neurology 1970;20:599–606.
50. Bauer M, Rabins SF. Trichlorethylene toxicity. Review. Int J Derm 1977;16:113–116.
51. Buxton PH, Hayward M. Polyneuritis cranialis associated with industrial trichloroethylene poisoning. J Neurol Neurosurg Psychiatry 1967;30:511–518.
52. Selby G. Diseases of the Fifth Cranial Nerve. In PJ Dyck, PK Thomas, EH Lambert, R Bunge (eds), Peripheral Neuropathy. Philadelphia: Saunders, 1984;1224–1299.
53. Mitchell ABS, Parsons-Smith BG. Trichloroethylene neuropathy. Br Med J 1969;1:422–423.
54. Albin RL, Albers JW, Greenberg HS et al. Acute sensory neuropathy-neuronopathy from pyridoxine overdose. Neurology 1987;37:1729–1732.
55. Feldman RG, Chirico-Post J, Niles C et al. Blink reflex as a measure of trichloroethylene exposure in individual and population studies [abstract]. Neurology 1989;39(Suppl 1):181.
56. Kimura J. The Blink Reflex. In J Kimura (ed), Electrodiagnosis in Diseases of Nerve and Muscle: Principles and Practice. Philadelphia: Davis, 1983;323–351.
57. Ruijten MW, Verberk MM, Salle HJ. Nerve function in workers with long term exposure to trichloroethene. Br J Ind Med 1991;48:87–92.
58. Cavanagh JB, Buxton PH. Trichloroethylene cranial neuropathy: is it really a toxic neuropathy or does it activate latent herpes virus? J Neurol Neurosurg Psychiatry 1989;52:297–303.
59. Herskowitz A, Ishii N, Schaumburg HH. N-hexane neuropathy: a syndrome occurring as a result of industrial exposure. N Engl J Med 1971;285:82–85.
60. Korobkin R, Asbury AK, Sumner AJ et al. Glue-sniffing neuropathy. Arch Neurol 1975;32:158–162.
61. Allen N, Mendell JR, Billmaier DJ et al. Toxic polyneuropathy due to methyl n-butyl ketone: an industrial outbreak. Arch Neurol 1975;32:209–218.
62. Buiatti E, Cecchini S, Ronchi O et al. Relationship between clinical and electromyographic findings and exposure to solvents, in shoe and leather workers. Br J Ind Med 1978;35:168–173.

63. DiVincenzo GD, Hamilton ML, Kapalan CJ, Dedinas J. Characterization of the Metabolites of Methyl *n*-Butyl Ketone. In PS Spencer, HH Schaumburg (eds), Experimental and Clinical Neurotoxicology. Baltimore: Williams & Wilkins, 1980;846–855.

64. Altenkirch R, Mager J, Stoltenburg G et al. Toxic neuropathies after sniffing a glue thinner. J Neurol 1977;214:137–152.

65. Scelsi R, Poggi P, Fera L et al. Industrial neuropathy due to *n*-hexane. Clinical and morphological findings in three cases. Clin Toxicol 1981;18:1387–1393.

66. Ruff RL, Petito CK, Acheson LS. Neuropathy associated with chronic low level exposure to *n*-hexane. Clin Toxicol 1981;18:515–519.

67. Chang CM, Yu CW, Fong KY et al. *N*-hexane neuropathy in offset printers. J Neurol Neurosurg Psychiatry 1993;56:538–542.

68. Spencer PS, Schaumburg HH, Sabri MI, Veronesi B. The enlarging view of hexacarbon neurotoxicity. CRC Crit Rev Toxicol 1980;7:279–357.

69. Paulson GW, Waylonis GW. Polyneuropathy due to *n*-hexane. Arch Intern Med 1976;136:880–882.

70. Lalloo M, Cosnett JE, Moosa A. Benzine-sniffing neuropathy. S Afr Med J 1981;59:522–524.

71. Tenenbein M, deGroot W, Rajani KR. Peripheral neuropathy following intentional inhalation of naphtha fumes. Can Med Assoc J 1984;131:1077–1079.

72. Kuwabara S, Nakajima M, Tsuboi Y et al. Multifocal conduction block in *n*-hexane neuropathy. Muscle Nerve 1993;16:1416–1417.

73. Oh SJ, Kim JM. Giant axonal swelling in "huffer's" neuropathy. Arch Neurol 1976;33:583–586.

74. Chang YC. Neurotoxic effects of *n*-hexane on the human central nervous system: evoked potential abnormalities in *n*-hexane polyneuropathy. J Neurol Neurosurg Psychiatry 1987;50:269–274.

75. Governa M, Calisti R, Coppa G et al. Urinary excretion of 2,5-hexanedione and peripheral polyneuropathies in workers exposed to hexane. J Toxicol Environ Health 1987;20:219–228.

76. Sumner AJ. Physiological Consequences of Distal Axonopathy. In PS Spencer, HH Schaumburg (eds), Experimental and Clinical Neurotoxicology. Baltimore: Williams & Wilkins, 1980;220–224.

77. Yokoyama K, Feldman RG, Sax DS et al. Relation of distribution of conduction velocities to nerve biopsy findings in *n*-hexane poisoning. Muscle Nerve 1990;13:314–320.

78. Mutti A, Ferri F, Lommi G et al. *N*-Hexane-induced changes in nerve conduction velocities and somatosensory evoked potentials. Int Arch Occup Environ Health 1982;51:45–54.

79. Iida M. Neurophysiological studies in *n*-hexane polyneuropathy in the sandal factory. Electroenceph Clin Neurophysiol 1982;36(Suppl):671–681.

80. Sumner AJ, Asbury AK. Physiological studies of the dying-back phenomenon: Muscle stretch afferents in acrylamide neuropathy. Brain 1975;98:91–100.

81. Griffin JW. Hexacarbon neurotoxicity. Neurobehav Toxicol Teratol 1981;3:437–444.

82. Spencer PS, Schaumburg HH, Raleigh RL et al. Nervous system degeneration produced by the industrial solvent methyl *n*-butyl ketone. Arch Neurol 1975;32:219–222.

83. Couri D, Milks MM. Hexacarbon neuropathy: tracking a toxin. Neurotoxicology 1985;6:65–71.
84. O'Donoghue JL, Krasavage WJ. Identification and Characterization of Methyl *N*-Butyl Ketone Neurotoxicity in Laboratory Animals. In PS Spencer, HH Schaumburg (eds), Experimental and Clinical Neurotoxicology. Baltimore: Williams & Wilkins, 1980;856–862.
85. Kantarjian AD, Shaheen AS. Methyl bromide poisoning with nervous system manifestations resembling polyneuropathy. Neurology 1963;13:1054–1058.
86. Horan JM, Kurt TL, Landrigan PJ et al. Neurologic dysfunction from exposure to 2-t-butylazo-2-hydroxy-5-methylhexane (BHMH): a new occupational neuropathy. Am J Public Health 1985;75:513–517.
87. Harkonen H. Styrene, its experimental and clinical toxicity. A review. Scand J Work Environ Health 1979;4:104–100.
88. Seppalainen AM. Neurotoxicity of styrene in occupational and experimental exposure. Scand J Work Environ Health 1978;4(Suppl 2):181–183.
89. Murata K, Araki S, Yokoyama K. Assessment of the peripheral, central, and autonomic nervous system function in styrene workers. Am J Ind Med 1991;20:775–784.
90. Cherry N, Gautrin D. Neurotoxic effects of styrene: further evidence. Br J Ind Med 1990;47:29–37.
91. Rosen I, Haeger-Aronson B, Rehnstrom S et al. Neurophysiological observations after chronic styrene exposure. Scand J Work Environ Health 1978;4(Suppl 2):184–194.
92. Cohr KH, Stokholm J. Toluene. A toxicologic review. Scand J Work Environ Health 1979;5:71–90.
93. Boor JW, Hurtig HI. Persistent cerebellar ataxia after exposure to toluene. Ann Neurol 1977;2:440–442.
94. Lazar RB, Ho SU, Melen O et al. Multifocal central nervous system damage caused by toluene abuse. Neurology 1983;33:1337–1340.
95. Maas EF, Ashe J, Spiegel P et al. Acquired pendular nystagmus in toluene addiction. Neurology 1991;41:282–285.
96. Filley CM, Heaton RK, Rosenberg NL. White matter dementia in chronic toluene abuse. Neurology 1990;40:532–534.
97. Goto I, Matsumura M, Inoue N. Toxic polyneuropathy due to glue sniffing. J Neurol Neurosurg Psychiatry 1974;37:848–853.
98. Hormes JT, Filley CM, Rosenberg NL. Neurologic sequelae of chronic solvent vapor abuse. Neurology 1986;36:698–702.
99. Bolla KI, Schwartz BS, Agnew J et al. Subclinical neuropsychiatric effects of chronic low-level solvent exposure in US paint manufacturers. J Occup Med 1990;32(8):671–677.
100. Cherry N, Hutchins H, Pace T et al. Neurobehavioural effects of repeated occupational exposure to toluene and paint solvents. Br J Ind Med 1985;42:291–300.
101. Rose F. Health risks and organic solvents. Occup Health Rev 1991;February-March:20–23.
102. Bleecker ML, Bolla KI, Agnew J et al. Dose-related subclinical neurobehavioral effects of chronic exposure to low levels of organic solvents. Am J Ind Med 1991;19:715–728.
103. Matikainen E, Jantunen J. Autonomic nervous system dysfunction in workers exposed to organic solvents. J Neurol Neurosurg Psychiatry 1985;48:1021–1024.

104. Arlien–Soborg P, Bruhn P, Gyldensted C et al. Chronic painters' syndrome. Chronic toxic encephalopathy in house painters. Acta Neurol Scand 1979;60:149–156.

105. Baker EL,Jr., Smith TJ, Landrigan PJ. The neurotoxicity of industrial solvents: a review of the literature. Am J Ind Med 1985;8:207–217.

106. Antti-Poika M. Overall prognosis after chronic organic solvent intoxication. Int Arch Occup Environ Health 1982;51:127–138.

107. Fagius J, Gronqvist A. Functions of peripheral nerves and signs of polyneuropathy in solvent-exposed workers at Swedish steelworks. Acta Neurol Scand 1978;57:305–316.

108. Seppalainen AM. Neurophysiological findings among workers exposed to organic solvents. Acta Neurol Scand 1982;92(Suppl):109–116.

109. Seppalainen AM. Solvents and peripheral neuropathy. Prog Clin Biol Res 1986;220:247–253.

110. Seppalainen AM, Antti-Poika M. Time course of electrophysiological findings for patients with solvent poisoning. Scand J Work Environ Health 1983;9:15–24.

111. Seppalainen AM, Husman K, Martinson C. Neurophysiological effects of long-term exposure to a mixture of organic solvents. Scand J Work Environ Health 1978;4:304–314.

112. Elofsson S, Gamberale F, Hindmarsh T et al. Exposure to organic solvents: a cross-sectional epidemiological investigation of occupationally exposed car and industrial spray painters with special reference to the nervous system. Scand J Work Environ Health 1980;6:239–272.

113. Juntunen J, Hupli V, Hernberg S et al. Neurological picture of organic solvent poisoning in industry. Int Arch Occup Environ Health 1980;46:219–231.

114. Halonen P, Halonen JP, Lang HA et al. Vibratory perception thresholds in shipyard workers exposed to solvents. Acta Neurol Scand 1986;73:561–565.

115. Gregersen P, Angels B, Nielsen TE et al. Neurotoxic effects of organic solvents in exposed workers: an occupational, neuropsychological, and neurological investigation. Am J Ind Med 1984;5:201–225.

116. Floden U, Edling C, Axelson O. Studies of psychoorganic syndromes among workers with exposure to solvents. Am J Ind Med 1984;5:287–295.

117. Maizlish NA, Fine LJ, Albers JW et al. A neurological evaluation of workers exposed to mixtures of organic solvents. Br J Ind Med 1987;44:14–25.

118. Grasso P, Sharratt M, Davies DM et al. Neurophysiological and psychological disorders and occupational exposure to organic solvents. Fd Chem Toxic 1984;22:819–852.

119. Spencer PS, Schaumburg HH. Organic solvent neurotoxicity. Facts and research needs. Scand J Work Environ Health 1985;11(Suppl 1):53–60.

120. van Vliet C, Swaen GMH, Meijers JM et al. Prenarcotic and neurasthenic symptoms among Dutch workers exposed to organic solvents. Br J Ind Med 1989;46:586–590.

121. van Vliet C, Swaen GMH, Slangen JJM et al. The organic solvent syndrome. A comparison of cases with neuropsychiatric disorders among painters and construction workers. Int Arch Occup Environ Health 1987;59:493–501.

122. Gade A, Mortensen L, Bruhn P. "Chronic painter's syndrome." A reanalysis of psychological test data in a group of diagnosed cases, based on comparisons with matched controls. Acta Neurol Scand 1988;77:293–306.

123. LeQuesne PM. Acrylamide. In PS Spencer, HH Schaumburg (eds), Experimental and Clinical Neurotoxicology. Baltimore: Williams & Wilkins, 1980;309–325.
124. Hashimoto K, Aldridge WN. Biochemical studies on acrylamide, a neurotoxic agent. Biochem Pharmacol 1970;19:591–590.
125. Gold BG, Griffin JW, Price DL. Slow axonal transport in acrylamide neuropathy: different abnormalities produced by single-dose and continuous administration. J Neurol Sci 1985;5:1755–1768.
126. Shenk Z, Mendell JR. Acrylamide and 2,5-hexanedion neuropathies: abnormal bidirectional transport rate in distal axons. Brain Res 1981;219:397–405.
127. Kaji R, Liu Y, Duckett S et al. Slow recovery of central axons in acrylamide neuropathy. Muscle Nerve 1989;12:816–826.
128. Fullerton PM. Electrophysiological and histological observations on peripheral nerves in acrylamide poisoning in man. J Neurol Neurosurg Psychiatry 1969;32:186–192.
129. Spencer PS, Schaumburg HH. A review of acrylamide neurotoxicity: II. Experimental animal neurotoxicity and pathologic mechanisms. Can J Neurol Sci 1974;1:152–159.
130. Spencer PS, Schaumburg HH. Central Peripheral Distal Axonopathy—The Pathology of Dying-back Polyneuropathies. In H Zimmerman (ed), Progress in Neuropathology. Vol. III. New York: Grune & Stratton, 1976;253–250.
131. Keogh JP. Classical syndromes in occupational medicine: dimethylamino-propionitrile. Am J Ind Med 1983;4:479–489.
132. Pestronk A, Keogh J, Griffin JG. Dimethyaminopropionitrile intoxication: a new industrial neuropathy [abstract]. Neurology 1979;29:540.
133. Garland TO, Patterson MWH. Six cases of acrylamide poisoning. Br Med J 1967;4:134–138.
134. Griffin JW, Price DL. Proximal Axonopathies Induced by Toxic Chemicals. In PS Spencer, HH Schaumburg (eds), Experimental and Clinical Neurotoxicology. Baltimore: Williams & Wilkins, 1980;613–630.
135. Davis CS, Johnson MK, Richardson DJ. Organophosphorus Compounds. In JL O'Donoghue (ed), Neurotoxicity of Industrial and Commercial Chemicals. Vol. II. Boca Raton, FL: CRC, 1985;1–24.
136. Koller WC, Klawans HL. Organophosphorous Intoxication. In PJ Vinken, GW Bruyn, (eds), Handbook of Clinical Neurology, Vol 37. Amsterdam: North Holland, 1979;541–562.
137. Gutmann L, Besser R. Organophosphate intoxication: pharmacologic, neurophysiologic, clinical, and therapeutic considerations. Semin Neurol 1990;10:46–51.
138. Wadia RS, Chitra S, Amin RB et al. Electrophysiological studies in acute organophosphate poisoning. J Neurol Neurosurg Psychiatry 1987;50:1442–1448.
139. Grob D. Anticholinesterase Intoxication in Man and its Treatment. In GB Koelle (ed), Cholinesterase and Anticholinesterase Agents. Handbuch der Experimentellen Pharmakologie, Vol. 15. Berlin: Springer, 1963;989–1027.
140. Stewart WG, Anderson EA. Effect of a cholinesterase inhibitor when injected into the medulla of the rabbit. J Pharmacol Exp Ther 1968;162:309–318.
141. Osterloh J, Lotti M, Pond SM. Toxicologic studies in a fatal overdose of 2,4-D, MCPP, and chlorpyrifos. J Analytical Pharmacol 1983;7:125–129.

142. Wills JH. Toxicity of Anticholinesterases and Treatment of Poisoning. In AG Karczman (ed), Anticholinesterase Agents. Vol. I. International Encyclopedia of Pharmacology and Therapeutics, Section 13. Oxford: Pergamon, 1970;355–471.

143. Senanayake N, Karalliedde L. Neurotoxic effects of organophosphorus insecticides. N Engl J Med 1987;316:761–763.

144. Senanayake N, Johnson MK. Acute polyneuropathy after poisoning by a new organophosphate insecticide. N Engl J Med 1982;306:155–157.

145. Aring CD. The systemic nervous affinity of triorthocresyl phosphate (Jamacia ginger palsy). Brain 1942;65:34–47.

146. Smith HV, Spalding JMK. Outbreak of paralysis in Morocco due to orthocresyl phosphate poisoning. Lancet 1959;2:1019–1021.

147. Morgan JP, Penovich P. Jamaica ginger paralysis. Arch Neurol 1978;35:530–532.

148. LeQuesne PM, Maxwell IC. Effects of edrophonium bromide on neuromuscular transmission in a healthy human subject. Neurotoxicology 1981;2:675–685.

149. Jager KW, Roberts DV, Wilson A. Neuromuscular function in pesticide workers. Br J Ind Med 1970;27:273–278.

150. Blaber LC, Bowman WC. Studies on the repetitive discharges evoked in motor nerve and skeletal muscles after injection of anticholinesterase drugs. Br J Pharmacol 1963;20:326–344.

151. Selevan SG, Lindbohm M-L, Hornung RW et al. A study of occupational exposure to antineoplastic drugs and fetal loss in nurses. N Engl J Med 1985;313:1173–1178.

152. Van den Neucker K, Vanderstraeten G, De Muynck M et al. The neurophysiologic examination in organophosphate ester poisoning. Case report and review of the literature. Electromyogr Clin Neurophysiol 1991;31:507–511.

153. Stalberg E, Hilton-Brown P, Kolmodin-Hedman B. Effect of occupational exposure to organophosphorus insecticides on neuromuscular function. Scand J Work Environ Health 1978;4:255–261.

154. LeQuesne PM. Neuropsychological investigations of subclinical and minimal toxic neuropathies. Muscle Nerve 1978;1:392–395.

155. Bischoff A. The ultrastructure of tri-ortho-cresyl phosphate-poisoning. Acta Neuropathol 1967;9:158–174.

156. Cavanagh JB. The toxic effects of tri-ortho-cresyl phosphate on the nervous system. J Neurol Neurosurg Psychiatry 1954;17:163–172.

157. Davis CS, Richardson RJ. Organophosphorus Compounds. In PS Spencer, HH Schaumburg (eds), Experimental and Clinical Toxicology. Baltimore: Williams & Wilkins, 1980;527–544.

158. Lotti M, Becker CE, Aminoff MJ. Organophosphate polyneuropathy: pathogenesis and prevention. Neurology 1984;34:658–662.

159. Johnson MK. The primary biochemical lesion leading to the delayed neurotoxic effects of some organophosphorus esters. J Neurochem 1974;23:785–789.

160. Kaplan JG, Rosenberg N, Pack D et al. Sensory neuropathy associated with Dursban (chlorpyrifos) exposure. Neurology 1993;43:2193–2196.

161. Barton EN, Gilbert DT, Raju K et al. Arsenic: the forgotten poison? West Indian Med J 1992;41:36–38.

162. Poklis A, Saady JJ. Arsenic poisoning: acute or chronic? Suicide or murder? Am J Forensic Med Pathol 1990;11:226–232.
163. Manzo L, Blum K, Sabbioni E. Neurotoxicity of Selected Metals. In K Blum, L Manzo (eds), Neurotoxicology. New York: Marcel Dekker, 1985;385–404.
164. Windebank AJ. Metal Neuropathy. In PJ Dyck, PK Thomas, JW Griffin, PA Low, JF Poduslo (eds), Peripheral Neuropathy. Philadelphia: Saunders, 1993;1549–1570.
165. Cavanagh JB. Neurotoxic Effects of Metal and Their Interaction. In CL Galli, L Manzo, PS Spencer (eds), Recent Advances in Nervous System Toxicology. NATO ASI Series. New York: Plenum, 1984;177–202.
166. Moyer TP. Testing for arsenic. Mayo Clin Proc 1993;68:1210–1211.
167. Donofrio PD, Wilbourn AJ, Albers JW et al. Acute arsenic intoxication presenting as Guillain-Barré-like syndrome. Muscle Nerve 1987;10:114–120.
168. Heyman A, Pfeiffer JB, Willett RW et al. Peripheral neuropathy caused by arsenic intoxication. N Engl J Med 1956;254:401–409.
169. Jenkins RB. Inorganic arsenic and the nervous system. Brain 1966;89:479–498.
170. Chhuttani PN, Chopra JS. Arsenic Poisoning. In PJ Vinkin, GW Bruyn (eds), Handbook of Clinical Neurology. Amsterdam: Elsevier, 1979;199–216.
171. Gherardi RK, Chariot P, Vanderstigel M et al. Organic arsenic-induced Guillain-Barré syndrome due to melarsoprol: a clinical, electrophysiological, and pathological study. Muscle Nerve 1990;13:637–645.
172. Oh SJ. Electrophysiological profile in arsenic neuropathy. J Neurol Neurosurg Psychiatry 1991;54:1103–1105.
173. Beritic T. Lead neuropathy. CRC Crit Rev Toxicol 1984;12:149–213.
174. Conradi S, Ronnevi LO, Norris FH. Motor neuron disease and toxic metals. Adv Neurol 1982;36:201–231.
175. Feldman RG, Hayes MK, Younes R et al. Lead neuropathy in adults and children. Arch Neurol 1977;34:481–488.
176. Needleman HL, Gunnoe C, Leviton A. Deficits in psychologic and classroom performance of children with elevated dentine lead levels. N Engl J Med 1979;300:689–695.
177. Seto DSY, Freeman JM. Lead neuropathy in childhood. Am J Dis Child 1964;107:337.
178. Aub JC, Fairhall LT, Minot AS et al. Lead poisoning. Medicine 1925;4:1–250.
179. Oh SJ. Lead neuropathy: case report. Arch Phys Med Rehabil 1975;56:312–317.
180. Buchthal F, Behse F. Electrophysiology and nerve biopsy in men exposed to lead. Br J Ind Med 1979;36:135–147.
181. Singer R, Valciukas JA, Rosenman KD. Peripheral neurotoxicity in workers exposed to inorganic mercury compounds. Arch Environ Health 1987;42:181–184.
182. Ehle AL. Lead neuropathy and electrophysiological studies in low level lead exposure: a critical review. Neurotoxicology 1986;7:203–216.
183. Seppalainen AM. Lead poisoning: neurophysiological aspects. Occup Neurol 1982;66:177–184.
184. Catton MJ, Harrison MJG, Fullerton PM et al. Subclinical neuropathy in lead workers. Br Med J 1970;2:80–82.
185. Aashby JS. A neurological and biochemical study of wearly lead poisoning. Br J Ind Med 1980;37:133–140.

186. Bordo BM, Filippini G, Massetto N et al. Electrophysiological study of subjects occupationally exposed to lead and with low levels of lead poisoning. Scand J Work Environ Health 1982;8(Suppl 1):142–147.

187. Seppalainen AM, Hernberg S. Sensitive technique for detecting subclinical lead neuropathy. Br J Ind Med 1972;29:443–449.

188. Seppalainen AM, Tola S, Hernberg S et al. Subclinical neuropathy at "safe" levels of lead exposure. Arch Environ Health 1975;30:180–183.

189. Schwartz J, Landrigan PJ, Feldman RG et al. Threshold effect in lead-induced peripheral neuropathy. J Pediatr 1988;112:12–17.

190. Seppalainen AM, Hernberg S, Kock B. Relationship between lead levels and nerve conduction velocities. Neurotoxicology 1979;1:313–332.

191. Triebig G, Weltle D, Valentin H. Investigations on neurotoxicity of chemical substances at the workplace. V. Determination of the motor and sensory nerve conduction velocity in persons occupationally exposed to lead. Int Arch Occup Environ Health 1984;53:189–203.

192. He F, Zhang S, Li G et al. An electroneurographic assessment of subclinical lead neurotoxicity. Int Arch Occup Environ Health 1988;61:141–146.

193. Nielsen CJ, Nielsen VK, Kirkby H et al. Absence of peripheral neuropathy in long-term lead-exposed subjects. Acta Neurol Scand 1982;65:241–247.

194. Krigman MR, Bouldin TW, Mushak P. Lead. In PS Spencer, HH Schaumburg (eds), Experimental and Clinical Neurotoxicology. Baltimore: Williams & Wilkins, 1980;490–507.

195. Whitaker JA, Austin W, Nelson JD. Edathamil calcium disodium (versenate) diagnostic test for lead poisoning. Pediatrics 1962;(82)29:384–388.

196. Baloh RW. Laboratory diagnosis of increased lead absorption. Arch Environ Health 1974;28:198–208.

197. Sack GHJ. Acute intermittent porphyria. JAMA 1990;264:1290–1293.

198. Moore MR, McColl KEL, Rimington C, Goldberg SA. Disorders of Porphyrin Metabolism, New York: Plenum, 1987;18–155.

199. Craven PC, Morrelli HF. Chelation therapy. West J Med 1975;122:277–278.

200. Beattie AD. Diagnostic and therapeutic uses of d-penicillamine in lead poisoning. Postgrad Med J 1974;50(Suppl 2):17–20.

201. Klaassen CD. Heavy Metals and Heavy-Metal Antagonists. In AG Gilman, LS Goodman, A Gilman (eds), The Pharmacological Basis of Therapeutics. New York: Macmillan, 1980;1615–1638.

202. Campbell AMG, Williams ER, Barltrop D. Motor neuron disease and exposure to lead. J Neurol Neurosurg Psychiatry 1970;33:877–885.

203. Conradi S, Ronnevi L-O, Nise G et al. Long-time penicillamine treatment in amyotrophic lateral sclerosis with parallel determination of lead in blood, plasma and urine. Acta Neurol Scand 1982;65:203–211.

204. Albers JW, Kallenbach LR, Fine LJ et al. Neurological abnormalities associated with remote occupational elemental mercury exposure. Ann Neurol 1988;24:651–659.

205. Chang LW. Mercury. In P Spencer, H Schaumburg (eds), Experimental and Clinical Neurotoxicology. Baltimore: Williams & Wilkins, 1980;508–526.

206. Feldman RG. Neurological manifestations of mercury intoxication. Acta Neurol Scand 1982;66(Suppl 92):201–209.

207. Berlin M. Mercury. In L Friberg, GF Nordberg, VB Vouk (eds), Handbook on the Toxicology of Metal. New York: Elsevier, 1986;387–445.

208. Shapiro IM, Sumner AJ, Spitz LK et al. Neurophysiological and neuropsychological function in mercury-exposed dentists. Lancet 1982;1:1147–1150.
209. Henderson R, Shotwell HP, Krause LA. Analysis for total, ionic, and elemental mercury in urine as basis for a biologic standard. Am Ind Hyg Assoc J 1974;35:576–580.
210. Langolf GD, Chaffin DB, Henderson R et al. Evaluation of workers exposed to elemental mercury using quantitative tests of tremor and neuromuscular function. Am Ind Hyg Assoc J 1978;39:976–984.
211. Matthes FT, Kirschner R, Yow MD et al. Acute poisoning associated with inhalation of mercury vapor. Pediatrics 1958;22:675–688.
212. Markowitz L, Schaumburg HH. Successful treatment of inorganic mercury neurotoxicity with n-acetyl-penicillamine despite an adverse reaction [abstract]. Neurology 1980;30:1000–1001.
213. Bakir F, Rustam H, Tikriti S et al. Clinical and epidemiological aspects of methylmercury poisoning. Postgrad Med 1980;56:1–10.
214. Hopmann A. Acute quecksilbergdampfvergiftungen. Zentralbl. Gewerbehygu Unfallverhutung 1927;14:422–420.
215. Hanninen H. Behavioral effects of occupational exposure to mercury and lead. Acta Neurol Scand Suppl 1982;66:167–175.
216. Waldron HA. Did the Mad Hatter have mercury poisoning? Br Med J 1983;287:1961.
217. Kark RAP. Clinical and Neurochemical Aspects of Inorganic Mercury Intoxication. In PJ Vinken, GW Bruyn (eds), Handbook of Clinical Neurology, Vol. 36. Intoxications of the Nervous System, Part 1. Amsterdam: Elsevier, 1979;147–197.
218. Cavanagh JB. Long term persistence of mercury in the brain. Br J Ind Med 1988;45:649–651.
219. Verberk MM, Salle HJA, Kemper CH. Tremor in workers with low exposure to metallic mercury. Am Ind Hyg Assoc J 1986;47:559–562.
220. Goetz CG, Cohen MM. Neurotoxic Agents. In AB Baker, LH Baker (eds), Clinical Neurology. Vol. 2. Philadelphia: Lippincott, 1990;9.
221. Agocs MM, Etzel RA, Parrish RG et al. Mercury exposure from interior latex paint. N Engl J Med 1990;323:1096–1101.
222. Iyer K, Goodgold J, Eberstein A et al. Mercury poisoning in a dentist. Arch Neurol 1976;33:788–790.
223. Albers JW, Cavender GF, Levine SP et al. Asymptomatic sensorimotor polyneuropathy in workers exposed to elemental mercury. Neurology 1982;32:1168–1174.
224. Kern F, Roberts N, Ostlere L et al. Ammoniated mercury ointment as a cause of peripheral neuropathy. Dermatologica 1991;183:280–282.
225. Adams CR, Ziegler DK, Lin JT. Mercury intoxication simulating amyotrophic lateral sclerosis. JAMA 1983;250:642–643.
226. Barber TE. Inorganic mercury intoxication reminiscent of amyotrophic lateral sclerosis. J Occup Med 1978;20:667–669.
227. Ehrenberg RL, Vogt RL, Smith AB et al. Effects of elemental mercury exposure at a thermometer plant. Am J Ind Med 1991;19:495–507.
228. Richter ED, Peled N, Luria M. Mercury exposure and effects at a thermometer factory. Scand J Work Environ Health 1982;8(Suppl 1):161–166.
229. Vroom FQ, Greer M. Mercury vapor intoxication. Brain 1972;95:305–318.

230. Von Burg R, Rustam H. Electrophysiological investigations of methyl mercury intoxication in humans. Evaluation of peripheral nerve by conduction velocity and electromyography. Electroencephalogr Clin Neurophysiol 1974;37:381–392.
231. Kurland LT, Faro SN, Seidler H. Minimata disease. The outbreak of a neurologic disorder in Minimata, Japan, and its relationship to the ingestion of seafood contaminated by mercuric compounds. World Neurol 1960;1:370–391.
232. Damluji SF, Tikriti S. Mercury poisoning from wheat. Br Med J 1972;2:804–800.
233. LeQuesne PM, Damluji SF, Rustam H. Electrophysiological studies of peripheral nerves in patients with organic mercury poisoning. J Neurol Neurosurg Psychiatry 1974;37:333–339.
234. Bank WJ. Thallium. In PS Spencer, HH Schaumburg (eds), Experimental and Clinical Neurotoxicology. Baltimore: Williams & Wilkins, 1980;570–577.
235. Passarge C, Weink HH. Thallium-polyneuritis. Fortschr Neurol Psychiatr 1965;33:477–470.
236. Andersen O. Clinical evidence and therapeutic indications in neurotoxicology, exemplified by thallotoxicosis. Acta Neurol Scand Suppl 1984;70:185–192.
237. Kalantri A et al. Electrodiagnosis in thallium toxicity: a case report. Muscle Nerve 1988;968.
238. Watnade I. Organotins (triethyltin). In PS Spencer, HH Schaumburg (eds), Experimental and Clinical Neurotoxicology. Baltimore: Wilkins & Williams, 1980;545–557.
239. Blaker WD, Krigman MR, Thomas DJ et al. Effect of triethyl tin on myelination in the developing rat. J Neurochem 1981;36:44–52.
240. Besser R, Kramer G, Thumler R et al. Acute trimethyltin limbic-cerebellar syndrome. Neurology 1987;37:945–950.
241. Graham DI, DeJesus TV, Pleasure DE et al. Triethyltin sulfate-induced neuropathy in rats. Electrophysiologic, morphologic and biochemical studies. Arch Neurol 1976;33:40–48.
242. Dyck PJ, Oviatt KF, Lambert EH. Intensive evaluation of referred unclassified neuropathies yields improved diagnosis. Ann Neurol 1981;10:222–226.
243. Albers JW. Inflammatory Demyelinating Polyradiculopathy. In WF Brown, CF Bolton (eds), Clinical Electromyography. Stoneham, MA: Butterworth's, 1987;209–244.

CHAPTER 9

Cumulative Trauma Disorders

Alan R. Berger, M.D.

Steven Herskovitz, M.D.

Within the last decade, there has been an epidemic rise in the number of worker's compensation claims for occupation-related upper-extremity pain and dysfunction. The clinical symptoms and signs are not stereotypic, and the exact nature of the clinical syndrome remains unclear. It is referred to by many names, including cumulative trauma disorders (CTDs), repetitive strain injuries, overuse syndromes, and occupational cervicobrachial disorders; the nomenclature reflects a widespread belief in the causal relationship between clinical symptoms and repetitive arm and wrist movements. In 1981, CTDs accounted for about 18% of all occupational illness, or about 23,000 cases. In 1989, these disorders accounted for 52% of all reported occupational illnesses, totaled 146,900 cases, and resulted in medical costs exceeding 22 billion dollars.[1] Since 1989, CTDs have continued to account for more than 50% of all occupational illnesses reported in the United States (Bureau of Labor Statistics).[2,3] Some estimate that by the year 2000, 50% of the American workforce will be affected.[4]

The contributing factors underlying this massive increase in compensation claims remain controversial. Many investigators attribute it to recent increases in repetitive hand and arm movements that have resulted from specialization and partial automation of the workplace. They note that jobs reported to be associated with CTDs have in common highly repetitive upper-extremity movements.[3] Proponents of the CTD concept believe that, similar to the way metal eventually fatigues and gives way after repeated use, so does the human upper extremity succumb to the cumulative effects of repeated microtrauma.[5] Injury is often ascribed to faulty ergonomics. This has led to the development of a new specialist whose job it is to analyze the manner in which humans perform their work, in order to detect a causal relationship between potentially injurious musculoskeletal activity and resultant worker dysfunction and disability.

The CTD concept is not without critics. Some investigators, albeit the minority, believe that the current explosion of worker's compensation claims is the result of medical and media hype, which has sensitized workers to view each bout of arm pain as a potential crippling injury.[6] The remarkable feature is not the frequency of musculoskeletal complaints but the fact that workers now perceive job-related soreness equivalent to being disabled, wrongfully injured, and potentially crippled.[7] Some believe that the labeling of poorly understood pain symptoms with pejorative names such as cumulative trauma disorders, repetitive strain injury, and overuse syndromes implies causality, pathology, and pathogenesis that are not yet proved. This change in workers' perception often propels them into the worker's compensation system, in which financial compensation requires the worker to be an advocate of his or her own disability. Some physicians believe that the current epidemic is an example of social iatrogenesis, with little firm data to suggest that work-related movements, which in their basic elements are usual and comfortable, are injurious, no matter how often performed.[6–8]

In 1979, Congress responded to the growing number of workers' complaints by enacting the Occupational Safety and Health Act, with the aim of preventing industrial injuries. Employers were required not only to record, on Occupational Safety and Health Administration (OSHA) logs, incidents of low back pain, which had come to be regarded as an occupational injury, but also episodes of upper-extremity pain. OSHA was empowered to issue citations and fines to employers with an unacceptably high rate of reportable incidents, and workers were encouraged to anonymously report perceived OSHA infractions. In 1986, following a consensus meeting, the National Institute for Occupational Safety and Health (NIOSH) issued the following statement: "When job demands...repeatedly exceed the biomechanical capacity of the worker, the activities become trauma inducing. Hence, traumatogens are workplace sources of injuries affecting the musculoskeletal system."[9] It was with this statement that OSHA targeted CTDs as a national concern and embraced the ergonomic concept that repetitive movements could be detrimental to workers' health. Union health and safety officials and the media were quick to warn their members and the general public of the potential dangers of CTDs.[10,11] The economic impact on individual companies has been dramatic. Insurance premiums, once 1–5% of payroll, have, in some cases, reached 30%. These costs, reflected in the price of goods and services, have placed affected businesses at a competitive price disadvantage, not only in the United States but in world markets not subjected to escalating worker's compensation costs.

What Are Cumulative Trauma Disorders?

Almost every painful musculoskeletal condition that affects the hand, wrist, shoulder, or neck, and that occurs in workers engaged in repetitive movements, has been classified as a CTD. Many reports in the occupational and hand surgery literature make little attempt to identify distinct musculoskeletal or neurologic entities, all complaints being considered the injurious consequence of repetitive, forceful movements. Other reports identify a number of different musculoskeletal conditions that potentially result from cumulative trauma.[12] The same job task may produce different clinical syndromes in different workers (see below). Specific medical syndromes reported as CTDs include cervical tension syndrome,[12-15] rotator cuff and biceps tendinitis,[16,17] lateral epicondylitis,[17] tenosynovitis,[18] ganglions of the wrist and hand, Dupuytren's contracture, and peritendinitis crepitans.[17] Nerve entrapment syndromes include carpal tunnel syndrome (CTS),[19-24] ulnar neuropathy at the wrist and elbow,[25,26] cervical radiculopathy,[27,28] and thoracic outlet syndrome.[29] Workers who use vibrating hand tools are clearly at risk for local vascular and digital nerve dysfunction.[30-33] Prolonged use of vibrating hand tools has also been alleged to be responsible for focal median nerve dysfunction within the carpal tunnel.[23,34-36] In many instances, the diagnostic criteria used to identify the above entities is either poorly described or varies considerably according to report.

In some cases, the reported pain syndrome does not fit into any of the above recognized diagnoses. Such patients complain of poorly localized arm or shoulder pain. Symptoms far outweigh signs and include any combination of muscle aches, subjective hand and arm swelling, subjective color and temperature changes, paresthesias, movement-induced pain, emotional irritability or depression, and sleep disturbance. There is often a paucity of objective abnormalities. Weakness, objective sensory loss, limitation of passive joint movement, and changes in skin color or temperature are noticeably absent. Results of laboratory studies, including muscle enzyme levels, radiographs, and electrodiagnostic studies, are usually normal.

An intriguing and yet unexplained feature of some CTDs is the tremendous disability that may result. This is especially so in cases in which a specific medical diagnosis cannot be made. Periods of complete rest, and administration of nonsteroidal antiinflammatory drugs, tricyclic antidepressants, and analgesic medications are often ineffective. Despite long periods of rehabilitative therapy, many workers are not only unable to return to their original job but also to other positions that require upper-extremity use. Even activities of daily living may occasionally be too arduous to perform.[37]

The variability of clinical symptoms among different workers and the lack of evident tissue damage have led many to question the link between arm activity and clinical disability. Few doubt that workers engaged in activities that require vigorous arm use experience frequent regional musculoskeletal discomfort. The current controversy centers around two issues: Are repetitive arm and wrist movements that are inherently comfortable and nonfatiguing harmful, and does the current escalation of worker's compensation claims reflect a true increase in the frequency and severity of work-related injury or is it a socioeconomic phenomenon fueled by the current medical climate and recent liberal compensation rulings?

Critics of the CTD concept point to a number of medical and epidemiologic inconsistencies in medical reports detailing CTDs:

1. A multitude of *different* musculoskeletal and nerve entrapment syndromes have been reported in workers performing similar activities (lack of specificity of association).
2. Remarkably different prevalence rates of CTDs have been reported in different industrial plants that perform identical manual tasks (lack of consistency of association). [6,37–39]
3. Despite marked functional disability, there may be few objective physical or laboratory abnormalities to indicate actual tissue injury.
4. There is often no statistically significant relationship between clinical complaints and objective evidence of musculoskeletal or neurologic injury. Conclusions about the causality of CTDs have often been made without statistical justification.[6]
5. The control population is frequently not representative of the workers in question.[20]
6. Many studies have ignored potential confounding factors, other than job activity, that may influence a patient's decision to become a claimant. Psychosocial issues, such as job content and satisfaction, family stress, and personality traits, are known to frequently play a major, and often predominant, role in determining the prevalence of CTDs and the level of worker disability.[40–42]
7. The results of "personal observations or anecdotal experience" have been used to support the association between repetitive activities and upper extremity dysfunction. For example, Birkbeck and Beer[21] report that 79% of their 588 patients with CTS were employed in a job that required repetitive movements. As no control population was available for comparison, this high prevalence may merely have reflected the pattern of employment common in their catchment area of Northamptonshire, England.

Both proponents and critics of the CTD concept are fervent in their respective beliefs. As can be expected when medical opinion is divided, inconsistencies are found in judicial decisions. In 1972, the Missouri Appellate Court ruled on the task-relatedness of CTS; the case involved a women who claimed injury from 2 weeks of "repetitive flexion under pressure" while manufacturing luggage.[43] Both a neurologist and general surgeon, who claimed to be practicing occupational medicine, reported that

CTS represented the result of cumulative trauma. The court ruled that CTS was a compensable occupational injury resulting from excessive repetitive activity.[44]

Within a few years, however, the Delaware Appellate Court reached an opposite conclusion regarding CTS. In this case, the court refused to overturn a worker's compensation denial regarding the alleged development of CTS from use of a heavy vibrating air gun. The deciding medical testimony centered around the lack of similar disease in other workers employed in the same fashion. The court decided that the patient must have had a predisposing susceptibility and that "for a hazard to occasion a compensable occupational disease claim...the hazard must not exist in employment generally or in everyday life."[43,45]

Does a Critical Review of the Literature Support the Cumulative Trauma Disorder Concept?

Documentation of occupational repetitive arm and shoulder movements goes back many years. Hammer[46] reported that tobacco workers performed 1,500–2,000 manipulations per hour. Tichauer[47] described the job of inserting at about 500 movements per shift and Arndt[48] reported that mail sorters may perform more than 64,000 keystrokes per day. A good typist may depress the keys of the keyboard seven to eight times per second, the average knitter may make 1,000 stitches per hour, and poultry cutters may perform more than 12,000 cuts per shift to bone turkeys.[21,49,50] The automation of industry and the popularity of the office personal computer have resulted in workers spending a good portion of their day performing repetitive movements.

Worker's compensation claims have often been used as instruments of medical surveillance.[51,52] The reported number of compensation claims for alleged occupational illness is impressive. Jensen and associates[53] used compensation claims from 26 states to estimate a 1979 incidence rate of almost 24 claims per 100,000 manufacturing workers. Armstrong and colleagues[49] reported 130 cases of upper extremity disorders per 100 worker-years in poultry employees; in Michigan, 30–34% of all OSHA claims between 1980 and 1982 were for repetitive motion disorders.[50,53] It is OSHA's contention that CTDs are not a new phenonemon and that previously low claim rates reflect underrecognition and underreporting.

Compensation claims have been used to contrast demographic differences between injured workers and the nonindustrial population. The implication is that if, for a particular medical condition, the demographics of affected workers differ from those seen when the general population is affected, then something related to the occupational task must be involved. For example, the incidence of compensation claims for CTS in

Washington State workers during the years 1984–1988 was 1.7 cases per 1,000 workers, higher than that expected in the general population.[54] The finding that the claimants were younger and more likely to be male than expected from other studies[55] was used to implicate repetitive motion as a causative factor.[56]

The clinical significance of worker's compensation claims should be interpreted with caution, however. The factors that enter into a worker's decision to initiate a compensation claim are multiple and include not only the absolute nature of the injury but also his or her perception of the significance of the illness including culpability, personality issues, and matters of job satisfaction.[40–42] The questionable accuracy of many compensation diagnoses prevents an acceptance at face value. Therefore, before the clinical significance of any apparent demographic differences can be ascertained, the diagnostic accuracy of each compensation claim must be verified through a case-by-case analysis of the specific medical details. Without such attention, the number of worker's compensation claims reflects the prevalence of workers' complaints but gives little reliable indication of underlying pathogenesis.

Armstrong and colleagues at the University of Michigan have been instrumental in popularizing a pathogenetic association between ergonomic insults and CTDs. In 1979, Armstrong and Chaffin[57,58] reported the relationship between CTS and repeated wrist flexion with power pinch in 18 women involved in the fabrication of automobile seat covers. Similar findings were found among workers in a poultry plant[49] and in a large study involving 574 volunteers from a number of different industrial plants.[59,60] In these latter studies, job tasks were divided into four categories depending on degree of force and repetition. Using worker questionnaires and follow-up clinical examinations, the investigators reported substantially more complaints and identifiable disease, particularly CTS, in the high-force/high-repetition group. Subsequent studies by these and other authors have identified the following ergonomic factors as potentially injurious: repetition, forceful exertions (e.g., pinch), awkward positions (e.g., ulnar deviation of the wrist, arms extended from the body or elevated), vibration, and low temperatures.

The studies of Armstrong and Silverstein were an integral part of the information base that OSHA used in formulating an initial policy regarding CTDs. CTS was clearly identified as a key CTD and cumulative trauma as a critical pathogenetic factor. Much of OSHA's policy regarding CTDs was driven by the ergonomic studies linking CTS to occupational activity. By extension, if CTS were an occupational hazard, then other musculoskeletal disorders encountered in the occupational setting were likely to also be a result of repetitive activity. A critical analysis of the CTD concept therefore centers around CTS. As stated by Hadler,[6] "...among the putative CTDs, carpal tunnel syndrome is the only entity associated with a damaging pathoanatomic outcome that has sufficient prevalence to be studied systematically. In the absence of damage, neither worker's compensation insurance nor the execution of the Occupational Safety and Health statute need pertain. If carpal tunnel syndrome did not qualify as a CTD, the policymakers at NIOSH and OSHA would be at a loss to argue for the CTD concept."

The current widespread acceptance of the pathogenetic relationship between repetitive movement and CTS and the resultant growing number of OSHA regulations and citations regarding perceived ergonomic infractions mandate a critical reappraisal of the CTD concept, and CTS in particular.

CARPAL TUNNEL SYNDROME: IS IT AN OCCUPATIONAL ILLNESS?

Of all the disorders believed to be related to cumulative trauma, CTS should be the one best able to be identified objectively. This is because of the high specificity and sensitivity that nerve conduction studies have in documenting focal median nerve entrapment.[61-63] Several large studies have suggested that diagnosing CTS by symptoms or signs alone, without electrodiagnostic confirmation, is fraught with inaccuracies. A large retrospective study of CTS from the Mayo Clinic documented a CTS prevalence rate of 1 per 1,000 patients, many of whom lacked classic symptoms and signs.[55] Katz and associates[64] investigated the sensitivity, specificity, and positive/negative predictive values of different clinical symptoms and signs in the diagnosis of CTS. Symptoms and signs proved to be remarkably nonspecific and at times misleading when used alone, despite a CTS prevalence rate of 40%.[6] At lower prevalence rates, as would be expected in the random occupational setting, the diagnostic utility of clinical symptoms and signs becomes much less reliable.[6,64] It seems reasonable, therefore, that for an occupational medicine report regarding CTS to be deemed authoritative, the clinical suspicion of CTS should be confirmed by electrodiagnostic studies. This is not to imply that *all* cases of CTS can be conclusively identified by electrodiagnostic evaluation. Certainly there exists a subgroup of patients with CTS who have neuropathic symptoms yet normal electrophysiology. These patients tend to have early or mild nerve entrapments; with time and progression of their entrapment they usually develop corroborating electrophysiologic abnormalities. It is our opinion that in examining the medical literature addressing the association between CTS and repetitive movements, the greatest weight should be placed on those studies that contain consistent clinical and electrophysiologic evidence of CTS.

The strength of the association between cumulative trauma and the development of CTS will be analyzed with regard to the following commonly accepted epidemiologic parameters:[50,56]

1. The demonstration of a clear association between risk factors and CTS.

2. The demonstration of a temporal relationship between repetitive movement and development of CTS.

3. The demonstration of a dose-response relationship between activity and CTS.

4. The demonstration that other intervening or confounding factors are lacking.

5. The demonstration of a high biological plausibility.

Unfortunately, many of the relevant reports are cross-sectional and case control studies; large-scale cohort studies with well-defined measures of exposure and health effect are lacking.[50]

THE ASSOCIATION BETWEEN REPETITIVE ACTIVITY AND CARPAL TUNNEL SYNDROME

Many studies have reported an association between upper-extremity symptoms and repetitive arm use. Oxenburgh[65] surveyed 46 keyboard operators who complained of arm symptoms, compared them to 238 "noninjured" control subjects, and found that a far greater percentage of those with symptoms operated their keyboards for more than 6 hours a day. This study can be criticized, however, because of its poor case definition and lack of attention to possible confounding factors. Masear and associates[19] analyzed medical claim reports over a 12-year period from an Illinois meat-packing plant and found that carpal tunnel release occurred in about 15% of workers involved with boning activities, compared to 4% of loading dock and sanitation workers. Electrodiagnostic confirmation was obtained in 82% of cases. More than half required bilateral surgery; those with unilateral disease usually had involvement of the dominant hand. The authors concluded that the repetitive, forceful activity of meat cutting was a risk factor in the development of CTS. It is not clear to us that this is true. The study was retrospective, with the medical details obtained from a review of plant medical records. There was no control group to determine the baseline level of median nerve abnormalities. The authors refer to a similar plant in another state that had only three carpal tunnel releases during the time the Illinois plant had 68. In addition, postsurgical follow-up showed that 46% of patients continued to have mild intermittent wrist pain, 39% had persistent numbness, and 78% continued to complain of hand weakness. What seems clear is that meat cutters had more surgical procedures than other plant workers, not that they had more CTS. The reasons behind their higher surgical rate may have involved psychosocial issues not addressed by this study. Falck and Aarnio[66] reported 17 Finnish butchers who cut with their right hand but forcefully grabbed the meat with their left. Since CTS usually occurs in the dominant hand in the nonindustrial population, it was remarkable that in these workers, four right hands but nine left hands were affected. In bilateral cases, the right hand was always less affected than the left. The authors concluded that the vigorous use of the nondominant hand explained the high frequency of CTS.

Feldman and associates[20] examined workers in a microelectronics assembly plant using a combination of clinical examination, nerve conduction studies, thermography, and quantitative sensory testing. They categorized job tasks into high- and low-risk groups; workers in high-risk jobs were more likely to have symptoms of CTS (numbness, hand weakness, Phalen's sign). Only finger numbness and tingling reached statistical significance in comparison to the low-risk population. Nerve conduction studies were performed at first visit and repeated one year later. Unfortunately, the control subjects used were not plant workers engaged in nonrepetitive tasks but "nonaffected persons of the same age group." Thus, the significance of their finding that 1.2% and 8.4% of conduction velocities and latencies, respectively, were abnormal on the first visit is unclear. Repeat electrodiagnostic studies were informative, however. No deterioration was found in median sensory latencies, the physiologic parameter one would expect to be most likely to worsen in progressive median nerve entrapment. Although median motor latencies showed a shift toward abnormal, these changes were mild and never reached statistical significance. As such, although it is clear that those workers involved with highly repetitive activities had more complaints, it is uncertain whether their complaints were truly due to CTS.

Punnett and colleagues[67] reported that the prevalence of CTS in women working in a garment sewing shop was three times that of hospital workers. Among garment workers, CTS prevalence varied according to task, being highest in those who stitched linings (highly repetitive movements of the wrist and fingers) and least among those who did hand ironing (more arm than wrist/fingers movement). Chiang and coworkers[68] reported that workers in a Taiwanese frozen food–processing plant who performed repetitive wrist movements were 14 times more likely to have CTS than were other workers. Wieslander and colleagues[23] performed a case referent study of hospitalized patients who underwent carpal tunnel release and report an association between CTS and use of vibrating hand tools and repetitive wrist movements. Patients were divided into three risk groups based on duration of exposure: less than 1 year, between 1 and 20 years, and greater than 20 years. Statistical significance was reached only in the small group of patients who used vibrating tools for greater than 20 years. Case referent studies are often susceptible to selection bias; the authors deemed this bias to be unlikely in this study.

If these studies are accurate, CTS prevalence is remarkably increased in workers who are involved in repetitive wrist movements or those who use vibrating hand tools. How prevalent is CTS in the industrial setting? A look at several large studies suggests that it may be surprisingly low. The results of these studies should be compared to the prevalence of CTS in the general population of 1 per 1,000 people found by the Mayo Clinic for inhabitants of

Rochester, Minnesota. Three reports investigated the prevalence and causes of upper extremity complaints in 512 Finnish industrial workers; out of all three studies, CTS was found definitively in one worker.[69-71] An analysis of worker's compensation claims from a microelectronic plant found no cases of CTS among 960 compensation claims over 6 years,[18] while a different study reported only 30 claims of CTS in 2 years in an aircraft manufacturing plant that employed 20,000 workers.[24] In this latter study, when the type of manual activities performed by the 30 patients with CTS was compared to that of other nonaffected plant employees, a statistically significant association was seen between CTS and use of vibrating hand tools but not with the "performance of repetitive motion tasks." If prevalence rates from the Minnesota population are accurate, the aircraft engine plant had less CTS than might be expected (i.e., 40 cases).

Three primarily electrodiagnostic studies bear mentioning. Schottland and associates[72] performed nerve conduction studies on 93 randomly selected poultry workers; the control group consisted of 85 job applicants to the same poultry plant. No statistically significant difference in median nerve conduction was found between the two groups, except in the right median sensory latency in female poultry workers; when age was controlled for, however, this difference substantially lessened. This study failed to show any definite physiologic evidence that poultry workers were at increased risk of median nerve entrapment compared to control subjects. Nathan and colleagues[73] used the inching technique to identify a focal area of median sensory latency prolongation. This technique has been reported to have a high degree of sensitivity and specificity.[74] Electrodiag-nostic studies were performed on 471 industrial workers from 27 different occupations. Workers were categorized into five different risk groups based on the degree of resistance and repetition that their job required. Median nerve conduction abnormalities were detected in 39% of workers. Since there was no control group for comparison it was unclear whether this value was outside the normal range for the study population. Of note, however, no relationship was found between nerve conduction abnormalities, occupational risk group, or level of hand activity. Many of these workers were restudied 5 years later. Not only did sensory conductions not deteriorate but it was again found that task and impaired median nerve conduction were not associated.[75]

Stetson and colleagues[76] compared median and ulnar motor and sensory studies in industrial workers performing repetitive tasks (symptomatic and asymptomatic groups) and control subjects comprised of plant managers. Industrial workers were reported to have significantly lower median sensory amplitudes and prolonged distal latencies compared to the control subjects. Interestingly, the ulnar nerve, as well as the median, was affected in the repetitive risk group. Median sensory amplitudes and median midpalm-to-wrist amplitudes were found to be significantly lower in symptomatic than in asymptomatic workers' hands. The authors concluded that the differences in median conduction studies demonstrated in the worker population reflected "the effect of differing lifetime occupational exposure to highly forceful and repetitive hand exertions." Unfortunately, this study is substantially flawed. Distal latencies are related to hand size and sensory amplitudes to finger circumference, both of which are greater in men than women. The control group contained 41% women while the asymptomatic worker group had only 198 women (p < 0.001). In addition, the workers were significantly taller than controls, probably due to the increased number of men. The authors controlled for age in their analysis but not for sex (and therefore height and finger circumference) despite the highly significant differences between groups. The reported differences between workers and control subjects were therefore probably due to differences in body habitus between groups rather than occupational task, a conclusion supported by the finding of concommitant abnormalities in ulnar latencies and amplitudes.

The Temporal Relationship Between Carpal Tunnel Syndrome and Repetitive Movements

There are no convincing studies that satisfactorily prove the temporal relationship between activity and onset of CTS. Ryan[50A] looked at the association between upper-extremity symptoms and the degree of arm use in Australian keyboard operators, at baseline and after 1 week of intensive overtime. After the 1 week of overtime work, there was a marked increase in the number of complaints of wrist and forearm pain. This increased level of pain persisted in eight of the nine operators still employed at 6 weeks and in four of the five operators remaining at 20 weeks, despite a reduction in workload. Although this study suggests a temporal relationship between arm symptoms and use, there is no indication that any of these operators had CTS. The persistence of pain despite rest raises questions of complicating psychosocial issues.

Determining the onset of median nerve dysfunction and its relationship to manual activity is difficult if pre-employment nerve conduction studies are not available. Most would agree that hand use is, at the least, an aggravating factor. Patients with CTS commonly complain of worsening symptoms while driving, knitting, or playing racquet sports. This does not prove, however, that repetitive use *caused* the nerve entrapment, and the fact that CTS symptoms occasionally respond to a change in job activity does not indict the activity as a causative factor.

The Dose-Response Relationship Between Carpal Tunnel Syndrome and Repetitive Activity

A number of reports have suggested a dose-response relationship between CTS and putative hand/wrist activities. Many of these studies have critical flaws and therefore add little to our understanding. Margolis and Kraus[22] gave symptom questionnaires to supermarket checkers and found a correlation between symptoms and number of hours on the job, years working, and use of laser scanners. None of their questionnaire parameters were validated for screening CTS, and nerve conduction studies were not performed. Dimberg and associates[77] examined the frequency of occurrence of arm symptoms in hourly versus salaried Volvo car employees. In 1981–1983, the percentage of workers reporting to the medical department with arm symptoms was two times as great in hourly as in salaried workers; 7% had hand symptoms. The frequency of complaints appeared related to their level of physical stress. As with the previous study, little can be gleaned regarding CTS. It has already been stated how perilous it is to try to diagnose CTS by symptom questionnaire alone.

A number of often-cited, ergonomically based studies have been published by Silverstein and colleagues[59,60] based on their analysis of 547 workers from a number of different industrial plants. Job tasks were classified as low force/low repetition, low force/high repetition, high force/low repetition, and high force/high repetition based on videotaped analysis of arm movements. The authors reported that CTS was correlated with high-force/high-repetition tasks and that repetition was a greater risk factor than force. Hadler[6] has criticized these studies based on his analysis of the original data contained in Silverstein's doctoral dissertation.[78] According to Hadler's analysis, workers in all four groups had a greater frequency of musculoskeletal complaints involving the neck, shoulder, elbow, and forearm than that anticipated in the general population. This suggested to him that awareness and recall were enhanced in these workers. Only symptoms involving the hand and wrist reached statistical significance; subjects in the high-force/high-repetition group had more hand/wrist complaints. However, when these patients were clinically examined for objective evidence of disease, no statistically significant difference was seen between risk groups. Electrodiagnostic studies were not employed. Thus, despite the fact that the high-force/high-repetition group had more complaints, no objective clinical evidence was found that they had any more *disease* than their low-risk counterparts.

THE ISSUE OF OTHER CONFOUNDING FACTORS

Most questionnaire surveys of industrial workers omit or only minimally address the many psychosocial issues that can potentially influence a patient's perception of pain and its significance. Those studies that directly addressed psychosocial issues have found a correlation between the likelihood of a worker seeking compensation and the level of life stress, job dissatisfaction, and specific personality features.[79–81]

Linton and Kamwendo[40] administered a battery of questionnaires to medical secretaries that addressed job satisfaction and musculoskeletal complaints. A "poorly" experienced psychologic work environment was related to a higher frequency of neck and shoulder pain. Aspects of work content and social support at work were related to pain, but there was no clear relationship with work demand. This study demonstrates the importance of psychosocial issues in the reporting of musculoskeletal pain, particularly those aspects pertaining to the work environment.

The impact of psychosocial issues in the workplace is now recognized by the World Health Organization (WHO). A report issued by the WHO in 1989 stated the following: "...Although various physical aspects may affect the health of VDT [video display terminal] users and are, to a large extent, inseparable from psychosocial effects, they have been addressed in a previous report. This report takes the view that, in the prevention of VDT-related health problems, psychosocial factors are at least as important as the physical ergonomics of work stations and the working environment."[42]

Events in Australia during the early 1980s illustrate the complex relationship between psychosocial issues and medical illness. An epidemic of upper-extremity pain occurred in which workers, predominantly women in the data processing and entry fields, presented to their physicians with incapacitating arm pain. Clinical or laboratory evidence of tissue damage was almost never present; electrodiagnostic studies were invariably normal. The condition was termed "repetitive strain injury" (RSI), reflecting a presumed but unproved causal relationship with repetitive arm movements. Beginning in 1980–1981, there was a rapid and progressive increase in the number of worker's compensation claims for RSI. The medical community was divided regarding its cause. Many considered it a cumulative trauma disorder; some went as far as to assign grades to the different stages of disability.[82] It became a common perception among workers that the slightest arm discomfort should not be ignored, lest it progress to irreversible damage. Many others, however, believed that the epidemic was a self-perpetuating cycle, fed by pervasive medical and media attention.

At the height of the RSI epidemic, many different occupations were affected. The experience of Telecom Australia is representative.[83] Telecom Australia was a statutory government authority that employed almost 90,000 people throughout Australia. In 1981, there were 109 claims for RSI among all Telecom workers. At the peak of the epidemic in 1985, the number of claims rose to 1,783; total cases during 1981–1985 numbered 3,976. There was an unusually high frequency of incapacity; 76% of cases resulted in lost work time. RSI claims were greatest among telephonists, followed by clerical workers and then telegraphists, despite an inverse relationship within these groups with regard to keystroke frequency. Inexplicably, the total number of RSI claims showed substantial regional variation, being higher in western Australia and least in New South Wales, despite no real differences in task mechanics. In addition, the workers from western Australia lost about 14 times more days of work and cost $194 more than the average worker elsewhere. By 1985, the epidemic had begun to decline and the numbers of worker's compensation claims began to approach preepidemic levels.

Several salient features about the epidemic in Australia have emerged. Despite the initial anxiety regarding irreparable tissue damage, none was ever found, and there was no consistent relationship with potential ergonomic insults. It is now believed that the Australian epidemic was, in part, fueled by inappropriately labeling the workers' regional arm pain "repetitive strain injury." This label, picked up by the media and unions, implied causality (i.e., repetition) without proof, tissue injury where none was ever proved, and culpability where none existed. The heightened worker concern, on a background of job dissatisfaction and other psychosocial factors, created a mass hysteria, in which the medical community readily took part.[84–87] Could a similar phenomenon be happening with the current cumulative trauma epidemic in the United States?

STUDIES OF BIOLOGICAL PLAUSIBILITY

Of all the different considerations mentioned above, probably the strongest link between repetitive wrist/finger activity and CTS lies in its biologic plausibility. A number of reports have detailed the changing anatomic relationship between median nerve and finger flexor tendons during wrist flexion and extension. When the wrist is in the neutral position, tension on finger flexor tendons remains restricted to the tendons themselves. Wrist flexion compresses the median nerve between flexor tendons and flexor retinaculum, while with wrist extension, the nerve is stretched over the flexor tendons and head of the radius bone.[50,88,89] Magnetic resonance imaging (MRI) studies of carpal tunnel dimensions during wrist flexion demonstrate a reduction in available space between median nerve, flexor tendons, and retinaculum.[90] Smith and associates[88] described how the median nerve was subjected to the greatest compression when the flexor profundus tendons of the second and third fingers were subjected to force while the wrist was flexed.

Wrist flexion and extension have been associated with changes in intracanal pressure recordings. Brain and associates[91] reported that pressures within the carpal tunnel were increased by 100 mm Hg with wrist flexion and 300 mm Hg with wrist extension. Patients with CTS have long been suspected of having increased carpal tunnel pressures at rest, somewhere about 30 mm Hg, with normal being 7–8 mm Hg.[89,92,93] When rat sciatic nerve was exposed to pressures at or above 30 mm Hg in a special chamber, venous congestion, endoneurial edema, and increased endoneurial collagen resulted. It was postulated that these changes, over time, could result in a cycle of progressive nerve edema and ischemia.[94,95] In patients with CTS, not only is canal pressure above normal at rest but once elevated by wrist movement, pressures continue to remain high, in contrast to what occurs in normal individuals.[93] The underlying cause of the increased canal pressures is not clear but may be a consequence of chronic edema and fibrosis of the flexor tendon synovium.[96] True tenosynovitis is rare, however; histologic analysis of flexor tendon synovium from patients with CTS shows neither acute nor chronic inflammatory changes.[97] Repetitive hand and wrist activity has been theorized to promote synovial edema and fibrosis, leading to elevated carpal tunnel pressures. Intermittent pressure spikes may occur during wrist flexion and extension, possibly creating a damaging cycle of edema, rising pressure, vascular compromise, and eventually nerve compression.

Some reports have suggested that measuring wrist dimensions and carpal tunnel size could identify subjects at risk of developing CTS. Bleecker[98] reports that workers with CTS had smaller cross-sectional areas on CT than did normal individuals, a finding not substantiated by Winn and Habes.[99] Gordon and colleagues[100] report that the ratio of the canal's anteroposterior-to-mediolateral diameters predicted those in whom CTS symptoms were likely to develop. Wyles and Rodriquez[101] were unable to replicate these findings. At present, the utility of anatomic measurements to predict CTS remains uncertain.

HADLER'S EXPERIENCE WITH CUMULATIVE TRAUMA DISORDERS AND CARPAL TUNNEL SYNDROME

Nortin Hadler is a rheumatologist at the University of North Carolina at Chapel Hill. He steadfastly opposes the CTD concept and likens it to the recent experience in Australia with RSI. He has written two books on the subject,[6,45] has testified extensively before OSHA regarding CTDs, and has been intimately involved in analyzing the Australian epidemic.

In 1978, Hadler[102] reported the results of his intensive clinical investigation of women employed in a knitting mill in rural Virginia. These women were subjected to highly repetitive hand activities for a minimum of 20 years. Although radiographic and clinical changes in hand structure were found to correlate with task activity, there were no cases of CTS or other nerve entrapments. No comment could be made regarding workers who may have left employment because of arm discomfort ("survivor effect").

The following "epidemics" in the United States illustrate the consequences of stubbornly ascribing workers' discomfort to cumulative trauma.[6] In each case, plant physicians and local surgical consultants steadfastly adhered to the belief that cumulative trauma was responsible for workers' symptoms, despite many medical inconsistencies. This perspective prevented them from seeing the other confounding factors that impacted on the symptom complex.

1. Oscar Meyer, Inc., operated two pork-processing plants, in Illinois and Iowa. Before 1978, only an occasional instance of carpal tunnel release occurred in the Illinois plant, but between 1978 and 1983 the surgical rate increased precipitously. Eventually 20% of the female workers and 15% of the male workers came to surgery. The epidemic was attributed to an increase in overtime hours for meat cutters, although nothing else changed

about the job.[19] Hadler[6] points out several features that should have alerted the plant physicians and their consultants that something other than cumulative trauma was occurring. Both the onset and termination of the epidemic were abrupt. In 1983, when the Illinois plant had 68 carpal tunnel releases, a sister plant in Iowa, with a similar workforce, had only three. Finally, although nerve conduction studies were abnormal in about 15% of their workforce, a pre-employment electrodiagnostic screening program found the same frequency of abnormalities. The prevalence of median nerve entrapments therefore did not differ between workers and community members. Finally, at the time of the epidemic, labor-management relations were strained; employees were not only ripe to become claimants but also to proceed with any and all recommended surgical therapies.

2.   In 1986, an epidemic of worker's compensation claims for upper-extremity pain and incapacity occurred at US West Communications. Many telecommunication companies, including US West, had recently introduced a new keyboard for directory 32 assistance, the Version II console. Although US West workers in Denver and Phoenix experienced a similar precipitous rise in the prevalence of compensation claims, their respective medical and rehabilitative courses were very different. In Phoenix, the illness was transient and relatively benign; in Denver, the workers suffered incapacitating pain, underwent multiple surgical procedures, and had an excessive amount of lost time from work.[6] Eventually, 30 claimants from Denver filed a class action suit against the keyboard manufacturer, alleging that their arm pain was a result of the keyboard's faulty ergonomic design and that irreparable tissue damage had occurred.

A look at the demographics of the epidemic showed that the majority came from those US West subsidiaries in Arizona and Colorado, with later increases in Oregon and Washington. Other areas of the country, however, remained remarkably spared, although their workers used a similar keyboard. In Denver, workers diagnosed with CTDs were seen by company physicians and a small group of outside local consultants. When workers' symptoms were refractory to conservative medical therapy, multiple diagnostic procedures were performed; most showed totally normal results. Despite the fact that the consultants could find no objective evidence of disease and none could agree on a diagnosis, a host of different surgical remedies were undertaken, mainly without success. In Phoenix, relatively few workers underwent surgical procedures, although referrals were also made to outside surgeons. Patients were mainly treated in-house and attention was paid to worker education, counseling, and schedule modification. The great majority of patients returned to work. After much investigation it eventually became obvious that the ergonomics of the keyboard was not the primary factor behind the rise in compensation claims.

This case illustrates the danger of the medical and industrial establishment steadfastly attributing pathogenesis to cumulative trauma despite obvious medical contradictions. It is doubtful that these physicians, when caring for a patient from the general population, would have undertaken the many surgical remedies that they did in the absence of objective clinical and laboratory evidence of disease. Instead of stepping back and examining the inconsistencies of the cases, the physicians maintained the belief that an unidentified injury had occurred, one with few clinical signs and normal laboratory results. The physicians' ineffectiveness was in stark contrast to those in Phoenix, where relatively minor therapeutic modifications were remarkably effective.

3.   The Pepperidge Farm Company experience is similar to that of US West Communications. Pepperidge Farm operated two plants, one in Downingtown, Pennsylvania, and the other in Downers Grove, Illinois. Both plants were cited by OSHA after workers complained of arm pain allegedly from the repeated action of placing a cookie atop its base. Sixty-eight workers from the Downingtown plant were given 190 different diagnoses. Despite normal electrodiagnostic studies in almost all, 42 surgical procedures were performed, including 33 carpal tunnel releases. The Downers Grove plant had a similar complaint rate, yet few underwent surgical procedures and the workers did well.[6] This case again illustrates the medical consequences that occur when physicians, wedded to the CTD concept, forsake basic medical tenets in search of an elusive medical entity.

CONCLUSIONS ABOUT CARPAL TUNNEL SYNDROME AND CUMULATIVE TRAUMA DISORDERS

There are a growing number of reports purporting an association between repetitive motion and CTS and an apparent groundswell of acceptance by the medical, occupational, and legal system of the CTD concept. OSHA continues to issue new regulations that render employers culpable for newly reported CTS in the workplace. One would think, given the modest amount of scientific protest, that the relationship between repetitive upper-extremity activity, CTDs, and CTS in particular would be incontrovertible. Although a review of the occupational literature raises a strong suggestion of such an association, it also poses many key questions and objections. The literature relied on is often flawed by use of poorly validated symptom surveys, faulty epidemiologic methods, or lack of electrodiagnostic confirmation. While activity can exacerbate, potentiate, and possibly even precipitate symptoms of CTS, questions remain about whether normal subjects, exposed to activities that are repetitive, yet comfortable and noninjurious in their basic elements, are at risk for development of CTS. Of all the purported CTDs, CTS should be the one most clearly proved to be associated with repetitive activity. After examination of the available literature, the strength of association between CTS and occupational activity remains unclear. Before new, restrictive industrial regulations are enacted, it seems reasonable to attempt to obtain a definite answer through large-scale prospective cohort investigations, with appropriate baseline electrodiagnostic studies.

There seems little doubt, just from the sheer number of reports, that workers involved with repetitive upper-extremity activity have an increased number of musculoskeletal complaints. What other factors, besides repetitive motion or cumulative trauma, could contribute to the epidemic rise in worker's compensation claims? Are these workers' complaints different from the aches and pains that are common to the general population? Large population-based studies have shown that regional discomfort involving the arm, shoulder, and neck is present in 5–10%[103] of the population at any one time. Most people conservatively treat their own discomfort, usually by modifying their activity, and never become a patient (or a claimant). Is it that workers, forced by their employment to continue with the repetitive activity, eventually suffer tissue damage that does not respond to rehabilitative measures?

The factors that propel a worker to become a claimant are multiple, the nature and severity of the arm pain being only one. As the Australian experience indicates, outside forces can influence workers' perceptions of a pain's significance and their desire for financial compensation. Much in the current rise in CTD claims and the resultant media and medical attention is reminiscent of the Australian experience.

The logistics of the worker's compensation system is intimately linked with the CTD; it potentially influences not only a decision about whether to become a claimant but also the likelihood that rehabilitative efforts will be successful. The idea of compensatory injury dates back nearly a century, during which time financial awards were given only to the obviously injured; in recent times disability, without evident injury, has become compensable. The award is contingent on the work relatedness of the illness and its effect on wage earning. Since loss of wage earning and its perceived equivalent, loss of work capacity, is difficult to quantify, the magnitude of compensation is often based on the extent of injury.[8] Administrative and medical disagreement often involves estimating the degree of disability by the extent of tissue injury, and the extent of tissue injury by the reported degree of functional disability.

Many believe that the current worker's compensation system, despite its noble aim, victimizes rather than benefits the injured worker. When obvious tissue injury is absent, workers may be forced to convince skeptical company physicians of their disability. If symptoms do not respond to conservative in-house measures, the patient has the right to outside medical consultation. Eventually, the patient may be shuffled between in-house physicians, outside medical consultants, and union or company administrators. Instead of facilitating the rehabilitative process and a return to work, the compensatory process forces workers to become advocates of their own disability. Disappointment, anger, and resentment are the usual emotional consequences, often accompanied by an inability to resume employment. If an award is made, it may be continued for the duration of the worker's incapacity. In many cases, based on actuarial estimates, the insurance company opts for a considerable lump sum settlement in exchange for release of liability ("permanent partial payment or redemption"). Thus, some workers will obtain a sizable financial gain as a result of their medical impairment. The degree to which this plays into a worker's decision varies. Certainly, other factors, such as job satisfaction, individual personality traits, and the degree the worker feels he or she has have been injured and entitled to compensation, play major roles.

In summary, there continue to be many questions regarding the relationship between repetitive movements, regional arm pain, and the rising number of compensation claims. Our concern is that there appears to be a level of general acceptance regarding pathogenesis that is not yet supported by a critical examination of the literature. Before the CTD concept becomes "embedded in stone," we believe it is imperative that methodologically sound, prospective studies be performed and that these be critically analyzed, similar to what we would do when faced with any new disease epidemic.

References

1. Holbrook TL, Grazier K, Kelsey J, Stauffer R. The Frequency of Occurrence, Impact, and Cost of Selected Musculoskeletal Conditions in the United States. Chicago: American Academy of Orthopedic Surgeons, 1984;1–87.
2. Bureau of Labor Statistics. Occupational Injuries and Illnesses in the United States by Industry 1989. US Department of Labor, Bulletin 2379.Washington, DC: US Government Printing Office, 1991.
3. Rempel DM, Harrison RJ, Barnhart S. Work-related cumulative trauma disorders of the upper extremity. JAMA 1992;267:838–842.
4. Mallory M, Bradford H. An invisible workplace hazard gets harder to ignore. Business Week 1989;January 30:92–93.
5. Sjogaard G. Work-induced muscle fatigue and its relation to muscle pain. In Conference Proceedings: Occupational Disorders of the Upper Extremity. Ann Arbor, MI: University of Michigan, March 29–30, 1990.
6. Hadler NM. Coping With Arm Pain in the Workplace. In NM Hadler (ed), Occupational Musculoskeletal Disorders. New York: Raven, 1993.
7. Hadler NM. Cumulative trauma disorders. An iatrogenic concept. J Occup Med 1990;32:38–41.
8. Hadler NM. Illness in the workplace: the challenge of musculoskeletal symptoms. J Hand Surg 1985;10A:451–456.
9. Association of Schools of Public Health/National Institute for Occupational Safety and Health. Proposed National Strategies for the Prevention of Leading Work-related Diseases and Injuries: Part 1. Washington, DC: Association of Schools of Public Health, 1986:19.
10. LeGrande D. Carpal tunnel syndrome: it hurts, it cripples. CWA News 1989;48:6–7.

11. The New York Times. August 21, 1988:1,8.
12. Viikari-Juntura I. Neck and upper limb disorders among slaughterhouse workers: an epidemiologic and clinical study. Scand J Work Environ Health 1983;9:283–290.
13. Waris P. Occupational cervicobrachial syndromes: a review. Scand J Work Environ Health 1979;3:3–14.
14. Hagberg M, Weegman D. Prevalence rates and odds ratios of shoulder-neck diseases in different occupational groups. Br J Ind Med 1987;44:602–610.
15. Onishi N, Nomura H, Sakai K, Yamamoto T et al. Shoulder muscle tenderness and physical features of female industrial workers. J Hum Ergol (Tokyo) 1976;5(2):87–102.
16. Herberts P, Kadefors R, Hogfors C, Sigholm G. Shoulder pain and manual labor. Clin Orthop 1984;191;166–178.
17. Thompson AR, Plewes LW, Shaw EG. Peritendinitis, crepitants and simple tenosynovitis: a clinical study of 54 cases in industry. Br J Ind Med 1951;8:150–158.
18. Hymovich L, Lindholm M. Hand, wrist, and forearm injuries: the result of repetitive motions. J Occup Med 1966;8:573–574.
19. Masear VR, Hayes JM, Hyde AG. An industrial cause of carpal tunnel syndrome. J Hand Surg 1986;11A:222–227.
20. Feldman RG, Travers PH, Chirico-Post J, Keyserling WM. Risk assessment in electronic assembly workers: carpal tunnel syndrome. J Hand Surg 1987;12A:849–855.
21. Birkbeck MQ, Beer TC. Occupation in relation to the carpal tunnel syndrome. Rheumatol Rehabil 1975;14:218–221.
22. Margolis W, Kraus JF. The prevalence of carpal tunnel syndrome symptoms in female supermarket checkers. J Occup Med 1987;12:953–956.
23. Wieslander G, Norback D, Gothe CJ, Juhlin L. Carpal tunnel syndrome (CTS) and exposure to vibration, repetitive wrist movements, and heavy manual work: a case-referent study. Br J Ind Med 1989;46:43–47.
24. Cannon LJ, Bernacki EJ, Walter SD. Personal and occupational factors associated with carpal tunnel syndrome. J Occup Med 1981;23:255–258.
25. Massey EW, Riley TL. Nontraumatic mononeuropathies: a review. Milit Med 1981;146;30–36.
26. Spaans F. Occupational Nerve Lesions. In PJ Vinken, GW Bruyn (eds), Handbook of Clinical Neurology. Vol. 7. New York: Elsevier, 1970;326–343.
27. Partridge REH, Andersson JAD, McCarthy MA, Duthie JJR. Rheumatic complaints among workers in iron foundries. Ann Rheum Dis 1968;27:441–443.
28. Partridge REH, Duthie JJR. Rheumatism in dockers and civil servants: a comparison of heavy manual and sedentary workers. Ann Rheum Dis 1968;27:559–567.
29. Feldman RG, Goldman R, Keyserling WM. Classical syndromes in occupational medicine. Peripheral nerve entrapment syndromes and ergonomic factors. Am J Ind Med 1983;4:661–681.
30. Takeuchi T, Futatsuka M, Imanishi H, Yamada S. Pathological changes observed in the finger biopsy of patients with vibration-induced white finger. Scand J Work Environ Health 1986;12:280–283.
31. Sakurai T, Matoba T. Peripheral nerve responses to hand-arm vibration. Scand J Work Environ Health 1986;12:432–434.

32. Alaranta H, Seppalainen AM. Neuropathy and the automatic analysis of electromyographic signals from vibration exposed workers. Scand J Work Environ Health 1977;3:128–134.

33. Lundborg G, Dahlin LB, Danielsen N, Hansson HA et al. Intraneural edema following exposure to vibration. Scand J Work Environ Health 1987;13:326–329.

34. Garkkila M, Pyykko I, Jautti V, Aatola S et al. Forestry workers exposed to vibration: a neurological study. Br J Ind Med 1988;45:188–192.

35. Savage R, Burka FD, Smith J, Hopper I. Carpal tunnel syndrome in association with vibration white finger. J Hand Surg 1990;15B:100–103.

36. Koskimies K, Farkkila N, Pyykko I, Jautt V et al. Carpal tunnel syndrome in vibration diesease. Br J Ind Med 1990;47:411–416.

37. Miller MH, Topliss DJ. Chronic upper limb pain syndrome (repetitive strain injury) in the Australian workforce: a systematic cross sectional rheumatological study of 229 patients. J Rheumatol 1988;15:1705–1712.

38. McDermott FT. Repetition strain injury: a review of current understanding. Med J Aust 1986;144:196–200.

39. Hocking B. Epidemiological aspects of "repetition strain injury" in Telecom Australia. Med J Aust 1987;147:218–222.

40. Linton SJ, Kamwendo K. Risk factors in the psychosocial work environment for neck and shoulder pain in secretaries. J Occup Med 1989;31:609–613.

41. Dimberg L, Olafsson A, Stefansson E, Aagaard H et al. The correlation between work environment and the occurrence of cervicobrachial symptoms. J Occup Med 1989;31:447–453.

42. World Health Organization. Work with visual display terminal: psychosocial aspects and health. J Occup Med 1989;31:957–968.

43. Warren BH vs General Motors Corporation, 344 Atlantic Reporter, Second Series (Delaware) 1975;248–251.

44. Collins K vs Neevel Luggage Manufacturing Company, 481 Southwestern Reporter, Second Series (MO App. DKC) 1972;548–555.

45. Hadler NM. Medical Management of the Regional Musculoskeletal Diseases. Orlando: Grune & Stratton, 1984.

46. Hammer A. Tenosynovitis. Med Rec 1934;140:353–355.

47. Tichauer E. Some aspects of stress on the forearm and hand in industry. J Occup Med 1966;8:63–71.

48. Arndt R. The development of chronic trauma disorders among letter sorting machine operators. Paper presented at American Industrial Hygiene Conference, Portland, 1981.

49. Armstrong TJ, Foulke JA, Joseph BS, Goldstein SA. Investigation of cumulative trauma disorders in a poultry processing plant. Am Ind Hyg Assoc J 1982;43:103–116.

50. Armstrong TJ, Silverstein BA. Upper-Extremity Pain in the Workplace—Role of Usage in Causality. In NM Hadler (ed), Clinical Concepts in Regional Musculoskeletal Illness. Orlando: Grune & Stratton, 1987;333–354.

50A. Ryan GA, Bampton M. Comparison of data process operators with and without upper limb symptoms. Community Health Studies 1988;12:63–68.

51. Park RM, Nelson NA, Silverstein MA, Mirer FE. Use of medical insurance claims for surveillance of occupational disease. An analysis of cumulative trauma in the auto industry. J Occup Med 1992;34:731–737.

52. Tanaka S, Seligman P, Halperin W, Thun M et al. Use of worker's compensation claims data for surveillance of cumulative trauma disorders. J Occup Med 1988;30:488–491.
53. Jensen R, Klein B, Sanderson L. Motion-related wrist disorders traced to industries, occupational groups. Mon Labor Rev 1983;13–16.
54. Franklin GM, Haug JA, Heyer N, Checkoway H et al. Occupational carpal tunnel syndrome in Washington State, 1984–1987. Am J Public Health 1991;81:741–746.
55. Stevens JC, Sun S, Beard CM, O'Fallon WM et al. Carpal tunnel syndrome in Rochester, Minnesota, 1961–1980. Neurology 1988;38:134–138.
56. Rosenbaum RB, Ochoa JL. Activity, Occupation, and Carpal Tunnel Syndrome. In RB Rosenbaum, JL Ochoa (eds), Carpal Tunnel Syndrome and Other Disorders of the Median Nerve. Boston: Butterworth, 1993;233–249.
57. Armstrong TJ, Chaffin DB. Carpal tunnel syndrome and selected personal attributes. J Occup Med 1979;21:481–486.
58. Armstrong TJ, Chaffin DB. Some biomechanical aspects of the carpal tunnel. J Biomech 1979;12:567–570.
59. Silverstein BA, Fine LJ, Armstrong TJ. Hand-wrist cumulative trauma disorders in industry. Br J Ind Med 1986;43:779–784.
60. Silverstein BA, Fine LJ, Armstrong TJ. Occupational factors and carpal tunnel syndrome. Am J Ind Med 1987;11:343–358.
61. Louis DS, Hankin FM. Symptomatic relief following carpal tunnel decompression with normal electroneuromyographic studies. Orthopedics 1987;10:434–436.
62. American Association of Electrodiagnostic Medicine, American Academy of Neurology, American Academy of Physical Medicine and Rehabilitation. Practice parameter for electrodiagnostic studies in carpal tunnel syndrome: summary statement. Muscle Nerve 1993;16:1390–1391.
63. AAEM Quality Assurance Committee. Literature review of the usefulness of nerve conduction studies and electromyography for the evaluation of patients with carpal tunnel syndrome. Muscle Nerve 1993;16:1392–1414.
64. Katz JN, Larson MG, Sabra A, Krarup C et al. The carpal tunnel syndrome: diagnostic utility of the history and physical examination findings. Ann Intern Med 1990;112:321–327.
65. Oxenburgh M. Musculoskeletal injuries occurring in word processing operators. In Proceedings of the 21st Annual Conference of the Ergonomics Society of Australia and New Zealand. Sydney, 1984;137–143.
66. Falck B, Aarnio P. Left-sided carpal tunnel syndrome in butchers. Scand J Work Environ Health 1983;9:291–297.
67. Punnett L, Robins JM, Wegman DH, Keyserling WM. Soft tissue disorders in the upper limbs of female garment workers. Scand J Work Environ Health 1985;11:417–425.
68. Chiang HC, ChenSS, Yu HS, Ko YC. The occurrence of carpal tunnel syndrome in frozen food factory employees. Kaohsiung J Med Sci 1990;6:73–80.
69. Kuorinka I, Koskinen P. Occupational rheumatic disease and upper limb strain in manual jobs in a light mechanical industry. Scand J Work Environ Health 1979;5(Suppl 3):39–47.
70. Luopajarve T, Kuorinka I, Virolainen M. Prevalence of tenosynovitis and other injuries of the upper extremities in repetitive work. Scand J Work Environ Health 1979;5(Suppl 3):38–55.

71. Viikari-Juntara E. Neck and upper limb disorders among slaughterhouse workers. Scand J Work Environ Health 1983;9:283–290.
72. Schottland JR, Kirschberg GJ, Fillingim R, Davis VP et al. Median nerve latencies in poultry processing workers: an approach to resolving the role of industrial "cumulative trauma" in the development of the carpal tunnel syndrome. J Occup Med 1991;33:627–631.
73. Nathan PA, Meadows KD, Doyle LS. Sensory segmental latency values of the median nerve for a population of normal individuals. Arch Phys Med Rehabil 1988;69:499–501.
74. Kimura J. The carpal tunnel syndrome: Localization of conduction abnormalities within the distal segment of the median nerve. Brain 1979;102:619–635.
75. Nathan PA, Keniston RC, Myers LD, Meadows KD. Obesity as a risk factor for slowing of sensory conduction of the median nerve in industry. J Occup Med 1992;34:379–383.
76. Stetson DS, Silverstein BA, Keyserling WM, Wolfe RA et al. Median sensory distal amplitude and latency: comparisions between non-exposed managerial/professional employees and industrial workers. Am J Ind Med 1993;24:175–189.
77. Dimberg L, Andersson G, Hagert CG et al. Symptoms of the neck and upper limb—an epidemiological, clinical, and ergonomic study performed at Volvo. Volvo Flygmotor, Sweden, 1985.
78. Silverstein BA. The Prevalence of Upper Extremity Cumulative Trauma Disorders in Industry (dissertation). Ann Arbor, MI: University of Michigan, 1985;1–262.
79. Kalimo R, El-Batawi MA, Cooper C (eds). Psychosocial Factors at Work. Geneva: World Health Organization, 1987.
80. MacKay CJ, Cooper CL. Occupational Stress and Health: Some Current Issues. In CL Cooper, IT Robertson (eds), International Review of Industrial and Organizational Psychology. Chicago: Wiley, 1987.
81. Ryan GA, Bampton M. Comparison of data process operators with and without upper limb symptoms. Community Health Stud 1988;12:63–68.
82. Browne CD, Nolan BM, Faithfull DK. Occupational repetition strain injuries. Guidelines for diagnosis and management. Med J Aust 1984;140:329–332.
83. Hocking B. Epidemiological aspect of "repetition strain injury" in Telecom Australia. Med J Aust 1987;147:218–222.
84. Ryan A, Pimble J et al. Repetition strain injury and the influence of the work environment. Presented to the ANZAAS 55th Congress, Melbourne, August 26–30, 1985.
85. Starr S, Shute SJ, Thompson CR. Relating posture to discomfort in VDT use. J Occup Med 1985;27:269–271.
86. Ferguson D. An Australian study of telegraphists' cramp. Ind Med 1971;28:280–285.
87. Wallace M. Factors Associated with Occupational Pain in Keyboard Users. In M Wallace (ed), Occupational Pain (RSI). Melbourne: Brain Behavior Institute, La Trobe University, 1986;15–18.
88. Smith EM, Sonstegard DA, Anderson WH Jr. Carpal tunnel syndrome: contribution of flexor tendons. Arch Phys Med Rehabil 1977;58:379–385.

89. Gelberman R, Hergenroeder P, Hargens A, Lundborg G et al. The carpal tunnel syndrome. A study of carpal tunnel pressures. J Bone Joint Surg [Am] 1981;61:380–383.

90. Skie M, Zeiss J, Ebraheim NA, Jackson WT. Carpal tunnel changes and median nerve compression during wrist flexion and extension seen by magnetic resonance imaging. J Hand Surg 1990;15A:934–939.

91. Brain WR, Wright A, Wilkinson M. Spontaneous compression of both median nerves in carpal tunnel. Lancet 1947;1:277–282.

92. Lundborg G, Gelberman R, Minteer-Convery M, Lee VF et al. Median nerve compression in the carpal tunnel: the functional response to experimentally induced controlled pressure. J Hand Surg 1982;7:252–259.

93. Szabo RM, Chidgey LK. Stress carpal tunnel pressure in patients with carpal tunnel syndrome and normal patients. J Hand Surg 1989;14A:624–627.

94. Myers RR, Miziain AP, Powell HC, Lanpert PW. Reduced nerve blood flow in hexachlorophene neuropathy. Relationship to elevated endoneurial fluid pressure. J Neuropathol Exp Neurol 1982;41:391–399.

95. Lundgorg G. Nerve Iniury and Repair. New York: Churchill Livingstone, 1988.

96. Faithfull DK, Moir DH, Ireland J. The micropathology of the typical carpal tunnel syndrome. J Hand Surg 1986;11B:131–132.

97. Kerr DC, Sybert DR, Albarracin NS. An analysis of the flexor synovium in idiopathic carpal tunnel syndrome: report of 625 cases. J Hand Surg 1992;17A:1028–1030.

98. Bleecker ML. Medical surveillance for carpal tunnel syndrome in workers. J Hand Surg 1987;12A:845–848.

99. Winn FJ, Habes DJ. Carpal tunnel area as a risk factor for carpal tunnel syndrome. Muscle Nerve 1990;13:254–258.

100. Gordon C, Johson EW, Gatens PF, Ashton JJ. Wrist ratio correlation with carpal tunnel syndrome in industry. Am J Phys Med Rehabil 1988;67:270–272.

101. Wyles JM, Rodriquez AA. The predictive value of wrist dimension measurement in median sensory latencies in carpal tunnel syndrome. Muscle Nerve 191;14:902–903.

102. Hadler NM, Gilling DB, Imbus HR, Levitin, PM et al. Hand structure and function in an industrial setting: influences of three patterns of stereotyped, repetitive usage. Arthritis Rheum 1978;21:210–220.

103. Cunningham LS, Kelsey JL. Epidemiology of musculoskeletal impairments and associated disability. Am J Public Health 1984;74:574–579.

CHAPTER 10

Brain and Spinal Cord Injuries in the Workplace

James P. Kelly, M.A., M.D.
Neil L. Rosenberg, M.D.

Traumatic injuries occur commonly in the workplace but usually result in relatively minor injuries. Even when injuries occur that affect the head or neck, only mild injuries causing transient pain and some lost work time usually result. This chapter discusses those more serious injuries that affect the brain and spinal cord—the epidemiology, at-risk occupations, and prevention strategies.

Occupational Traumatic Brain Injury

The most celebrated case of work-related traumatic brain injury (TBI) is the penetrating brain injury of Phineas Gage, whose frontal lobes were severely damaged by an explosion that drove a tampering iron through his skull.[1] This chapter focuses on nonpenetrating, or closed head injuries (CHI), in the workplace. We discuss injuries to the neck as well, rather than considering brain injury in isolation, since cervical and cranial injuries commonly occur together. Information regarding the occurrence and nature of occupational brain injury is scarce, and there is little scientific evidence that industrial methods intended to prevent or minimize brain injuries actually work. The reduction of activity by government watchguarding agencies in the 1980s has contributed to a paucity of data for measuring the success of safety interventions.

We have chosen not to include a lengthy discussion of injuries due to motor vehicle accidents, even though this remains one of the leading causes of morbidity and mortality from TBI in the occupational setting. We focus on issues related to head injuries in common occupational work settings found in industrialized nations, such as manufacturing, construction, and farming, and discuss in detail how the neurologic sequelae impact on the workplace.

EPIDEMIOLOGY

Approximately 5.5 million work-related injuries occurred in the United States during 1986, according to the U.S. Department of Labor Bureau of Labor Statistics, *Occupational Injuries and Illnesses in the United States by Industry*.[2] The incidence of occupational injuries of all types was 7.7 per 100 full-time workers during that year. Nearly half of these injuries were severe enough to cause time off from work or special activity restrictions beyond the day the injury occurred. While this report offers detailed statistics on occupational injury incidence rates by industry, it does not distinguish types of injury. An occupational injury was defined only as "any injury which results from a work-related accident or from exposure involving a single incident in the work environment."[2] Injuries were recorded if the accident resulted in death, lost work time, medical treatment other than first aid, loss of consciousness, restriction of work or motion, or transfer to another job.

Since no network exists for hospital reporting of brain injuries in the United States, it is impossible to accurately state the incidence figures for TBI in general, let alone for work-related TBI. No epidemiologic studies of civilian brain injury in the United States were published before 1980. National estimates of all head injuries based on trauma incidence studies published in the 1980s range from 175 per 100,000 to 367 per 100,000 (Table 10.1). These figures vary widely since methods of case selection and definitions of TBI are not uniform. Most U.S. studies find a male-female ratio of 2 to 1, with men suffering a three to five times higher mortality than women. The vast majority of brain injuries result from transportation-related accidents, such as motor vehicle accidents involving drivers, passengers, and pedestrians, as well as motorcyclists and bicyclists.

While most of these studies reported statistics on rates of fatality, severity of injury, male-female ratios, and category of injury (e.g., transport, falls, assaults), none included statistics on the relation of injury to occupation. Our medical reporting of trauma cases all too often omits details such as the setting in which the injury occurred. Two earlier studies from England[10] and Australia[11] found that 14% and 11%, respectively, of the total number of head (which may or may not involve brain) or spinal injuries, or both, occurred at work. In the English study, fully half of the injuries were due to falls and one-fourth to falling objects. These numbers

TABLE 10.1
Epidemiologic Studies of Head Injury in the United States

Authors	Location	Years Studied	Number of Cases	Rate/ 100,000
Annegers et al., 1980 [3]	Olmstead County, NM	1965–1974	3,587	193
Kalsbeck et al., 1981 [4]	United States, national	1974	422,000	200
Klauber et al., 1981 [5]	San Diego County, CA	1978	5,055	294
Cooper et al., 1981 [6]	Bronx, NY	1980–1981	1,209	249
Jagger et al., 1984 [7]	Virginia	1978	735	175
Kraus et al., 1984 [8]	San Diego County, CA	1981	1,862	180
Whitman et al., 1984 [9]	Chicago	1979–1980	782	367

are similar to those for occupational spinal cord injury (see later in chapter), and distinctly different from those of head injuries in the nonoccupational setting, where the largest number of closed head injuries occur from motor vehicle accidents. In the Australian report, the occupational groups at highest risk of head trauma (32%) were laborers and craftsmen, but the nature of the injuries was not discussed.

In 1980, the U.S. Bureau of Labor Statistics[12] published the results of a survey of workers who suffered nonfatal head injuries on the job. The data were gathered from 20 states during a 3-month period from July–September 1979. A total of 1,033 workers involved in reported head injury accidents were included in this survey, which was generated from data obtained through a detailed questionnaire. This report states that most impact injuries to the head suffered on the job occurred in workers who were not wearing head protection. In fact, only 16% of workers who sustained head injuries were wearing hard hats at the time. Common explanations as to why head protection was not used included statements that such protection was not required for the type of work being performed or that such a practice was not practical.

This survey was not confined to traumatic brain injury, thus avoiding the problem of defining head injury. The questionnaire included all blows to the head and allowed the respondent to describe the injury sustained. Salient findings of the survey included the following[12]:

1. Of the workers sustaining head injuries, 89% were male.
2. The most common industries involved were manufacturing (42%) and construction (21%).

3. Most head-injured workers (56%) were 20–35 years of age.
4. The most common causes were falling (36%), swinging (19%), or flying objects (12%) striking the head.
5. While lacerations and contusions were the most common extracranial injuries, fully 25% of the accidents involved concussion.

The Bureau of Labor Statistics published a similar summary of results in a separate report, entitled "Accidents Involving Face Injuries."[13] Again, manufacturing and construction were the industries most commonly involved, and flying, swinging, or falling objects striking the face were the most common causes of injury.

PROTECTIVE HEADGEAR

Federal guidelines for the use of protective equipment and clothing are contained within the Occupational Safety and Health Administration (OSHA) Standards and Interpretations, which is now incorporated into the Code of Federal Regulations.[14] The intent of these rules is to protect workers employed in areas where head injuries may occur from falling objects, from direct impact, or from electrical shock and burns. The employer is required to comply with these federal regulations by reducing the risk of injury through modifications of the workplace environment as well as by providing appropriate protective headgear. Failure to comply may result in a citation following an OSHA compliance inspection, or the employer may be sued by an injured employee.

Helmets worn by workers are expected to meet the specifications of the American National Standards Institute (ANSI), which periodically updates its standards. The most recent publication for personnel protection is *Protective Headwear for Industrial Workers—Requirements*.[15] These requirements establish helmet types and classes, specify physical and performance characteristics, and outline testing methods that protective headwear must pass.

ANSI established standards for three classes of protective headgear (ANSI Z289.9-1986):

1. *Class A.* Class A helmets are intended to reduce the force of impact of falling objects and to reduce the danger of contact with exposed low-voltage conductors. Representative sample shells are proof-tested at 2,200 volts (phase to ground).
2. *Class B.* Class B helmets are intended to reduce the force of impact of falling objects and to reduce the danger of contact with exposed high-voltage conductors. Representative sample shells are proof-tested at 20,000 volts (phase to ground).
3. *Class C.* Class C helmets are intended to reduce the force of impact of falling objects. This class offers no electrical protection.

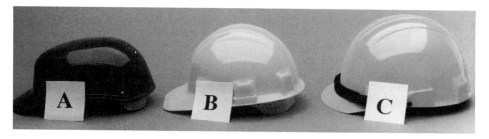

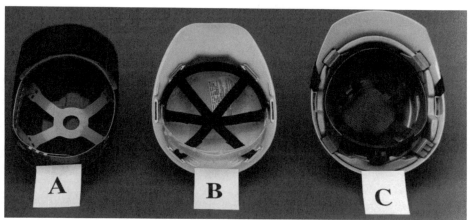

FIGURE 10.1   A. Bump cap. B. Standard hard hat. C. Larger and more protective hard hat.

"Bump caps" (Fig. 10.1A) are lightweight hats intended to offer protection against minor bumps and lacerations, but they are not designed to comply with the above standards and should not be used as substitutes for industrial safety helmets.

Safety helmets, or hard hats (Fig. 10.1B), are typically constructed with a durable, resilient plastic shell and an energy-absorbing interior suspension with an adjustable headband. Various added features, such as protective padding or accessories for cold weather, face protection, and ear protections, can be obtained on certain models. Industrial hard hats are intended primarily for protection from penetration of small falling objects that would strike the top of the head, such as nails, bolts, and rivets. They offer some protection against light bumps but only minimally reduce the force of impact from a severe blow to the top of the head. Hard hats offer far less protection against side- or rear-impact blows. Only recently have manufacturing companies included chin straps for fastening the helmet and offered added protection against off-center blows. However, most hard hat models do not require the use of a chin strap in their "user instructions." One hard hat model offers better impact absorption and more head area protection than conventional models (Fig. 10.1C).

Safety helmet manufacturers conduct product testing on random samples of their helmets as part of their quality assurance programs in compliance with ANSI standards. Independent agencies offer a voluntary program of helmet testing, which provides an outside analysis of a manufacturer's quality assurance program and helmet testing procedures.

To meet ANSI standards, helmets must pass three tests:[15]

1. An 8-lb contoured missile is dropped from a height of 5 ft onto the top of a helmet. Special sensing devices must indicate a transmission of less than 850 lb through to the head form.
2. A 1-lb pointed penetrator dropped from a height of 10 ft must not penetrate more than 3/8 in. into the helmet shell.
3. "Leaking" of electrical current must meet a specified minimum criterion for each class A and class B helmet.

ACUTE CARE

While it is not the intention of this chapter to provide a detailed description of emergency procedures in acute head and spinal trauma, a brief review is warranted. Thorough reviews of this subject matter are available elsewhere.[16-18] On-site health care providers should be familiar with standard emergency treatment of injuries and would be least prepared if they are certified in basic life support and first aid techniques. Physicians who are likely to be called on for on-site evaluation of injured workers should be periodically updated on emergency trauma care. The best means of keeping abreast of new treatment approaches for a wide variety of traumatic injuries is through certification in advanced trauma life support (ATLS). Courses are offered periodically at medical centers across the United States under the sponsorship of the American College of Surgeons.[19]

Most occupational head injuries result in laceration and contusions of the scalp or face. Careful examination of the external injuries may offer valuable information about underlying brain lesions, as in penetrating injuries or depressed skull fractures. No attempt should be made at the scene of the injury to lift bone fragments or to remove foreign objects penetrating the skull or facial bones as they may serve to tamponade underlying lacerated blood vessels.

Life-threatening hemorrhage and airway compromise must be rapidly assessed and treated in cases of severe injury. Cardiopulmonary status must be stabilized and basic life support measures undertaken when necessary. As with any bodily trauma, resuscitation and stabilization of vital signs must precede more detailed examination of nervous system function. Head injuries that affect brain function must be distinguished from extracranial lacerations and contusions. An individual who exhibits any mental status alteration following a blow to the head should be considered to have suffered a traumatic brain injury. The vague overinclusiveness of the term *head injury* is gradually giving way to the more precise descriptiveness of TBI.

MILD HEAD INJURY

The least severe brain injuries are typically referred to as concussions or mild head injuries.[20] It is well established that one need not be rendered unconscious to have suffered a brain injury.[21] Transient confusion and amnesia resulting from the impact or subsequent events (posttraumatic amnesia), or both, are common consequences of TBI. Amnesia for events leading up to the impact (retrograde amnesia) is less common and usually denotes a more serious injury. Unconsciousness occurs when both cerebral hemispheres or the brain stem reticular activating system are affected.

Guidelines that have been established for the management of concussion in sports[22] are useful for any setting in which concussion occurs. Recent evidence suggests that worrisome neuropathologic changes are often hidden following concussion, only to surface minutes or hours later or following a second head injury occurring a short time after the first injury. A grading scale for concussion and suggested guidelines for the immediate evaluation of the injured workers are offered (Tables 10.2 and 10.3). The main purpose of such a concussion grading scale is to identify features of concussion that require close monitoring to emphasize the need to avoid a second head injury while postconcussion symptoms persist (Table 10.4).

EVALUATION OF THE HEAD-INJURED WORKER

The evaluation of the head-injured worker must follow along lines of any emergency care for the trauma victim. Evidence of injury from general examination is obviously of importance. A general sense of the force of the blow should be obtained by history from the patient and from any eyewitnesses. Damage to any clothing or protective apparel should also be taken into consideration.

The usefulness of skull x-rays in this setting has come under scrutiny.[23] If computed tomographic (CT) scanning is available on an emergency basis, there is no added benefit to skull x-rays, since CT scanning can be used to detect fractures that are sometimes obscured by standard x-ray techniques. The superiority of magnetic resonance imaging (MRI) scanning over CT scanning in detecting evidence of intracranial pathology from trauma is now well established.[24–26] However, MRI is typically not available on an emergency basis, and CT has proved quite useful in detecting lesions of surgical importance.

Since approximately 10% of work-related head injuries also involve injuries of the neck,[12] a work-up of any neck pain or associated neurologic complaints must be thoroughly performed. Any evidence of cervical myelopathy must be addressed as a possible neurosurgical emergency. The

TABLE 10.2
Grading Scale for Concussion in the Workplace

The history of recent head trauma outside the work setting (e.g., recreational injury or motor vehicle accident), should be considered in the "return to work" section for each grade of concussion (see Table 10.3).

Grade 1
Confusion without amnesia
No loss of consciousness
Remove from job pending on-site evaluation prior to return to work

Grade 2
Confusion with amnesia
No loss of consciousness
Remove from job and disallow return for that day

Grade 3
Loss of consciousness
Remove from job and and transport to appropriate medical facility

TABLE 10.3
Guidelines for Return to Work

Grade 1
Remove from job. Examine immediately and every 5 minutes thereafter for the development of amnesia or postconcussive symptoms at rest and with exertion. May return to work if amnesia does not appear and no symptoms are seen for at least 20 minutes.

Grade 2
Remove from job for the remainder of the day. Examine frequently for signs of evolving intracranial pathology. Reexamine the next day. May return to work only after 1 full week without symptoms.

Grade 3
Transport from field to nearest hospital by ambulance (with cervical spine immobilization if indicated). Thorough neurologic evaluation emergently. Hospital confinement if signs of pathology are detected. If findings are normal, instructions to family for overnight observation. May return to work only after 2 full weeks without symptoms.

majority of neck injuries will most likely be of the "whiplash" variety. These are typically managed by ruling out significant bony pathology or malalignment by cervical spine x-ray series.

REHABILITATION

Rehabilitation of individuals who suffer traumatic brain injury typically begins in the acute care setting, with physical therapy often providing passive range of motion exercises for the comatose patient. Transfer to a rehabilitation floor or freestanding facility is arranged after the patient's condition is medically stable and he or she is able to engage in multidisci-

TABLE 10.4
Neurobehavioral Sequelae of Head Trauma

Cognitive
Attention and concentration deficits
Inflexible or stimulus-bound thinking
Memory disorders
Speech and/or language impairment
Impaired abstraction and judgment capabilities
Decreased speed, accuracy, and consistency of information processing
Defective reasoning processes
Diminished mental stamina
Distractibility
Perceptual
Decreased acuity or increased sensitivity in vision, hearing, or tactile sensation
Vestibular dysfunction and vertigo
Spatial disorientation
Disorders of smell and taste
Physical
Headache
Weakness
Incoordination or clumsiness
Easy fatigability
Affective/emotional
Apathy or lack of motivation
Impulsivity
Anxiety
Loss of insight or denial of disability
Irritability
Impatience
Poor frustration tolerance
Dependency

---

plinary therapy. This is typically provided by a team of health care professionals in physical, speech, occupational, and recreational therapy, as well as nursing. The best outcomes are reported by those facilities in which all therapies are coordinated and guided by neuropsychological principles that rely on the accurate medical and neuropsychological assessment of the patient's deficits and strengths.[23,27] Compensatory mechanisms are encouraged, as are emotional coping skills and new learning strategies to optimize the individual's potential for recovery. Consistency and frequent communication among treatment team members are essential for the maximum benefit of the individual patient.

The person who suffers from mild TBI may also benefit from an outpatient therapy program that uses the same multidisciplinary treatment approach. However, the benefit of "cognitive retraining" using computer interface therapy alone has not been well established and seems to have gained widespread popularity without adequate evidence of its usefulness. Often some other form of cognitive "retraining" or cognitive stimulation is used in a multidisciplinary or transdisciplinary rehabilitation environment.[28,29]

The National Head Injury Foundation regularly publishes the *National Directory of Head Injury Rehabilitation Services*,[30] which is a useful guide to rehabilitation hospitals and other service providers in any given region of the country.

RETURN TO WORK

Several authors have reviewed aspects of return to work for head injury victims. In studies that have reviewed factors predicting an individual's ability to return to work, hospital length of stay and severity of brain injury (as determined by duration of coma or posttraumatic amnesia) have been found to be significant contributing factors to vocational outcome.[31] Age when injured[32] and behavioral or personality changes have also been shown to be related to the person's ability to return to work.[33]

Other important factors include the individual's ability to return to his or her previous job, provision of a work trial or possibly easier work, and a lengthy period of support as provided by a colleague that includes modification of job responsibilities. After suffering severe TBI, a minority of individuals return to work. Most studies find that about half return at some point, but many subsequently fail. The other half never even attempt to return to work in most studies. Even for those returning to work, problems such as memory dysfunction, motor slowness, more frequent errors, and attitude or behavior problems are common.[34] Modification of the job without interference with productivity or other workers often allows survivors of brain injury to return to work, even if at a lower level of productivity or accuracy.[35]

Features of supported work models for individuals with traumatic brain injury outline these important factors.[36]

A. Job placement
   1. Matching job needs to client abilities or potential
   2. Encouraging employer-client communications
   3. Encouraging family or caretaker-client communications
   4. Establishing travel arrangements or providing travel training
   5. Analyzing the job environment to identify potential obstacles
B. Job site training and advocacy
   1. Behavioral training of job skills
   2. Advocacy on behalf of the client
C. Ongoing assessment
   1. Supervisor evaluation data
   2. Client data
D. Job retention and follow-along
   1. Regular on-site visits to employers

2. Periodic reviews of supervisory evaluations
3. Client progress reports
4. Family or caregiver evaluations

Occupational Spinal Cord Injury

Like traumatic brain injury, spinal cord injury (SCI) is most commonly the result of a motor vehicle accident in the nonoccupational setting. Few studies have even addressed occupation in relation to spinal cord injury. The treatment of occupational SCI is the same as that of nonoccupational SCI and incorporates many of the principles of treatment of traumatic brain injury described previously. Although few studies have been published regarding the significance of the work environment to SCI or the reentry of the spinal cord-injured patient into the occupational setting, what data are available are reviewed.

OCCUPATIONAL STATUS AT TIME OF INJURY

National statistics[37] of spinal cord-injured individuals have revealed that the majority were employed in the competitive labor market (59.9%) or were students (19.7%) at the time of injury. Others were unemployed (12.5%), retired (3.4%), or homemakers (2.5%), and for some no information was available (2%).

A five-year study (1986–1990) of the Spinal Cord Injury Early Notification System (SCIENS) in Colorado and Wyoming is the first to look at specific occupations and their possible relation to SCI.[38] This study analyzed 522 reported cases of SCI. The two leading causes of SCI in these two states are motor vehicle accidents (56%) and falls (20%), which is true of the nation as a whole. Other causes include sports (9%), falling objects (3%), violence (7%), plane crash (1%), and all other causes (4%).

The majority of persons hurt in motor vehicle accidents are young and many are injured in the summer months. Persons injured through falls are in two distinct categories: younger individuals injured while in the occupational setting or during recreational activities and elderly people who fall in and around their homes.

FREQUENCY AND ETIOLOGIES OF OCCUPATIONAL SPINAL CORD INJURY

In one study, the workplace was found to be the setting for 14% of all cases of SCI, second only to incidents in transit (48%).[38] This number of occupational SCIs is consistent with findings in the few other studies that have looked at the frequency of occupational SCI.[39–43] In an epidemiologic study of SCIs in Denmark, 18% of SCI were related to industrial accidents, and most were due to falls.[39]

TABLE 10.5
Etiologies for Occupational and Nonoccupational Spinal Cord Injury

Etiology	Occupational (%)	Nonoccupational (%)
Motor vehicle accident	19	59
Fall	50	16
Hit by an object	19	1
Violence	5	9
Sports	1*	11
Other/unknown	6	4

*Snow skiing injuries.

In another study, 50% (37 of 74 cases) of occupational SCIs were due to falls, compared to only 15.9% of nonoccupational SCIs[44] (Table 10.5). A total of 566 cases of SCI were reviewed based on data gathered through the SCIENS for a period of 5.5 years (January 1, 1986, through June 6, 1991). Of the 566 cases, 74 (13.1%) were due to injuries sustained during the course of employment. In this study, only 18.9% of occupational SCIs resulted from motor vehicle accidents compared to 59.3% of nonoccupational SCIs. Other major etiologies for occupational SCI included being hit by a falling object (18.9%), gunshot wound (4%), lifting (2.8%), and one (1.4%) each of the following: skiing, stabbing, being struck in the head, and unknown.[44] These numbers are similar to those from a Texas study in which 15.5% of SCIs were related to "industrial" accidents, with 44% of these injuries being due to falls.[41]

OCCUPATIONS AT THE TIME OF SPINAL CORD INJURY

Although only 14% of all spinal cord injuries occurred in the occupational setting in the Colorado study,[38] workers in construction occupations sustained 41.9% of those injuries. Only minor differences were found between the nonoccupational and occupational groups in most other occupations (Fig. 10.2). Construction occupations were held by 14% of all men with SCI, even though these occupations account for less than 8% of the male workforce in Colorado. Despite the risk of working in the construction industry, those individuals who do not work at all (students, unemployed, retired) sustain over one-third of all SCIs that occur in Colorado.

AGE AND SEX DISTRIBUTIONS FOR OCCUPATIONAL
SPINAL CORD INJURY

Seventy of 74 (94.6%) occupational SCIs were sustained by men in the Colorado study.[44] Fewer (73.8%) of the nonoccupational SCIs were sustained by men, although men still dominated this group. Men dominate all age groups for both occupational and nonoccupational groups (Figs. 10.3

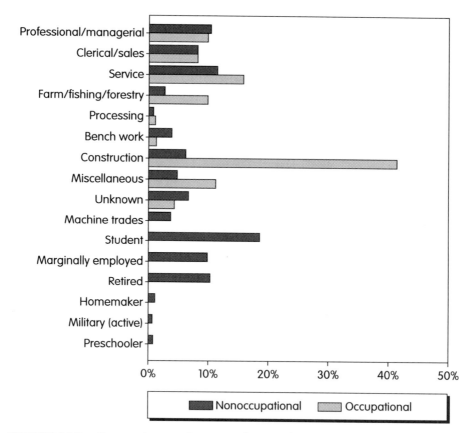

FIGURE 10.2 Occupations at the time of injury for both occupational and nonoccupational spinal cord injury.

and 10.4). Younger individuals dominate the SCI group in general; the occupational group tends to be slightly older, with a mean of 38.9 years versus 34.4 years for the nonoccupational group (Figs. 10.3 and 10.4).

LEVEL AND COMPLETENESS OF INJURY

Figures 10.5 and 10.6 show both the level of injury (cervical, thoracic, lumbar, sacral) and the "completeness" of the injury for both occupational and nonoccupational SCIs from the Colorado study.[44] The values between the two groups are comparable, with the exception of cervical and lumbar injuries, with a significantly lower number of cervical injuries and a significantly higher number of lumbar injuries in the occupational group. This is most likely due to the lower percentage of motor vehicle accidents in the occupational group (and thus fewer cervical injuries) and a greater number of falls, producing more lumbar injuries.

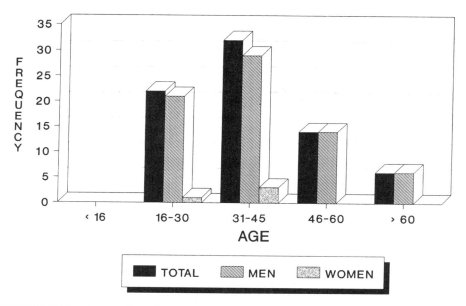

FIGURE 10.3   Age and sex for occupational spinal cord injury.

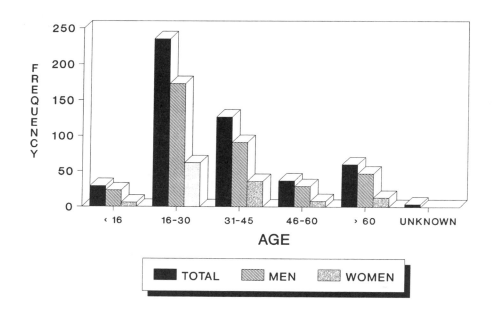

FIGURE 10.4   Age and sex for nonoccupational spinal cord injury.

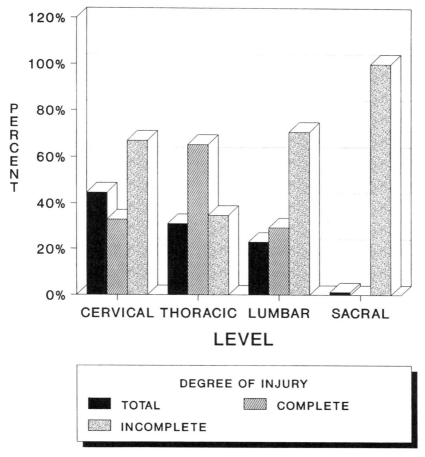

FIGURE 10.5   Level and completeness of injury in occupational Spinal Cord Injury.

Occupational Status Following Spinal Cord Injury

One of the major goals in the rehabilitation of individuals with SCI is securing gainful employment. Two studies have addressed return to work status following SCI.[37,45]

National statistics gathered over a 15-year period concerning patients with SCIs who were followed with regard to occupational status show several interesting trends.[45] Two-thirds of patients were either employed in the competitive labor market (63.7%), students (14.7%), or unemployed (17.6%) at the time of injury. At one year post-SCI 68.8% were unemployed, while only 11.5% were employed and 15.1% were students. The number of individuals employed in the competitive labor market gradually rose over time and peaked at 38% in year 12.

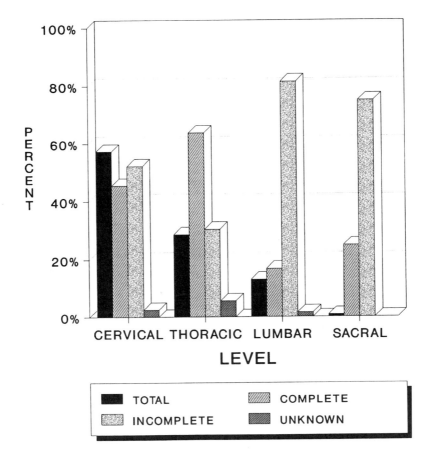

FIGURE 10.6   Level and completeness of injury in nonoccupational spinal cord injury.

In another study, employment was compared to level and complete-ness of injury.[37] The proportion of patients employed in the competitive labor market increased over time for each category, and not surprisingly employment was highest for incomplete paraplegics, followed by complete paraplegics, incomplete quadriplegics, and complete quadriplegics.[37]

Patients who returned to work within the first postinjury year gener-ally returned to a similar or identical position with their pre-injury employer. However, subsequent increases in employment were due almost exclusively to patients who returned to different positions with different employers, and to patients who were students when injured and who sub-sequently found employment. Other studies have been published on the types of jobs obtained by patients with SCI, income levels, and predictors of obtaining and sustaining postinjury employment.

PREVENTION OF OCCUPATIONAL SPINAL CORD INJURY

The importance of having occupational statistical information on SCI is to be able to direct prevention strategies in the workplace. Since little can be done to reverse a neurologic deficit after severe SCI, physicians need to be involved in educational programs in those occupations, such as the construction industry, in which the risk of SCI is highest.

References

1. Harlow, JM Recovery after severe injury to the head. Mass Med Soc 1968; 2:327–346.
2. Occupational Injuries and Illnesses in the United States by Industry 1986. U.S. Department of Labor Bureau of Labor Statistics, May 1988.
3. Annegers JF, Grabow HD, Kurland LT et al. The incidence, causes, and secular trends in head injury in Olmsted County, Minnesota, 1935–1974. Neurology 1980;30:912–919.
4. Kalsbeck WD, McLauren RL, Harris BSH et al. The national head and spinal cord injury survey: major findings. J Neurosurg 1981;53(S):19–31.
5. Klauber MR, Barrett-Connor E, Marshall LF et al. The epidemiology of head injury. A prospective study of an entire community: San Diego, California, 1978. Am J Epidemiol 1981;113:500–509.
6. Cooper JD, Tabaddor K, Hauser WA. The epidemiology of head injury in the Bronx. Neuroepidemiology 1983;2:70–88.
7. Jagger J, Levine J, Jane J et al. Epidemiologic features of head injury in a predominantly rural population. J Trauma 1984;24:40–44.
8. Kraus JF, Black MA, Hessel N et al. The incidence of acute brain injury and serious impairment in a defined population. Am J Epidemiol 1984;119:186–201.
9. Whitman S, Coonley-Hoganson R, Desai BT. Comparative head trauma experiences in two socioeconomically different Chicago-area communities. A population study. Am J Epidemiol 1984;119:570–580.
10. Kerr TA, Kay DW, Lassman LP. Characteristics of patients, type of accident, and mortality in a consecutive series of head injuries admitted to a neurosurgical unit. Br J Prev Soc Med 1971;25:179–185.
11. Selecki BR, Hoy RJ, Ness P. Neurotraumatic admissions to a teaching hospital: a retrospective survey. Part 2: Head injuries. Med J Aust 1968;55:582–585.
12. Accidents involving head injuries: U.S. Department of Labor Bureau of Labor Statistics, July 1980.
13. Accidents involving face injuries: U.S. Department of Labor Bureau of Labor Statistics, May 1980.
14. Code of Federal Regulations, Title 29.
15. Protective Headwear for Industrial Workers—Requirements. New York: American National Standards Institute, Publication No. ANSI Z89.1–1986.
16. Cooper PR (ed). Head Injury (3rd ed). Baltimore: Williams & Wilkins, 1993.
17. Fink ME. Emergency management of the head-injured patient. Emerg Clin North Am 1987;5:783–795.

18. Tyson GW. Head Injury Management for Providers of Emergency Care. Baltimore: Williams & Wilkins, 1987.
19. ATLS Program Office: American College of Surgeons, 55 East Erie Street, Chicago, IL 60611.
20. Levin HS, Eisenberg HM, Benton AL. Mild Head Injury. New York: Oxford University Press, 1989.
21. Kelly JP, Nichols JS, Filley CM, Lillehei KO, Rubinstein D, Kleinschmidt-DeMaster BK. Concussion in sports. JAMA 1991;266:2867–2869.
22. Colorado Medical Society: Report of the sports medicine committee: guidelines for the management of concussion in sports (revised). Denver: Colorado Medical Society, 1991.
23. Unger JM, Eisenberg RL, Bathelemy CR, Shaffer KA. Handbook of Head and Neck Imaging. New York: Churchill Livingstone, 1987.
24. Gentry LR, Godersky JC, Thompson B, Dunn VD. Prospective comparative study of the intermediate-field MR and CT in the evaluation of closed head trauma. Am J Neuroradiol 1988;150:673–682.
25. Jenkins A, Teasdale G, Hadley MDM, MacPhearson P, Rowan JO. Brain lesions detected by magnetic resonance imaging in mild and severe head injuries. Lancet 1986;2:445–446.
26. Levin H., Amparo EG, Eisenberg HM et al. Magnetic resonance imaging and computerized tomography in relation to the neurobehavioral sequelae of mild and moderate head injuries. J Neurosurg 1987;66:706–713.
27. Ben-Yishay Y, Silver SM, Piasetsky E, Rattok J. Relationship between employability and vocational outcome after intensive holistic cognitive rehabilitation. J Head Trauma Rehabil 1987;2:35–48.
28. Leland M, Lewis FD, Hinman S, Carrillo R. Functional retraining of traumatically brain injured adults in a transdisciplinary environment. Rehabil Counsel Bull 1988;31:289–297.
29. Novack TA, Roth DL, Boll TJ. Treatment alternatives following mild head injury. Rehabil Counsel Bull 1988;31:313–324.
30. National Directory of Head Injury Rehabilitation Services, National Head Injury Foundation, 1140 Connecticut Avenue, NW, Suite 812, Washington, DC 20036.
31. Rao N, Rosenthal M, Cronin-Stubbs D, Lambert R, Barnes P, Swanson B. Return to work after rehabilitation following traumatic brain injury. Brain Injury 1990;4:49–56.
32. McMordie WR, Barker SL, Paolo TM. Return to work (RTW) after head injury. Brain Injury 1990;4:57–69.
33. Brooks N et al. Closed head injury: psychological, social, and family consequences. Oxford, England: Oxford University Press, 1984.
34. Johnson R. Return to work after severe head injury. Int Disabil Studies 1987;9:49–54.
35. Welch M. Job modification relieves problems of head-injured persons at work. Occup Health Saf 1987;94:65–66.
36. Wehman P, Kreutzer J, Wood W, Morton MV, Sherron P. Supported work model for persons with traumatic brain injury: toward job placement and retention. Rehabil Counsel Bull 1988;31:298–312.
37. Stover SL, Fine PR (eds). Spinal Cord Injury: The Facts and Figures. Birmingham: University of Alabama, 1986.

38. Annual report of the spinal cord injury early notification system: Division of Prevention Programs, Colorado Department of Health, 1990.
39. Biering-Sorensen F, Pedersen V, Clausen S. Epidemiology of spinal cord lesions in Denmark. Paraplegia 1990;28:105–118.
40. Burke DC. Spinal cord injuries, 1976. Australia N Z J Surg 1977;47:166–170.
41. Carter RE Jr. Etiology of traumatic spinal cord statistics of more than 1,100 cases. Texas Med J 1977;73:61–65.
42. Cheshire DJE. The complete and centralised treatment of paraplegia. Paraplegia 1968–1969;6:59–73.
43. Kurtzke JF. Epidemiology of spinal cord injury. Exp Neurol 1975;48:163–236.
44. Rosenberg NL, Gerhart K, Whiteneck G. Occupational spinal cord injury: demographic and etiologic differences from nonoccupational injuries. Neurology 1993;43:1385–1388.
45. National Spinal Cord Injury Statistical Center, Annual Report no. 8. For the period October 1, 1989 through September 30, 1990.

CHAPTER 11

Work-Related Low Back Pain

Neil L. Rosenberg, M.D.
Brent Lovejoy, D.O.

Musculoskeletal disorders, particularly back pain, account for greater than $50 billion in annual costs in the United States,[1] affecting one million workers annually[2] and accounting for 20% of lost work-time injuries.[3] Clinical evaluation and management of individuals with back pain are particularly difficult for several reasons. First, there is heavy reliance on subjective reports by the patient, without objective findings. Second, physical examination of the low back has surprisingly limited reliability.[4] Third, it has been difficult to make specific recommendations for allowable exposure of the patient to work situations.

Low back pain creates a socioeconomic problem because of its cost and prevalence. As many as 50–80% of individuals in the United States suffer back pain sometime during their lives, and it is the most common cause of impaired activity in persons under 45 years of age.[5-9] More money is spent in the United States to compensate for back pain than for any other nonmalignant medical condition. According to the National Safety Council, back injuries account for 32% of compensable injuries and 42% of total compensation costs, including medical and medicolegal expenses.[10] The cost of disability increased in the United States between 1956 and 1975 by 2,700%,[11] and the total medical cost of back disorders in the United States is approaching $56 billion per year.[12] The direct costs alone (i.e., not including absenteeism and other indirect costs associated with absenteeism) for occupationally related back pain was $11.1 billion, with a mean cost per claim of $6,807,[13] although a small number of high-cost back pain cases tend to account for a significant proportion of the costs.[14,15]

Evaluation of Low Back Pain in the Injured Worker

There is a common misconception that an inciting event is responsible for back problems in most individuals. Low back pain is a symptom diagnosis,[16,17] and very few of the patients suffer from diagnoses that are scientifically valid, which include disk herniation, spondylolisthesis, fracture, tumor, infection, and rheumatologic diseases. This means that for the majority of patients the cause of back pain is unknown.

Patients who have sudden onset of acute low back pain generally recover in a short period of time.[18,19] In the majority of these patients, symptoms resolve in 6 weeks with little or no treatment, and at 6 months, approximately 80–90% of individuals who had acute symptoms return to work and require no further treatment. The remaining 10–20% of the patients account for most of the costs related to occupational low back pain.

Previously, the patient with chronic back pain was defined as one whose symptoms had not resolved by 3 months, but current thinking is that patients who do not recover by the sixth week have a chronic problem[20] and that they should be managed far more aggressively. This becomes more critical when one realizes that the patient with chronic low back pain will constitute 80–90% of the total costs for back pain.[10,21,22] Therefore, after 6 weeks, the physician should be aware that usual and ordinary recovery may not be occurring and that other problems may be preventing this patient from getting well. Some of these may be anatomic and some may be psychosocial.

The numerous potential diagnoses make the evaluation and treatment of low back pain extremely difficult and complex. Certain causes of back pain can be specifically diagnosed (Table 11.1), but it is estimated that in 85–88% of the cases of low back pain, the physician is unable to identify a specific anatomic cause.[23] This chapter will focus on those cases without a specific diagnosis. It is the responsibility of the evaluating physician to rule out the identifiable diseases. This must be done at an early stage so that working patients with back pain can be evaluated and set into a management program that allows for early return to work.

FOCUSED HISTORY

Immediate evaluation of the individual with acute back pain should be performed by a clinician skilled in the diagnosis and management of such cases. A thorough history should be taken, focusing on a clear description of the job that was being performed at the time of the injury. Other important historical data include prior work-related or non–work-related back injuries, prior back surgery, and recreational activities or hobbies.

PHYSICAL EXAMINATION

A complete physical examination needs to be performed on every patient who presents with either acute or chronic low back pain. Many other con-

TABLE 11.1
Clinical Classification of Low Back Pain

Degenerative spinal disorders
Etiology known
    Age-related spinal degeneration
    Herniated nucleus pulposus
    Spinal stenosis
Etiology less clear*
    Segmental instability
    Facet syndrome
    Disk disruption syndrome
Congenital spinal abnormalities
Spina bifida occulta
Segmental malformations
    Lumbarization: First sacral segment with appearance of lumbar vertebra (i.e., six lumbar segments).
    Sacralization: Fifth lumbar vertebra incorporated into sacrum (i.e., only four mobile vertebrae)
    Conjoined nerve roots: Possible cause of sciatica
Spondylolysis and spondylolisthesis
Spine trauma
Compression fracture
Other fractures
Fracture-dislocation
Inflammatory spinal disorders
Bacterial infections
    Staphylococcus
    Tuberculosis
Noninfectious spondylitis
    Ankylosing spondylitis
    Reiter's syndrome
    Spondylitis associated with inflammatory bowel disease
Fibromyalgia and myofascial pain syndrome

---

* Most common causes of work-related low back pain.

tributing factors to low back pain also need to be considered, including metabolic diseases, tumors, vascular diseases, infectious diseases, and rheumatologic disorders.

The physical examination consists of inspection, measurements, palpation, percussion, and neurologic and other specialized tests, and should always be performed with the patient undressed. It is helpful to develop a systematic approach to the examination because it reduces the time involved and ensures that no aspect of the exam will be omitted.

Observation is one of the most important aspects of the physical examination. This should include observation of pigmentation, abnormal bony prominences, evaluation of ranges of motion and what changes occur in the spine when the individual moves in flexion-extension, rotation, lateral bending, and standing and sitting.

Standing Posture

Fluidity of body movements both when standing and walking gives a measure of the severity of the pain. A guarded gait with scoliosis or other postural disturbance suggests more severe pain. Seated posture should also be evaluated, since some spinal problems can be worsened or improved with sitting.

Range of Motion

Patients should be examined for the following spine movements: flexion, extension, and lateral bending. Axial rotation should be tested with the patient standing.

Manual Muscle Testing

Walking on heels (testing L5 root), walking on toes (testing S1 root), and squatting (testing L2–4 roots) can be performed easily even before the patient sits down.

Recumbent Examination

One also needs to palpate the spine, abdomen, and surrounding soft tissue for tenderness or masses. Evaluation of the peripheral pulses can also be done at this time if a vascular lesion is suspected. A pelvic or rectal examination, or both, may also be performed if indicated, particularly in patients who are not responding to treatment. Palpation for tender points, as in fibromyalgia, or trigger points, such as those seen in myofascial pain syndrome, should also be done.[24]

NEUROLOGIC EXAMINATION

The neurologic examination may be done throughout the examination and in all positions. More detailed muscle strength testing and sensory and reflex testing should be performed in all patients with low back pain. Details of the neurologic examination are reviewed in Chapter 2.

NERVE TENSION SIGNS

Looking for sciatic stretch (nerve tension) signs is an important part of the examination. Since it is important for the patient to be relaxed during this part of the examination, we prefer to gently roll the limb to measure hip flexibility and then to test hip range of motion. This serves to relax the patient before straight leg–raising.

Straight Leg–Raising

This test has been described in many ways. It can be done simply by elevating the leg with the knee extended and the examiner's hand supporting the leg behind the ankle. The other hand should be placed on the pelvis to guard against pelvic movement. The test is considered positive when posterior leg pain is reproduced that is not related to tightness of the hamstring muscle group. Straight leg–raising can also be performed with the patient seated.

Lasegue's Sign

This test is performed by flexing the hip and knee joints 90 degrees. The knee is then extended to the point where sciatica is reproduced. Dorsiflexion of the foot may add information to the performance of this test.

Internal Hip Rotation

If sciatica is produced with straight leg–raising, the leg is then lowered to a level where sciatica is relieved. Next, the hip is then internally rotated. This test is positive if sciatica is reproduced.

Bowstring Test

This is a straight leg–raise test that is performed until sciatica is reproduced. The leg is then lowered to a level where the sciatica is relieved. Pressure is next applied behind the knee. The test is positive if sciatica is reproduced.

RADIOLOGIC STUDIES

For years x-rays have been used to evaluate patients to predict outcome and the possibility of injury. Large series, some involving review of up to 25,000 sets of x-rays, have been unable to determine which patients had or would be most likely to develop low back injuries.[25–28] Back x-rays are not indicated at the initial visit in the absence of major trauma.[29] Because so many unnecessary back x-rays are performed, patient education is essential to promote understanding and to prevent "doctor shopping" or the use of inappropriate practitioners.[30]

The method of diagnostic testing for spinal disorders should be chosen properly. Currently, the choices are magnetic resonance imaging (MRI), computed tomography (CT) scanning, and CT myelography or contrast CT. Before the advent of MRI, the Quebec Task Force for Spinal Disorders (QTFSD) performed an extensive review of the medical literature through 1985.[10] This study concluded that the only test that was useful based on controlled trials was CT in patients with confirmed spinal stenosis. Plain x-rays and myelography were not shown to be useful under the conditions of randomized, controlled trials.

With the advent of MRI, our knowledge of the spine has greatly improved, particularly in regard to age-related disk changes[31-34] and whether alterations seen are normal age-related changes or related to other factors.[35,36] Some studies compare CT with MRI. The comparison of diagnostic methods in correlation with surgical findings is important. The sensitivity of MRI was 97.1%, compared with 83.3% for CT; the MRI specificity of 100% was superior to that of CT, at 71.4%. Surface-coil MRI can be used as the initial diagnostic procedure for a suspected herniated lumbar disk. If necessary, invasive contrast studies and CT scans can be used to clarify an equivocal MRI finding.[37]

A study comparing MRI and contrast CT imaging of the spine with conventional myelography not only suggests that MRI will one day replace myelography but that it is also superior to CT.[38] The accuracy of MRI was 90.3%; the sensitivity, 91.7%; and the specificity 100%. The same findings for CT were 77.4%, 83.3%, and 71.4%. MRI had no complications versus 13.5% for contrast CT. The cost was less for MRI: $840 versus $1,060 for CT; the costs vary geographically and obviously change over time.

Despite its increased diagnostic capabilities, MRI has clear limitations. These are primarily related to the problem of correlating clinical signs and symptoms with the radiologic findings. Negative findings are obtained on all imaging studies in some patients with clear radicular signs or symptoms,or both. Furthermore, a significant percentage of normal, asymptomatic individuals have radiologic abnormalities, including frank disk herniation.[39-43] While MRI has greatly improved our imaging resolution and our understanding of the normal aging process of the spine, it has not altered the clinical decision process in dealing with the delayed-recovery patient and the question of whom to select for surgical intervention.

FUNCTIONAL TESTING

When radiologic studies fail to give useful information about diagnosis of low back pain, a rational approach to treatment must be developed by using information from outcome studies and objective functional testing.

It has been determined that the majority of work-related physical impairments in the United States are due to the loss of strength in either limb or lower back. Therefore, the measure of one's residual strength is essential in determining the extent of physical impairment.

Static strength is defined as "...the maximal force muscles can exert isometrically in a single voluntary effort."[44] This technique of strength assessment has several advantages: (1) the technique is relatively simple; (2) the subjects are at minimal risk of injuring themselves, since the exertion is isometric and completely voluntary; they are requested to increase their exertions slowly, and to stop if abnormal discomfort is felt; and (3) the measurement is repeatable with a high degree of reliability.

Several methods of functional testing can be used to evaluate a worker's capability of handling heavy loads safely. Some may have merit; but others are of questionable value. When choosing among the several methods of functional testing, the following questions should be asked: (1) Is the test safe to administer? (2) Does the test give reliable, quantitative values? (3) Is the test related to specific job requirements? (4) Is the test practical? (5) Does the test predict risk of further injury or illness?

There are four major methods of functional testing: (1) isokinetic testing, which measures the patient in a single axis while moving at a constant velocity; (2) isoinertial or isodynamic testing, where velocity is variable but the resistance is fixed; (3) isometric strength testing, which measures isometric lifting capacity; and (4) aerobic testing, done by maximum treadmill evaluation.

Other functional tests use a series of randomly weighted boxes. Patients lift the boxes to various heights and determinations are made regarding lifting capacity in various positions. The disadvantage of non-computerized testing is the inability to assess patient effort.

Computerized instrumentation measures volitional effort by use of coefficients of variance, calculating the range as stated in percentages and looking at the variability or reproducibility of subsequent measures. The patient's efforts can be graphed to identify consistency of effort (Fig 11.1).

Three different forms of functional testing that have been systematically studied are recommended: isoinertial or isodynamic testing, isometric strength testing, and aerobic capacity testing.

Isoinertial/Isodynamic Testing

Isoinertial/isodynamic testing has the advantage of being able to measure all three axes of motion of back function and can rank dysfunction as mild, moderate, or severe. Current computer programs are able to assess a patient's efforts to perform in a physiologic or nonphysiologic manner. One device that can test in this fashion is the B-200 isodynamic testing machine (Fig. 11.2). This device will allow ranking the patient by degree of dysfunction of the lumbosacral complex. The results also show whether the test was physiologic or had a nonphysiologic component. A second value is given for the patient's effort.

Isometric Strength Testing

The second computerized device used in functional testing tests isometric strength. This is the oldest form of functional testing and the most extensively studied. It has been shown to be safe, reliable, and reproducible. Guidelines have been developed by the National Institute for Occupational Safety and Health (NIOSH) that use normative data related to age, sex, and weight.

Isometric strength tests are preferred because of their safety. In an isometric test, the subject is required to increase the force exerted slowly until a level is reached that "feels" safe. No specific feedback or challenges are given during the testing. This procedure has been proposed in the American Industrial Hygiene Association (AIHA) Ergonomics guide as being safe and reliable.[45] It has been used in industrial studies testing over

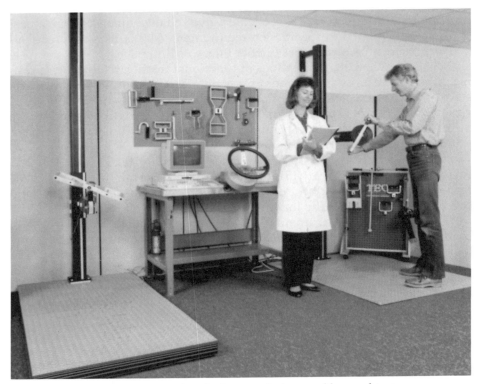

FIGURE 11.1A   Isometric testing device seen being used by a subject.

3,000 individuals, with no injuries reported. These studies have revealed that both frequency and severity rates of musculoskeletal problems were about three times greater for workers who were placed on jobs that required physical exertion above that demonstrated by them in the isometric strength test than for workers placed on jobs that had physical requirements well within their demonstrated capabilities on isometric testing.

It has been determined by research in muscle physiology, psychophysical principles, biomechanics, and job design that isometric strength tests simulating work tasks are the best measures of whether or not a person has the strength to perform a particular job.[46]

Isometric strength testing is safe, reliable, and reproducible, and one can test in an isometric mode that allows the physician to understand the patient's lifting capabilities in the sagittal plane. The sagittal plane is the most efficient and safest when lifting. Workers should be trained to work in this position. The importance of knowing the pressure on the L5-S1 disk is related to job safety. Pressures of 770 lb (action limit) or less are considered ideal. A job should be designed so that a worker's L5-S1 disk is not strained beyond 1,440 lb (maximum permissible limit); when pressures exceed these values, engineering controls or job modification should be instituted.

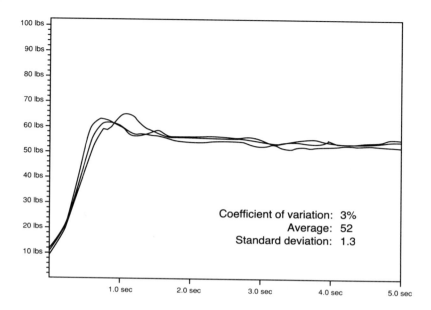

FIGURE 11.1B   A normal response on the isometric testing device with a demonstrated reproducible effort on three trials.

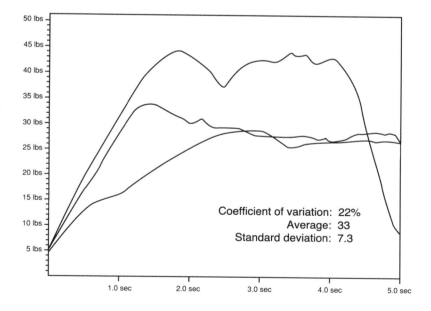

FIGURE 11.1C   Marked variation on three trials characteristic of nonphysiologic response. This lack of reproducibility suggests poor effort by the subject.

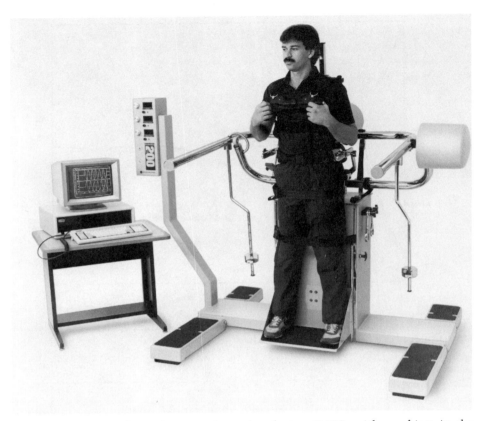

FIGURE 11.2A   Isodynamic strength testing device, B-200, with a subject in the testing position.

Two longitudinal studies have tested whether such testing is a valid indicator of potential risk of future injury. Together, these have involved nearly 12,000 workers in both light and heavy products industries.[47,48] To establish load limitations that correspond to actual lift loads in the workplace, research indicates that 15–30% of maximum voluntary contraction (MVC) ensures adequate protection from fatigue and stress that would compromise the healing process and allows return to normal function at the earliest possible time.[49]

Dynamic concentric contractions can probably be performed for long periods of time only if the intensity does not exceed 10–20% maximum isometric strength,[50] and it has been established that no reduction in strength occurs if the holding force is limited to 50% maximum strength.[51] With forces of 20–30% MVC, blood flow increased steadily during the activity.[52] At forces exceeding 30%, however, blood flow decreased and was completely arrested at 70%. There are also indications that stronger subjects are less able to maintain isometric contractions at the same per-

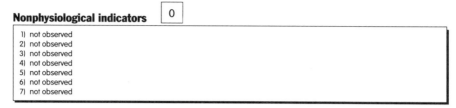

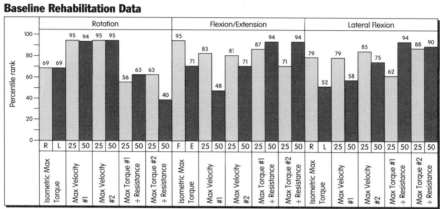

FIGURE 11.2B   Partial data from isometric strength testing in normal subject with normal percentile ranks in most test parameters and absence of "nonphysiologic" indicators.

centage of their maximal strength than are weaker subjects.[53,54] With a range of 15–30% MVC used as a guideline for initial reconditioning, individual strength test data should be analyzed to set the appropriate intensities within this range.[55–61]

Aerobic Capacity Testing

Aerobic capacity testing identifies the patient's true aerobic capacity, which may well be the most significant factor in predicting the outcome of back disorders.[62] If the aerobic capacity necessary for the patient to perform his or her job is known, the physician is able to classify work relative to the aerobic output. Matching the patient's aerobic capacity to that of the job allows us to properly match training procedures with the patient's needs.[63]

The basic principle of all aerobic graded exercise test protocols is a progressive increase in external work of large muscle groups to an end point of fatigue, or VO_2 max, or termination because of abnormal responses. The goal of the evaluation is to measure total body or ventilatory oxygen consumption, which is the amount of oxygen extracted from inspired air as the body performs work. Total body oxygen consumption can be estimated by the aerobic workload performed or by total exercise time.

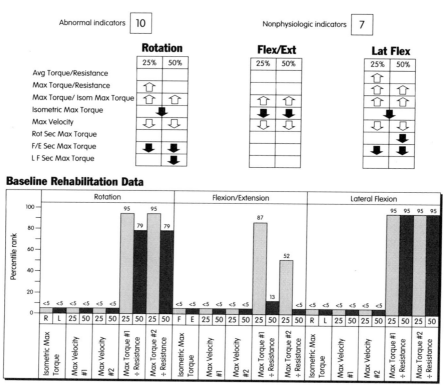

FIGURE 11.2C   Partial data from isometric strength testing with abnormal results in a subject with several "nonphysiologic indicators" suggesting lack of effort.

Another method of energy quantification is based on the metabolic equivalent (MET)—the energy requirement for basal homeostasis while awake, sitting. Aerobic capacity testing measures an individual's ability to use oxygen as may be needed for various levels of work. A person working at a sedentary job needs approximately 3.5 METs and needs to consume 7.5–12 METs to do a heavy or very heavy job.

Summary of Functional Testing

The objective data obtained from the results of these three methods of functional testing will allow design of a therapeutic program specifically for the individual being tested.

The absence of objective functional capacity measurements is a likely reason for much of the present confusion in low back care. The potential value of objective measurement of spine function leading to the same understanding of the spine as currently used in guiding treatment of the extremities has been recognized for some time, although practical and clinically useful technology has not been generally available.[64] Fortunately quantitative techniques for objectively documenting spine function are now available, as opposed to imaging techniques, which assess spinal degenerative processes. Disuse and the deconditioning syndrome are factors in long-term disability, and recent developments in the quantification of spinal range of motion,[65] trunk muscle strength,[66–68] endurance, and lifting capacity[69] present new options for low back assessment and treatment.

Objective measurement of lumbar function has been shown to be effective in evaluating and treating patients with nonspecific back pain. This approach contrasts with past reliance on patients' decreased pain symptoms as an indicator of recovery. Objective measurements rely instead on quantitative data, even with continued pain, to ascertain restoration of function.[64,69,70]

Back evaluations must address several issues. One issue is deciding which type of parameter best measures function. Absolute values of isometric torque in range of motion are initially indicated, but these alone may not adequately characterize function. Significant differences in isometric torque between patients with back pain and normal individuals have not been found in some studies. Differences in other studies have been found only after a period of prolonged rest, or only in certain planes of back movement.[71–73] There is also disagreement about how normal spinal range of motion can best be categorized and how changes in the measured range of motion actually reflect changes in back function.[71,73,74]

There is evidence that velocity is an important measure of back function and may serve as a reliable measure of low back impairment. Velocity of motion potentially greatly increases back loading. The reduction of motion and velocity by a patient represents a protective mechanism to guard against excessive loading and the resulting stimulation of nociceptors within the spinal structure.[75] Deutsch[76] used isodynamic strength testing to compare normal patients to those with low back pain. He found that velocity measures were the most sensitive performance indicators. Li and colleagues[77] used the same isodynamic evaluation to examine the relationships among resistance level, torque output, and velocity of movement. They concluded that the measured torque was not the sole indicator of strength, and that a stronger individual has a higher-velocity profile than a weaker individual for the same resistance. Thus, both velocity and torques have to be analyzed in the isodynamic mode of testing.

There are also increasing data that measurements of back function should be made in all three cardinal planes of back motion.[71,73,74] Two types of motion of the spine, translation and rotation, are normally coupled; that is, to a degree the two types of motion occur simultaneously. For example, in a flexion movement the vertebrae rotate in the sagittal plane and at the same time translate in the same plane. "Accessory motion" occurring during primary axis motion may be indicative of pathology and should be further researched as a possible determinant of effort levels and three-dimensional reproducibility.[78] Measuring the maximal isometric trunk strength of male adults, it was found that the torque generated was more coupled in lateral bending and axial rotation than in flexion and extension.[79] Overlap between the function tasks of trunk muscles indicates a need for coordination and control of the central nervous system in recruiting these muscles during task performance. This coordination control could be compromised by the onset of muscular fatigue, thus predisposing an individual to injury. The effect of fatigue was examined on motor output and movement patterns of isodynamic trunk movement in a normal male population.[80] The results showed that the reduction in functional capacity of the primary muscles is compensated by secondary muscle groups. It is postulated that this fatigue mechanism caused the spinal structure to be loaded in more injury-prone configurations. Based on the mechanism of dynamic fatigue, the following conclusions were postulated: (1) people who have to lift repeatedly in industry have to be trained for the task to reduce the risk for injury; (2) if fatigue occurs during a job, the person performing the job will perform the lifting or frequent bending in a more injury-prone pattern (i.e., lifting will take place with more twisting or lateral bending); and (3) the job has to be designed to reduce fatigue or overuse of trunk muscles and thereby reduce risk of injury.

Psychosocial Issues

Psychosocial issues, not necessarily physical capacity, are the most significant factors that differentiate those individuals who return to work from those who do not.[81,82] Psychosocial factors, including patient behavior, physician factors, employer factors, and legal/financial issues, play a major role in the final outcome in workers with low back pain and need to be addressed in an individual who is not recovering as expected.

Psychological issues have long been considered major factors in low back dysfunction.[81,83,84] Numerous psychological factors will predict return to work in the individual with low back pain, including one's personality traits, coping skills, and prior experiences with recovery from injury, and the postinjury management.[85] Psychological and other psychosocial issues that are associated with poor return to work outcome are listed in Table 11.2.

Appropriate psychological testing and consultation should be done soon after the injury, especially when there is evidence of nonorganic findings (symptoms perceived by the patient that have no anatomic, neurologic, or physical foundation),[86,87] obvious psychological factors, or subjective complaints that do not match the objective findings as observed on the physical examination.

Five findings are believed to typify nonorganic features:[86] (1) tenderness, either superficial or nonanatomic; (2) stimulation of the symptoms, through axial loading or rotation; (3) distraction, as noted in straight leg–raising; (4) regional symptoms such as weakness or sensory dysfunction; and (5) overreaction to stimuli unrelated to either anatomic or physiologic

TABLE 11.2
Psychosocial Factors Associated with Poor Return to Work Outcome

Psychological factors
Dissatisfaction with job
Depression
Personality disorder
Somatoform disorder
Social isolation
Substance abuse
Hostility
Neuroses
Legal/financial factors
Involvement in litigation
Physician factors
Ordering of additional tests
Employer factors
Dissatisfaction with care
No job rotation during recovery
Family history of disability
Unpleasant working environment
Symptom magnification
Fatigue at end of working day
Fear of subsequent injury
Monotonous and repetitive tasks

disorders.[86] If three of the five signs are observed, one should consider the fact that the patient is exhibiting nonorganic findings, which should alert the clinician to psychological or other problems unrelated to the patient's specific presenting complaint.

Nonorganic problems may involve malingering, the deliberate voluntary fabrication, or exaggeration of symptoms for secondary gain. Malingering is uncommon. Symptom magnification behavior, a more common phenomenon, tends to increase with prolonged disability and with involvement with litigation.[88]

Another useful tool in the identification of a psychological disorder is the pain drawing. As seen from the example in Fig. 11.3, this patient has depicted pain over his total body; however, his primary presenting symptoms were low back pain. The pain depicted is unrelated to any specific or significant anatomical dysfunction. The neurologic examination in this patient was within normal limits.[89]

Treatment and Prevention Strategies

The treatment of low back injuries can be divided into three phases based on the type and severity of the injury. Phase I deals with treatment during

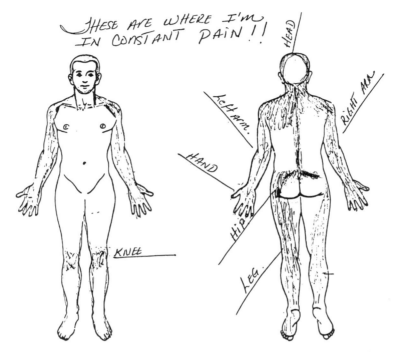

FIGURE 11.3   Pain drawing marked by a patient who presented initially with low back pain but whose pain drawing does not suggest a localized process. This drawing suggests that the patient has a psychogenic component or is suffering from a more widespread process, such as fibromyalgia.

the first 48 hours and uses primarily passive modalities. Phase II involves an educational process known as "back school," which is instituted early in treatment but also forms the core of prevention of future injuries. Phase III encompasses the major part of rehabilitation management, a sports-modeled rehabilitation program. These three phases overlap, but all are critically important in the management of occupational back injuries.

PHASE I: ACUTE TREATMENT MODALITIES

When the physician initially sees a patient with an acute back injury in the first 48 hours, therapy should consist of resting the patient for up to 48 hours. However, absolute bed rest is probably contraindicated. In fact, patients should be instructed to be up 30 minutes out of every 3 hours. This starts the sports-modeled rehabilitation process described below. If there is no evidence of neurologic disease following the initial evaluation, the patient should be so informed and told that the disorder is benign and will probably resolve rapidly. These patients should be told to expect rapid recovery if they follow the approach that will be outlined.

Treatment should not be limited to the use of passive physical modalities such as hot packs, ultrasound, manipulation, and massage. The only passive physical modality for which there is evidence of effectiveness is ice massage.[90,91] Active modes of treatment, including light stretching and walking, may also be used in this phase to the limit the patient is able to tolerate.

Manipulation

In the past 10–15 years, physical therapists and physicians have shown an increasing interest in the field of manipulation. Manipulation comes into play in the managment of the early acute injuries. Because manipulation has the ability to improve range of motion, improve function, and often reduce pain, it has become a very popular treatment in the first 4–6 weeks, with the maximum response occurring in the first to second week. The response seems to decrease after 4 weeks.[92]

A number of studies have investigated the effectiveness of manipulation for uncomplicated acute and chronic pain.[93–95] None of the studies have shown that repetitive or multiple manipulations have demonstrated effectiveness, and there is no evidence that the manipulation corrects or changes the underlying pathology. Additionally, the mechanism of manipulation is unknown.

Nonetheless, manipulation is a valid treatment if used in the early stages of an injury or back strain. The practitioner should know its limitations and be aware of potential serious side effects that can occur when manipulation is not handled properly.[96]

The back education program described below also should be instituted early in all cases, by using a formalized course, with instruction given by adequately trained therapists. It is important that the education of the patient begin with the initial examination so that he or she will have a clear understanding of the expectations of the physician and of what treatment will lie ahead.

Medication

Medications are often overused in the treatment of low back pain, especially narcotics and certain tranquilizers used as muscle relaxants. Physicians can help patients enhance their ability to recover from the low back problem without dangerous medications.[86] Nonnarcotic analgesics are adequate in almost all instances of acute low back pain. Narcotics should only be used in exceptional cases. Controlled-trial evidence of the effectiveness of nonsteroidal antiinflammatory agents in low back pain is lacking, despite their widespread use and the common belief of their effectiveness. In our experience, however, patients who are treated with aspirin, acetaminophen, or one of the other nonsteroidal antiinflammatory drugs do better than patients treated with narcotics or muscle relaxants. There is also no evidence based on controlled clinical trials that muscle relaxants are effective in the treatment of low back pain.

If the patient has used narcotics before conservative case management, the physician usually has a problem convincing him or her that these medications are not necessary. Before any constructive treatment can be given, the patient must be detoxified. This is often the time in the treatment when confrontation occurs and patients will drop out of a program, as the need for drugs may be greater than the need to resolve their low back problems.

Bed Rest

Until recently, bed rest has been the cornerstone of treatment for low back pain of either muscular or discogenic origin. Although bed rest has been greatly overused, with significant unnecessary loss of work and physical conditioning, patients are still being given instructions to take narcotics or muscle relaxants, or both, and to go to bed for up to 6 weeks. Clinical studies have clearly shown that if pain is nondiskogenic and there are no objective neurologic deficits, 2 days of bed rest are just as effective as 7 days. Others have suggested that constant bed rest is not necessary at all. In individuals with disk herniation, rest for up to 7 days is beneficial, but there is no indication that bed rest for more than that period has any added benefit.[97–99] In women, a loss of 6% of bone density in two weeks has been reported as a complication of bed rest;[100] this loss will not be recovered. In addition, strength declines 3% per day during bed rest. It has been shown that in people on prolonged bed rest problems develop, such as constipation, stiffness, and aching in the joints, that further delay recovery, and these individuals may suffer from memory loss and other psychological problems, all of which adversely affect the ability to get well.[100]

Surgery

It is believed by most surgeons that surgery should be contemplated only when there are appropriate objective findings, including abnormalities on MRI, CT scan, or myelogram that correlate with symptoms; positive physical examination (including sciatic tension signs); a positive history with radicular symptoms; and no contraindications for surgery.[100] Additionally, it is recommended that 6 weeks of conservative therapy be attempted before surgery, unless serious complicating factors are present that would make surgery necessary sooner. Major complicating factors that necessitate emergent surgical intervention are bladder and bowel dysfunction.

Recently, Nachemson[9] discussed his extensive experience with surgery in various causes of low back pain. With a ruptured or herniated disk, meaning a disk whose nucleus pulposus has broken through the restraining fibers of its anulus fibrosus, appropriate surgery produces a resolution of symptoms in up to 98% cases. With an incomplete herniation or a contained disk, meaning a disk still contained by a few of the outer fibers of the anulus or by the posterior longitudinal ligament, significantly fewer positive results will be seen. Surgery for a bulging disk or for just back pain without appropriate neurologic findings is unlikely to alter the outcome of the patient's symptoms.

Studies have shown that the primary advantage of surgery is an earlier return to work.[101] Four years after diagnosis, surgical and nonsurgical patients did equally well. After 10 years, 95% were doing well in both groups, and in only 2% did treatment fail, regardless of the modality.[101]

PHASE II: BACK EDUCATION PROGRAMS (BACK SCHOOL)

Back education programs teach people with injured backs the function of the back, how it gets injured, and how it gets well. These classes generally include slide presentations or other visual aids. Some innovative companies have devised back education programs for their own particular needs, using photographs taken within the company and demonstrations by their own workers.

The scientific community has been working diligently to evaluate the impact of back pain on society and attempt to improve its understanding. Studies from Canada have compared sophisticated back education programs with programs in which the injured workers were simply told by telephone that their job was waiting and that they were liked, and were asked to return to work as soon as possible.[102] Interestingly, it was found that the sophisticated back program made no difference in cost outcome compared to the latter telephone approach.[102] However, back education programs are still not totally without merit, and any patient who has sustained an injury may benefit from a back education program in the first 6–12 weeks after injury. Patients with back disorders are more receptive to back education at the time of their injuries than when uninjured.[103]

PHASE III: SPORTS-MODELED REHABILITATION

Sports-modeled rehabilitation is a program that uses the process of activation—that is, getting the patient physically active, so that he or she can become involved in normal daily activities, exercise, and ultimately return to work. Sports-modeled rehabilitation incorporates techniques that have been specifically developed for the rehabilitation of the injured athlete into the treatment and rehabilitation of the injured worker. This treatment approach uses the exercise equipment found in a health club or gym. It is important that each patient have a specifically designed program, keeping in mind his or her occupation and the physical capabilities needed for the specific job.

Once it has been established that the patient has no underlying neurologic disorder and does not require surgery, appropriate rehabilitation efforts can be instituted. The prescription for this rehabilitation needs to take into account that the treatment of the patient requires a team effort, in which physician, therapists, and often the employer and insurance carrier are part of the overall team to ensure proper management. In well-managed cases, all parties, including the patient, are well informed and a successful outcome is more likely.

The amount of training needed to recondition an individual depends on the length of "down time"—the time from injury to the return to full activity. Down time need not be the same for all fitness parameters. Whenever possible, the patient should attempt to maintain the condition and strength of healthy body parts while receiving treatment for the injured part. Conditioning should begin as soon as possible after injury to reduce the psychophysiologic dysfunction that occurs when problems continue for extended periods. Over time, pain behavior secondary to such dysfunction can decrease capacity more than the original injury itself and may contribute to the development of a chronic pain syndrome. If a chronic pain syndrome develops, it is difficult to determine whether disability is due to the pain symptoms or to disuse.[91]

Much confusion lies in the development of strength and conditioning programs. With strength training, as for aerobic training, it is recommended to begin with intensities lower than the individual's capacity, to prevent overstrain and delayed progression. Physical conditioning should match the physiologic demands of the activities the patient will experience on return to work. While strength training of specific muscle groups is important in rehabilitation, overall muscular endurance and aerobic conditioning are important in the early phases of a program to develop a strong "base." Once a strong base has been developed, the program can more safely move into strengthening the specific muscle groups for the individual's needs.

In 1977, the first prospective treatment study regarding back schools was done in Sweden, using 210 patients.[103] The patients were divided into three groups and three different methods of treatment for low back pain were used: (1) placebo, consisting of detuned microwave deep heat; (2) physical therapy, including manipulation and other modalities; and (3) the Swedish Back School and exercise. The study concluded that patients using the Swedish Back School, combined with exercise, returned to work 7 days sooner than patients who were treated with traditional physical therapy or placebo. The latter two groups returned to work at the same time, suggesting that standard conventional physical therapeutic modalities were no better than placebo.

Studies from Sweden have emphasized the need to evaluate and treat patients early after the injury. Aggressive intervention for the employee with a back injury should be performed in the first 4–6 weeks.[103] In addition, patients who have not responded in the first 6 weeks of more conservative treatment should be evaluated and treated aggressively as has been outlined, using functional testing, back school, and sports-modeled rehabilitation.

In another study, patients were evaluated and placed in the Swedish Back School, where fitness training was used to improve endurance. An early return to work was encouraged, ergonomic evaluations were performed in the workplace, and jobs were redesigned when necessary, so that employees could return to work at an earlier date than had been initially determined. Long-term disability was reduced by 50%, time lost by the employee was significantly reduced, and the cost savings were significant (A. Nachemson, unpublished study).

In 1979, Cady and coworkers[104] studied Los Angeles firefighters and evaluated them with respect to levels of fitness and endurance training. The incidence of back injury was reduced by 90% when only programs designed to increase cardiovascular fitness were used for wellness conditioning. The net effect of this was a 25% reduction in the worker's compensation costs.[105]

Most recently, a 4-year prospective study was done by Volvo, which showed that by using an activation program, male patients were able to return to work 7 weeks sooner and stayed at work 16 weeks longer over the next 2 years (A. Nachemson, unpublished study).

In the patient who has gone beyond the sixth week without resolution of symptoms, it is necessary to obtain a description of his or her job. This can be accomplished several ways: asking the company for a description of the job, including the physical factors; interviewing the patient and doing a detailed job description; and going to the workplace and evaluating the job, employing ergonomic principles. This means taking appropriate measurements and fitting the task to the individual, as opposed to making the individual fit the task, which may not be practical. This evaluation can be done by the physician, the occupational therapist, or an ergonomist. The physician should then review the job analysis to understand the demands of this patient's job. The physician can analyze the patient's physical impairment to see what it would take for the patient to return to work. The physician also needs to take a critical look at the physical therapy program, to make certain that its goals are consistent with what the patient needs to return to work.

The Strength and Conditioning
Exercise Prescription

Fitness has been recognized as an important factor in decreasing the incidence of low back injuries,[105] and a direct relationship between specific functional measures and subsequent back injury has been demonstrated.[103] The guiding philosophy of this functional restoration program is the restoration of joint mobility, muscular strength, endurance, and conditioning, as well as cardiovascular fitness, leading to a restoration of the ability to perform specific functional tasks such as lifting, bending, twisting, and tolerance of prolonged static positioning (i.e., sitting and standing).

Using the objective data, a strength and conditioning exercise prescription can be developed using the principles outlined above. Again, a specifically designed program is dictated following parameters that take into account the endurance and strength of the individual. In the acute phase, patients should not exercise strenuously, and pain control measures such as ice, heat, massage, ultrasound, electrical stimulation, or manipulation may be indicated. "Rest" should be interpreted as avoidance of abuse; general motion exercises are recommended, since all scientific evidence indicates the beneficial effect of motion on both symptoms and healing. In essence, early but moderate and gradual motion and loading improve healing in all the structures that build the back.[106] Endurance exercises that emphasize full range of motion and technique should be coordinated with flexibility exercises. With attention to the objective parameters measured in testing, the program should progress toward increasing efficiency.

Aerobic Conditioning

Aerobic conditioning or endurance training is the next phase of the sports-modeled rehabilitation program and uses concepts derived from studies of competitive athletes.[107,108] Movement into this phase of conditioning depends on assessment of the individual's endurance adaptations and symptomatic responses. While strength-training intensity and duration differ from those of endurance training, there is a distinct relationship between the two terms. A muscle that demonstrates the ability to generate greater maximum strength will have a greater ability to generate muscular endurance than its weaker counterpart, because it will need to use a smaller percentage of its maximum strength-generating ability. To maintain progression along the endurance-strength continuum, resistance should be increased. For this reason the overload principle has been modified to what is now called the principle of progressive resistance; this means increasing the resistance gradually as the body gets used to the new stress. When the muscle is stressed progressively beyond its normal demand, it responds positively and becomes stronger.

Strength Training

In beginning the strength-training protocol, the intensity again should be based on the individual's strength testing, to eliminate trial-and-error guesswork in setting progressive resistances. Studies on work physiology state that a person can work comfortably at about 40% of his or her maximum lifting capacity.[109] Loads of 60–80% of a muscle's force-generating capacity are sufficient to increase strength. When training with weights in dynamic contractions, one talks about "NRM" load (number of repetitions maximal load). Weight is chosen so that it can be lifted "N" times with proper technique, but it is too heavy to lift "N + 1" times.

When beginning strength training in an individual with a back injury, there is an established order of resistance and duration progression: Initially, one sets the intensity level at 40% maximum lifting capacity. This lower beginning intensity level is set based on the supposition that high repetitions and low weight should precede programs of higher resistance to allow adequate time for cellular adaptations to occur.[110] Once these adaptations have occurred, the higher intensities can be applied to make training more specific to the traditional concepts of strength.

Fleck and Schutt[111] published a comparative review of various weight training programs, but regardless of which method of training is used, strength effectively increases when the exercised muscles are overloaded. Moving from an endurance to a strength training program constitutes muscular adaptations specific to the manner and mode of exercise. Whereas high-repetition endurance training brings about an increase in energy-producing aerobic enzymes found in the mitochondria, high-resistance strength training leads to increased synthesis of contractual protein actin and myosin.

Hickson[112] showed that simultaneous strength and endurance training interferes with the development of strength. From recent studies, researchers suggest that short-term endurance training leads to some increase in strength and work output, with no change in oxidative capability.[113] Strength training alone does not seem to interfere with development of endurance.[114]

One of the goals of the strength phase is to increase absolute muscular endurance (AME), the ability to maintain a given, fixed, submaximal force output during work, relying primarily on aerobic metabolism, until exhausted.[2,114]

Key points to remember when developing a strength program are the following:

1. Load program design variables only to the point where the workout can be tolerated and recovery allowed.

2. Underestimate physical capacities rather than overestimating them when prescribing exercise to beginners.

3. Upgrade and evaluate the program on a regular basis to maintain exercise stimulus.

4. Keep in mind the type of advanced program for which you are preparing the individual and overload the variables in that direction (i.e., strength, local muscular endurance).

As was noted previously, studies have shown that when surgery is indicated, it is effective. However, in one controlled study, 64 patients with herniated disks were treated both surgically and nonsurgically with a sports-modeled approach and followed for an average of 31.1 months. It was found that 90% of the total group had a good or excellent outcome, with a 92% return to work rate. There was also very little difference between the surgical and nonsurgical groups in other areas, including sick leave. This study demonstrated that herniated nucleus pulposus of the lumbar intervertebral disks with radiculopathy can be treated very successfully with aggressive nonoperative care.[115] Hence, when programs are designed around functional training, even patients with surgical lesions can frequently be treated effectively.

One clinical study has shown that by using a clinically supervised strength and conditioning program for chronic low back symptoms, over a period of 6 months, patients showed an 80% decrease in the number of reported symptoms, a 40% decrease in pain symptoms based on an analogue pain scale, a 35% increase in anaerobic capacity, and a 40% improvement in aerobic conditioning.[116]

Conclusion

Low back pain is one of the most costly problems to treat and one of the most elusive to diagnose. Surgery is rarely indicated, but when individuals are carefully selected, it is generally successful.

The clinician must be ever mindful of the problems associated with the diagnosis of low back pain. Care must be taken to be certain that the case he or she is diagnosing is "occupational" rather than one stemming from a nonindustrial injury. This is of utmost importance when the physician is asked to apportion the injury or event between occupational and nonoccupational factors.[117] It is also important so that one can assess the workplace design, the work technique, and the produced work itself, in order to avoid recurrent episodes of pain and disability.[118]

Once the clinician has determined that an injury exists and the degree of injury has been quantified, it must be decided whether the injury should be treated surgically or nonsurgically. An appropriate treatment plan must then be formulated.

If the patient's examination meets the criteria for surgery and conservative management has not been beneficial, an operation should be performed. The clinician then needs to work closely with the surgeon to remain an active partner in the rehabilitation process, which will aid in the early return to work of the injured worker.

In the nonsurgical patient, a rational approach to care is needed. The ergonomics of the patient need to be identified, via the use of the measurements of his or her aerobic and strength capacities, as has been described. With this information the clinician is able to write the exercise prescription that will best fit the patient's needs, addressing the issues in treatment that will allow the patient to return to work at the earliest possible time and with maximum efficiency. While the patient is in therapy, functional testing is repeated regularly so that the patient and the clinician receive continuous feedback.

Further studies are needed to evaluate the long-term outcome of patients with occupational low back injuries. Methods of assessment, including the use of MRI and computerized functional testing equipment, should be evaluated, and continued evaluation of treatment modalities in larger series of patients is also needed.

References

1. National Institute for Occupational Safety and Health: Work Practices Guide for Manual Lifting. Washington, DC: Dept. of Health and Human Services, 1981.
2. Lamb DR. Physiology of Exercise. New York: Macmillan, 1978.
3. Dept. of Industrial Relations. Back Strains—Incidence Rates by Industry. In Work Injuries and Illnesses, California QIAQ, 1982;54:2–4.
4. Nelson MA, Allen P, Clamp SE et al. Reliability and reproducibility of clinical findings in low back pain. Spine 1979;4:97–101.
5. Andersson GBJ. Epidemologic aspects of low-back pain in industry. Spine 1981;6:53–60.
6. Kelsey JL, White AA, Pastides H, Bisbee GE. The impact of musculoskeletal disorders on the population of the United States. J Bone Joint Surg [Am] 1979;61A:959–964.
7. Nachemson AL. The lumbar spine: an orthopaedic challenge. Spine 1976;1:59–71.
8. White AA, Gordon SL. Synopsis: workshop on idiopthic low-back pain. Spine 1982;7:141–149.
9. Nachemson AL. Spinal disorders. Overall impact on society and the need for orthopedic resources. Acta Orthop Scand 1991;241(Suppl):17–22.
10. Spitzer WO, LeBlanc FE, Dupuis M. Scientific approach to the assessment and management of activity-related spinal disorders. A monograph for clinicians. Report of the Quebec Task Force on Spinal Disorders. Spine 1987;12(Suppl):S1–S59.
11. Social Security Statistical Supplement, Sup. Doc. Num. HE 3.3/3:979. Washington, DC: U.S. Government Printing Office, 1977–79.
12. Burton CV. The gravity lumbar reduction therapy program. J Musculoskel Med 1986;13:12–21.
13. Webster BS, Snook SH. The cost of compensable back pain. J Occup Med 1990;32:13–15.
14. Troup JDG, Martin JW, Lloyd DCEF. Back pain in industry: a prospective survey. Spine 1981;6:61–69.
15. Federspiel CF, Guy D, Kane D, Spengler DM. Expenditures for nonspecific back injuries in the workplace. J Occup Med 1989;31:919–924.
16. Nachemson A, Bigos SJ. The Low Back. In R Cruess, WRJ Rennie (eds), Adult Orthopaedics (Vol 2). New York: Churchill Livingstone, 1984;842–937.
17. Morris EW, Di PM, Vallance R, Waddell G. Diagnosis and decision making in lumbar disc prolapse and nerve entrapment. Spine 1986;11:436–439.

18. Wood PHN, Badley M. Epidemiology of Back Pain. In M Jayson (ed), The Lumbar Spine and Back Pain. London: Pitman, 1980;29–55.
19. Wiesel SW, Cuckler JM, Deluca F, Jones F, Zeide MS, Rothman RH. Acute low back pain: an objective analysis of conservative therapy. Spine 1980;5:324–330.
20. Frymoyer JW. Back pain and sciatica. N Engl J Med 1988;318:291–300.
21. Taugher NJ. Incidence of Industrial Back Injuries and the Significance to Our Community. Workmen's Compensation Data. Madison, State of Wisconsin, Department of Industrial Labor and Human Relations, 1973.
22. Miller HG. Compensable Back Injuries in Wisconsin 1938–1965. Accident Facts 1967. Chicago: National Safety Council, 1967;31.
23. Bigos SJ, Battie MC. Acute care to prevent back disability: ten years of progress. Clin Ortho Rel Res 1987;221:121–130.
24. Goldman B, Rosenberg NL. Fibrositis, fibromyalgia, and myofascial pain syndrome. Semin Neurol 1991;11(3):274–280.
25. Frymoyer JW, Pope MH, Clements JH, Wilder DG, MacPherson B, Ashikaga T. Risk factors in low back pain. An epidemiological survey. J Bone Joint Surg [Am] 1983;65A:213–218.
26. Redfield JT. The low back x-ray as a pre-employment screening tool in the forest products industry. J Occup Med 1971;13:219–226.
27. Magora A, Schwartz A. Relationship between the low back pain syndrome and x-ray findings. 2. Transitional vertebra (mainly sacralization). Scand J Rehab Med 1978;10:135–145.
28. Chaffin DB, Andersson GBJ. Occupational Biomechanics. New York: Wiley, 1984.
29. Deyo RA, Diehl AK. Lumbar spine films in primary care: current use and the effects of selective ordering criteria. J Gen Intern Med 1986;1:20–25.
30. Deyo RA, Diehl AK, Rosenthal M. Reducing x-ray utilization: can patient expectations be altered? [abstract]. Clin Res 1986;34:269A.
31. Tertti M, Paajanen H, Laato M, Alanen A, Salmi TT, Kormano M. Disc degeneration in magnetic resonance imaging. A comparative biochemical, histologic, and radiologic study in cadaver spines. Spine 1991;15:124–129.
32. Modic MT, Masaryk TJ, Ross JS, Carter JR. Imaging of degenerative disc disease. Radiology 1988;168:177–186.
33. Sether LA, Yu S, Haughton VM, Fischer ME. Intervertebral disc: normal age-related changes in MR signal intensity. Radiology 1990;177:385–388.
34. Yu S, Haughton VM, Sether LA, Wagner M. Criteria for classifying normal and degenerated lumbar intervertebral disks. Radiology 1989;170:523–526.
35. Riihimaki H, Mattsson T, Zitting A, Wickstrom G, Hannien K, Waris P. Radiographically detectable degenerative changes of the lumbar spine among concrete reinforcement workers and house painters. Spine 1990;15:114–119.
36. Battie MC, Videman T, Gill K et al. 1991 Volvo Award in clinical sciences. Smoking and lumbar intervertebral disc degeneration: an MRI study of identical twins. Spine 1991;16:1015–1021.
37. Forristall RM, Marsh HO, Pat NT. Magnetic Resonance Imaging and Contrast CT of the Lumbar Spine. Spine 1988;13(9):1049–1054.
38. Wiesz GM, Lamond MGB, Ditchener MB. Spinal imaging: will MRI replace myelography? Spine 1988;13(1):67–68.
39. Hult L. Cervical, dorsal and lumbar spinal syndromes. Acta Orthop Scand 1954;(Suppl 17):65–73.

40. Weinreb JC, Wolbarsht LB, Cohen JM, Brown CE, Maravilla KR. Prevalence of lumbosacral intervertebral disk abnormalities on MR images in pregnant and asymptomatic nonpregnant women. Radiology 1989;170:125–129.
41. Wiesel SW. The incidence of positive CAT scans in an asymptomatic group of patients. Spine 1984;9:549–551.
42. Boden SD, Davis DO, Dina TS, Patronas NJ, Wiesel SW. Abnormal magnetic-resonance scans of the lumbar spine in asymptomatic subjects. A prospective investigation. J Bone Joint Surg 1990;72:403–408.
43. Greenberg JO, Schell RG. Magnetic resonance imaging of the lumbar spine in asymptomatic adults. J Neuroimag 1991;1:2–9.
44. Roebuck JA, Kroemer KHE, Thompson WC. Engineering Anthropometry Methods. New York: Wiley, 1975.
45. Chaffin DB. Ergonomics guide for the assessment of human static strength. Am Ind Hyg Assoc J 1975;36:505–510.
46. Keyserling WM, Herrin GD, Chaffin DB. Isometric strength testing as a means of controlling medical incidents on strenuous jobs. J Occup Med 1980;22:332–336.
47. Chaffin DB. Human strength capability and low back pain. J Occup Med 1974;16:248–254.
48. Chaffin DB, Herrin GD, Keyserling WM. Pre-employment strength testing— an updated position. J Occup Med 1978;20:403–408.
49. Moritani T, deVries HA. Neural factors vs. hypertrophy in the time course of muscle strength gain. Am J Phys Med 1979;58:115–130.
50. Asmussen E. Growth in Muscular Strength and Power. In GL Rarick (ed), Physical Activity Human Growth and Development. New York: Academic, 1973;60.
51. Rohmert W. Problems in determining rest allowances. Part I. Use of modern methods to evaluate stress and strain in static muscular work. Appl Erg 1973;4.2:91–95.
52. Simonson E, Lind AR. Fatigue in Static Work. In E Simonson (ed), Physiology of Work Capacity and Fatigue. Springfield, IL: Thomas,1971;241.
53. Mundale MO. The relationship of intermittent isometric exercise to fatigue of hand grip. Arch Phys Med Rehabil 1970;51:532–539.
54. Thorstensson A, Hulten B, von Dobeln W, Karlsson J. Effect of strength training on enzyme activities and fibre characteristics in human skeletal muscle. Acta Physiol Scand 1976;96:392–398.
55. Frederick WS. Human Energy in Manual Lifting. Modern Materials Handling. March, 1959.
56. Snook SH. Group Work Capacity: A Technique for Evaluating Physical Tasks in Terms of Fatigue. Unpublished Report. Boston: Liberty Mutual Insurance Co., 1965.
57. Aquilano NJ. A physiological evaluation of time standards for strenuous work as set by stopwatch time study and two predetermined motion time data systems. J Indust Eng 1968;19:425–432.
58. Hamilton BJ, Chase RB. A work physiology study of the relative effects of pace and weight in a custom handling task. AIIE Transactions 1969;1:106–111.
59. Brown JF. Lifting as an Industrial Hazard—Ontario: Labour Safety Council of Ontario, Ontario Dept. of Labour, 1971.

60. Lind AR, Petrofsky JS, Betz W. A Comparative Study of Metabolic, Respiratory and Cardiovascular Characteristics of Fatigue During Lifting Tasks and Bicycle Ergometry. Final report, Dept. Of Health and Human Services (NIOSH) Contact CDC 00-74–8, 1977.
61. Garg A, Chaffin DB, Herrin GD. Prediction of metabolic rates for manual materials handling jobs. Am Ind Hyg Assoc J 1978;39:661–674.
62. Svensson HO, Vedin A, Wilhelmsson C, Andersson GBJ. Low-back pain in relation to other diseases and cardiovascular risk factors. Spine 1983;8:277–285.
63. Hartung GH, Smolensky MH, Harris RB et al. Effects of varied durations of training on improvement in cardiorespiratory endurance. J Hum Ergol 1977;6:61–68.
64. Mayer TG, Gatchel RJ, Kishino N et al. Objective assessment of spine function following industrial injury. Spine 1985;10:482–493.
65. Mayer TG, Tencer A, Kirstoferson S et al. Use of noninvasive techniques of quantification of spinal range-of-motion in normal subjects and chronic low-back dysfunction patients. Spine 1984;9:588–595.
66. Davis G, Gould J. Trunk testing using a prototype Cybex II isokinetic stabilization system. J Ortho Sports Phys Ther 1982;3:164–170.
67. Langrana N, Lee C, Alexander H et al. Quantitative assessment of back strength using isokinetic testing. Spine 1984;9:287–290.
68. Schmidt G, Herring T, Amundsen L et al. Assessment of abdominal and back extension function: a quantitative approach and results for chronic low-back patients. Spine 1983;8:211–219.
69. Mayer TG, Gatchel RJ, Mayer H et al. A prospective two-year study of functional restoration in industrial low back injury: an objective assessment procedure. JAMA 1987;258:1763–1767.
70. Mayer TG, Kishino N, Keeley J et al. Using physical measurements to assess low back pain. J Musc Skel Med 1985;2:44–59.
71. Berkson M, Schultz A, Nachemson A et al. Voluntary strengths of male adults with acute low back syndromes. Clin Orthop 1977;129:84–95.
72. Jackson CP, Brown M.D. Is there a role for exercise in the treatment of patients with low back pain? Clin Orthop 1983;179:39–45.
73. McNeil T, Warwick D, Andersson G et al. Trunk strengths in attempted flexion, extension and lateral bending in healthy subjects and patients with low-back disorders. Spine 1980;5:529–538.
74. Smith SS, Mayer TG, Gatchel RJ, Becker TJ. Quantification of lumbar function. Part I. Isometric and multispeed isokinetic trunk strength measures in sagittal and axial planes in normal subjects. Spine 1985;10:752–764.
75. Marras WS, Wongsam PE. Flexibility and velocity of the normal and impaired lumbar spine. Arch Phys Med Rehabil 1986;67:213–217.
76. Deutsch S. Comprehensive Evaluation of Back Function. Occupational Orthopaedic Center, Inc., Pawtucket, RI. Presented at the Isotechnologics 1988 User Applications Seminar, Dallas, June 1988.
77. Li F, Parnianpour M, Nordin M et al. A Database for Isodynamic Performances Against Three Resistance Levels in the Sagittal, Coronal and Transverse Planes. Presented at the Occupational and Industrial Orthopaedic Center, Hospital for Joint Diseases Orthopaedic Institute, New York 1987.
78. Seeds RH, Levene J, Goldberg HM. Normative data for Isostation B-100. J Ortho Sports Phys Ther 1987;9:141–155.

79. Parnianpour M, Nordin M, Frankel VH et al. Triaxial Coupled Isometric Trunk Measurements. Occupational and Industrial Center, Hospital for Joint Diseases Orthopaedic Institute, NY. Presented at the Orthopaedic Research Society Meeting, Atlanta, January 1988.

80. Parnianpour M. The Effect of Fatiguing on Isoinertial Trunk Flexion and Extension Movements on the Patterns of Movement and Motor Output (dissertation). Occupational Biomechanical Program, New York University, 1987.

81. Milhous R, Haugh LD, Frymoyer JW, Ruess JM, Gallagher RM, Wilder DG, Callas PW. Determinants of vocational disability in patients with low back pain. Arch Phys Med Rehab 1989;70:589–593.

82. Frymoyer JW, Cats-Baril W. Predictors of low back pain disability. Clin Orth Rel Res 1987;221:89–98.

83. Kelsey JL, White A III. Epidemiology and impact of low back pain. Spine 1980;5:133–142.

84. Taylor WP, Stern WR, Kubiszyn TW. Predicting patients' perceptions of response to treatment for low back pain. Spine 1984;9:313–316.

85. Peters P. Successful return to work following a musculoskeletal injury. AAOHN J 1980;38:264–270.

86. Waddell G, McCullock JA, Kummell E, Verner RM. Nonorganic physical signs in low back pain. Spine 1980;5(2):117–125.

87. Mooney F. Evaluating low back disorders in the primary care office. J Musculoskel Med 1989;6:18–35.

88. Matheson LN. Symptom Magnification Syndrome. In S Isernhagen (ed), Work Injury Prevention and Management. Frederick, MD: Aspen, 1988;257–282.

89. Ransford AP, Cairns D, Mooney V. The pain drawing as an aid to the psychological evaluation of patients with low back pain. Spine 1976;1:127–134.

90. Deyo RA. Conservative therapy for low back pain: distinguishing useful from useless therapy. JAMA 1983;250:1057–1062.

91. Bortz WM. The disuse syndrome. West J Med 1984;141:691–694.

92. MacDonald RS, Bell CMJ. An open controlled assessment of osteopathic manipulation in nonspecific low-back pain. Spine 1990;15:364–370.

93. Hadler NM. Diagnosis and Treatment of Backache. In NM Hadler (ed), Medical Management of the Regional Musculoskeletal Diseases. Orlando: Grune & Stratton, 1984;3–52.

94. Jayson MIV, Sims-Williams H, Young S, Baddeley H, Collins E. Mobilization and manipulation for low back pain. Spine 1981;6:409–416.

95. Sims-Williams H, Jayson MIV, Young SMS, Baddeley H, Collins E. Controlled trial of mobilization and manipulation for low back pain: hospital patients. Br Med J 1979;2:1318–1320.

96. Dan NG, Saccasan PA. Serious complications of lumbar spinal manipulation. Med J Aust 1983;2:672–673.

97. Deyo RA, Diehl AK, Rosenthal M. How many days of bed rest for acute low back pain? A randomized clinical trial. N Engl J Med 1986;315:1064–1070.

98. Holm S, Nachemson A. Variations in the nutrition of the canine intervertebral disc induced by motion. Spine 1983;8:866–874.

99. Videman R. Connective tissue and immobilization: key factors in musculoskeletal degeneration? Clin Orthop 1987;221:26–32.

100. Hirsch C. Efficiency of surgery in low back disorders: pathoanatomical, experimental, and clinical studies. J Bone Joint Surg [Am] 1965;47A:991–1004.

101. Weber H. Lumbar disc herniation: a controlled, prospective study with ten years of observation. Spine 1983;8:131–142.
102. Wood DJ. Design and evaluation. Spine 1987;12:77–82.
103. Bierling-Sorenson P. Physical measurements as risk indicators for low-back trouble over a one-year period. Spine 1984;9:106–119.
104. Cady LD, Bischoff DP, O'Connell ER, Thomas PC, Allan JH. Strength and fitness and subsequent back injuries in firefighters. J Occup Med 1979;21:269–272.
105. Cady LD, Thomas PC, Karwasky RJ. Program for increasing health and physical fitness of firefighters. J Occup Med 1985;27:110–114.
106. Nachemson A. Work for all. Clin Orthop 1983;179:77–82.
107. Tschiene P. The Distinction of Training Structure in Different Stages of Athlete's Preparation. Paper presented at the International Congress of Sports Sciences, Edmonton, Alberta, Canada. July 25–29, 1979.
108. Stone MH, O'Bryant H, Garhammer J. A hypothetical model for strength training. J Sports Med Phys Fitness 1981;21:342–351.
109. Bannister EW, Brown SR. The Relative Energy Requirements of Physical Activity. In EW Bannister, SR Brown (eds). Exercise Physiology. New York: Academic, 1968.
110. Jackson CGR, Dickinson A, Ringel SP. Cellular muscle area alterations following two modes of resistance exercise training in the same individual [abstract]. Med Sci Sports Exercise 1983;15:136.
111. Fleck SJ, Schutt RC. Types of strength training. Orthop Clin North Am 1983;14:449–458.
112. Hickson RC. Interference of strength development by simultaneously training for strength and endurance. Eur J Appl Physiol 1980;45:255–263.
113. Sharkey BJ. Training for Cross-Country Ski Racing. Champaign, IL: Human Kinetics, 1984.
114. deVries HA. Physiology of Exercise (3rd ed). Dubuque, IA: Brown, 1980.
115. Saal JA, Saal J S. Nonoperative treatment of herniated lumbar intervertebral discs with radiculopathy and outcome study. Spine 1989;14:431–437.
116. Reilly K, Lovejoy B, Williams R, Roth H. Differences between a supervised and independent strength and conditioning program with chronic low back syndromes. J Occu Med 1989;31:547–550.
117. Waddell G. Clinical assessment of lumbar impairment. Clin Orth Rel Res 1987;221:110–120.
118. Nordin M, Frankel VH. Evaluation of the workplace: an introduction. Clin Orth Rel Res 1987;221:85–88.

CHAPTER 12

Neurologic Disorders in Performing Artists

Richard J. Lederman, M.D., Ph.D.

The performing arts have been an integral part of human experience since the beginning of recorded history, serving as an expression of emotion, a means of paying homage and respect to deities, and a reflection of the human sense of awe of the environment. Music, dance, and dramatic arts are prominent features of all cultures; indeed, these activities are nurtured and encouraged among the youngest members of society. It is perhaps because the performing arts are so much a part of everyday experience that we have often failed to perceive them as an occupation. Even the words we choose to describe these activities (e.g., singing, dancing, acting, or playing) tend to portray a sense of leisure and relaxation rather than one of labor.

The medical problems of prominent members of the performing arts community have long been a subject of interest in professional as well as lay publications, certainly as much as those of other public figures.[1] Nonetheless, little attention has been paid to the collective health problems of performers as a group, with few exceptions, until very recently.[2] The emergence and rapid development of sports medicine as a discipline helped set the stage for the appearance of performing arts medicine as a specific area of interest, initially with a focus on health problems of dancers[3,4] and vocalists.[5-7] More recently, considerable attention has been paid to the medical problems of instrumentalists.[8,9] Neurologists have played a major role in this emerging field, and problems of special interest to the neurologist seem to be particularly prevalent among the ailments identified in performing artists.[9-12] In this chapter, these disorders are reviewed, looking at the scope and extent of the problem, the special methods of approaching the performer as a patient, and the most common neurologic disorders that may be seen in the performing artist; also, some recommendations are made for treatment and prevention.

Scope and Extent of the Problem

All segments of the performing arts community, including professional performers, students, and amateurs, are at risk for neurologic disorders. Approximately 200,000 professionals earn their living in the performing arts in the United States, representing less than 0.1% of the total population.[12] In addition, there are a large number of performing arts students and an even greater number of amateur performers. Although all of these individuals are subject to similar problems, it is our experience that professionals and full-time music students make up the bulk of those referred for problems related to playing.[13] Amateurs, however serious, appear to be affected less frequently, with certain exceptions, and account for only about 5% of our patients. This might be compared to sports medicine, in which amateurs, the so-called weekend athletes, account for an ever-increasing proportion of those injured in sporting activities.[14]

EPIDEMIOLOGIC STUDIES OF MUSICIANS

A number of attempts have been made to determine the prevalence of playing-related problems among performing artists, particularly among instrumental musicians. Caldron and associates[15] surveyed 250 non–wind instrumentalists via questionnaire; 59% reported some musculoskeletal problem related to instrumental playing. Since these were self-reported symptoms and diagnoses, considerable uncertainty remains about the actual disorder. Of the group surveyed, 58% were students and 41% were professional instrumentalists or teachers. Fry,[16] interviewing and performing limited examination on 485 professional orchestra musicians, found recurrent or persisting playing-related pain in 312, or 64%. The largest and most comprehensive survey to date was conducted by the International Conference of Symphony and Opera Musicians (ICSOM), in which instrumentalists in 48 orchestras were surveyed, again by questionnaire.[17] Of the 2,212 respondents, 76% indicated that they had at least one problem characterized as severe in its effect on performance. Fully 58% overall had a musculoskeletal problem, which would include most neurologic disorders.[18] In this survey, a greater percentage of women reported musculoskeletal problems than men (70% of females, 52% of males). This has been a consistent finding in surveys among performers as well as in epidemiologic surveys of musculoskeletal complaints in the general population.[19] Whether this represents a difference in susceptibility to injury or a difference in reporting remains uncertain. In the ICSOM survey, again as in others, differences in prevalence are also seen depending on the instrument. It must be remembered that in this study as well as in Fry's,[16] orchestra musicians were surveyed, meaning that only a small number of keyboard instrumentalists were included. Within the orchestra, string players appeared to be more susceptible to musculoskeletal problems than wind instrumentalists or percussionists. The study by Caldron and colleagues[15] did include keyboard instrumentalists and suggests that prevalence among this group is also high.

Several groups of student musicians have been studied as well. Fry[20] reports about 10% prevalence of playing-related pain among conservatory-level students in Australia. A questionnaire survey of college-level piano students found that 42% of 71 respondents had pain associated with playing.[21] Lockwood[22] surveyed a group of secondary school-aged musicians and found that 32% of 113 respondents had mild playing-related problems and 17% had more severe problems.

Manchester[23] reviewed the occurrence of problems in a well-defined population of music students at conservatory level, focusing on upper extremity symptoms. The incidence of hand problems in this group was 8.5 episodes per 100 students per year. Once again, female musicians appeared to be at greater risk, with an average incidence of 11.5 per 100 per year, compared to 5.7 for men. Further analysis indicated that keyboard instrumentalists had a slightly greater incidence rate than string players (13.2 and 9.6, respectively) and both groups had a considerably greater incidence rate than wind performers (3.9).

In one of the few surveys of amateurs, Newmark and Lederman[24] studied a group of participants in an intensive amateur chamber music camp and found that 72% developed a new playing-related problem, almost all of which could be characterized as musculoskeletal. The vast majority of these were transient and were clearly related to a relatively abrupt increase in amount and intensity of playing compared to the previous level.

In a study of choral conductors, Simons[25] found that 36% of 153 questionnaire respondents reported a musculoskeletal pain problem associated with that activity.

PREVALENCE OF INJURY IN DANCERS

Studies of musculoskeletal injury in dancers have also been carried out. However, the majority of these have been reports of clinical experience with no attempt to determine prevalence or incidence. Chmelar and associates[26] report on a group of university level and professional dancers who volunteered to participate in the study; no attempt was made to survey a larger group. Among these volunteers, 23% reported a major injury and 74% a less serious injury related to dancing. A large-scale survey of Japanese aerobic dance instructors and students found an injury prevalence rate of 72.4% and 22.8%, respectively.[27]

It is critical in interpreting the above prevalence data to have some idea about the prevalence of musculoskeletal complaints and disorders in the general population. One source of this is a study of musculoskeletal impairments among adults in the United States in the early 1970s.[19] Based on a detailed history and physical examination of almost 7,000 adults, this study reported a prevalence of musculoskeletal symptoms involving the shoulder in 6.7% and the fingers in 6.8% of the study population and physical signs of musculoskeletal impairment in 3.0% and 4.4%, respectively. Since the population studied ranged in age from 25–74 years, and since a steady increase in prevalence was seen with increasing age, the frequency of musculoskeletal symptoms in the performing artist population would seem to reflect a considerable excess. It is, of course, recognized that comparing data from different surveys is treacherous at best, and any conclusion from this comparison should be viewed cautiously.

PREVALENCE OF NEUROLOGIC DISORDERS

From these various studies, it can be seen that performance-related disorders are common and that the majority are musculoskeletal in the broadest sense. Among these, neurologic problems represent an uncertain proportion. Surveys by questionnaire cannot provide diagnostically accurate information and only by physician-reported series can one hope to obtain this type of data. A number of such reports are available but these have the disadvantage of selection bias related to referral patterns. In the series reported from the Massachusetts General Hospital[28] and the Cleveland Clinic,[29] neurologic problems account for approximately one-third of the disorders, with remarkable similarity between the two institutions. In a series from an orthopedic practice, heavily weighted toward acute trauma and musculoskeletal disorders, only 5% were found to have a neurologic problem.[30] Similarly, in the series of music students with upper-extremity problems reported by Manchester,[23] only a very small fraction of these injuries were identified as neurologic in origin.

Diagnostic Approach to the Performer

Do performing artists represent special problems for the neurologist and do they provide a unique challenge? Certainly, some differences from the average patient can be seen.

SPECIAL PROBLEMS IN TAKING THE HISTORY

As in many occupations, performers, and particularly musicians, may communicate in a special language. The history may be punctuated by words unfamiliar to some physicians as the performer attempts to describe the problem in terms of its effect on playing or on the production of music. Some knowledge of the physical demands of the performing art is also desirable. This would include insight into the rigors of the training process and recognition of the need of the performer and the student to maintain the highest possible standard of playing or performing, often achieved only by extraordinary concentration and effort. One also needs to have some understanding of the psychosocial and economic demands of the particular performing art. All of these may influence not only the type of problem that brings the performer to the neurologist but also the response of the performer to that problem.

Another feature often unappreciated by someone less familiar with the performing arts is the early age at which training for the profession begins. Most of us are not accustomed to seeing patients in their third or fourth decade who have been vigorously pursuing their career since early childhood. Thus, a 20-year-old conservatory student may have had a single-minded dedication to the instrument for 15 years and cannot glibly be told to give up playing because it seems to produce pain.

The evaluation of the performer who presents to the neurologist must include, as always, a detailed description of the symptoms and the circumstances under which they have developed as well as their temporal sequence and evolution. In the case of the instrumentalist, this information may have to include an enumeration and accounting of time spent in practice and performance as well as an analysis of techniques of practicing. The student who has been working on a particular passage by repeating it literally hundreds of times at an increasingly faster tempo or who has been working to strengthen one or another finger by specific exercises or etudes may be at special risk. Abrupt and substantial increases in practice time or in the "intensity" of practicing (e.g., an urgent need to learn a new piece or prepare for an important audition or recital) are often correlated with the time of onset of symptoms. Change in technique of playing prompted by consulting a new teacher or acquiring a new instrument may also be an important predisposing factor. It further behooves the neurologist to inquire about specific stresses that may be playing a role in the development of the problems being evaluated. Again, the physician unfamiliar with the intensity of competition in the conservatory, the potential interpersonal problems in the orchestra or ballet company, and the rigors of the touring actor, instrumentalist, or vocalist may miss important factors in the pathogenesis of or response to the observed physical problem.

EXAMINING THE PERFORMER

The examination of the performer, including the neurologic examination, is not generally different from that of other patients. It is usually desirable, however, and at times crucial to observe the patient while performing or playing. This may present some logistical problems, especially for the pianist, organist, or others with nonportable instruments, as well as for the dancer, who may require more space than is commonly available in the examining room. Despite these difficulties, critical information is often obtained from these observations. The neurologist cannot, of course, be expected to be expert in any, let alone all, instruments and performance techniques. What can be observed, however, is that the performer may assume certain positions, adopt specific postures, and use particular movements that may predispose to the problem being analyzed. Inefficient movements, excessive tension, and other ergonomically undesirable muscle activity can be recognized even in the absence of an understanding of the particular instrument or technique. Obviously, this is a skill that needs to be developed with experience. A special need for observing a performer exists when suspicion of occupational cramp is high. In this situation, the difficulty may occur only while the performer is carrying out that specific task or activity, and there can be no substitute for observation during its performance. Videotaping the performer while playing may be of great help in facilitating the analysis, allowing repeated review and serving as a baseline for later comparison.

LABORATORY STUDIES AND SPECIAL TECHNIQUES

The ancillary studies familiar to neurologists and other physicians may also need to be used in the course of the evaluation. Blood analysis, x-ray and other imaging procedures, radionuclide scans, and electrodiagnostic studies may all be performed at the discretion of the physician. Other less common and, in some cases, more controversial procedures, such as thermography, magnetic resonance spectroscopy, kinesiologic electromyography (EMG), and various motion analysis techniques, may all be helpful in some specific situations. Currently, insufficient experience is available to judge their potential benefits.

Neurologic Problems in Performers

The neurologic disorders seen in performing artists can arbitrarily be divided into three categories. The first includes those disorders that can be expected to occur as often in performers as in any other population group and that should have no greater effect on the performer than on any other patient. The second category includes disorders that would have no special predilection for performing artists but might, because of the special demands of the performing arts, have a greater impact on such an individual than on someone in other professions or occupations. The final group includes those disorders that appear to have an increased prevalence among performing artists compared to members of some other occupational groups. The latter are discussed in greatest detail.

DISORDERS THAT SIMILARLY AFFECT PERFORMERS AND NONPERFORMERS

Among the neurologic disorders that are not unusually frequent among performers and thus have no special impact on this group are the common forms of headache, epilepsy in almost all of its forms, the dementing disorders including Alzheimer's disease, strokes, the toxic and metabolic disorders of the nervous system, neoplastic disorders, and most infectious disorders. An exception to the latter would be human immunodeficiency virus (HIV) infection, which is briefly discussed below. While many of these neurologic diseases may have profound effects on the performer's career, they are no more likely to do so in this than in other groups and need not be considered in this context.

DISORDERS WITH SPECIAL IMPACT ON PERFORMERS

A few examples from the above categories can be considered to have some special relevance to the performer and can be discussed within the second category of neurologic disease. One type of seizure disorder, for instance, that may have specific relevance to the musician is musicogenic epilepsy. This very rare disorder is said to occur more often in those with musical talent.[31] A variety of triggering stimuli for this form of reflex epilepsy have been described, including specific sounds, types of instruments, and even the music of particular composers. Treatment may consist of anticonvulsant medications and sensory desensitization.[32] Psychotherapy has also been helpful in some cases.[33]

Although there is no reason to suspect that stroke has any special predilection for performing artists, some strokes may have a more damaging effect on a performer than on someone in another occupation. For instance, an instrumentalist with what appears to be a minor residual motor or sensory deficit might well be unable to continue a high level of performance, whereas most others with a similar degree of impairment could compensate and return to full effectiveness in a job with less rigorous sensorimotor requirements.

Another example of a stroke that might preferentially disable a musician would be one of those rare examples of specific disruption of musical function—the so-called amusias. A very small number of such patients have been described and the interested reader is referred to these carefully studied cases.[34,35]

HIV infection and resultant acquired immunodeficiency syndrome (AIDS) have had an especially severe impact on the performing arts community, presumably because of the higher prevalence of risk factors for AIDS among performing artists.[36] Central nervous system (CNS) involvement may take many forms, including primary HIV infection of the brain (HIV-associated dementia) and secondary infection with toxoplasmosis or cytomegalovirus. Malignant brain tumors, particularly CNS lymphoma, and progressive multifocal leukoencephalopathy are also being seen with increasing frequency. Spinal cord, peripheral nerve, and muscle disease have all been associated with AIDS.[37]

A substantial number of other neurologic diseases might have particularly damaging effects on performing artists, although they certainly do not appear to be any more common in this group than in others. Most of these affect in some way the control of motor function, which might be more readily tolerated in someone whose career does not depend on the highest level of sensorimotor function.

An example of this category is multiple sclerosis. An instrumental musician might well be able to continue performing despite relatively severe involvement of the lower extremities but would be quickly disabled by a sensorimotor abnormality in the upper extremity or, in wind players, by involvement of lip, tongue, or breath control. A brief case from the author's practice may serve as an example of this phenomenon.

> A 26-year-old right-handed clarinetist developed optic neuritis with complete recovery. Five years later he noted difficulty with the left leg and developed the Lhermitte's symptom. He continued to play in a symphony orchestra until 8 years later, when he began to have problems with sensory function and fine motor control in the right hand. This then progressed to the point at which he could no longer maintain his orchestral position. Magnetic resonance imaging (MRI) showed an area of abnormal signal intensity in the cervical spinal cord.

Parkinson's disease is another disorder that may exert relatively subtle effects on limb, lip, or voice control, perhaps quite tolerable in another occupation but disabling to a singer or instrumental musician. This disease often begins in the fifth or sixth decade, possibly at the peak of the performer's career, and the difficulty in movement may be hard to recognize in its early stages. The instrumentalist may complain of problems in rapid passage work or in trills, for example. At this point, the neurologist may well be hard pressed to identify any abnormality of motor function. The temptation must be resisted to reassure the musician that all is well. Observation of the instrumentalist's playing may sometimes facilitate recognition of a subtle deficit in fine motor control. In the absence of this, the most reasonable approach is to defer specific diagnosis and follow the patient with serial examinations. Once the diagnosis of Parkinson's disease has been established, the availability of highly effective medication may, of course, allow the performer to continue playing, although not infrequently the level of performance declines sufficiently to make this impossible.

Essential tremor is another movement disorder that can cause equally debilitating effects on motor performance. The tremor may affect bow control or vibrato in the string instrumentalist or vocal control in the singer. Again, this may be ameliorated with medication, including beta blockers and primidone. The potential for deleterious side effects in the performer must be given serious consideration in these cases.[38]

Amyotrophic lateral sclerosis (ALS) and other forms of motor neuron disease may begin with subtle dysfunction of the hand or the bulbar muscles, disabling the instrumentalist at an early stage. Myasthenia gravis may also disable the instrumentalist or singer early in its course. The wind player (or vocalist) may complain of difficulty in breath control or in maintaining embouchure,[39] and the string or wind player may have problems in maintaining support of the instrument. Once these disorders are suspected, the approach is the same as for nonperformers.

Idiopathic facial palsy (Bell's) is a relatively common disorder that, again, is no more likely to afflict performing artists than other individuals. Bell's palsy is, however, particularly disabling to the wind instrumentalist, who cannot maintain a seal because of the lip weakness. It is necessary to exclude symptomatic forms of facial palsy, such as those due to central nervous system, skull base, or extracranial tumors; infections or other destructive processes in the inner ear, and more widespread processes such as Lyme disease, multiple sclerosis, sarcoid, and Guillain-Barré syndrome. Use of steroids remains controversial despite a number of studies. Most instrumentalists will recover sufficient function to return to performance. Wind players have sometimes found ingenious ways of adapting, such as taping the paretic side of the lips closed or moving the instrument off center to allow earlier return to playing.

Trigeminal neuralgia is another cranial neuropathy that may have special importance for the wind instrumentalist. Again, one may have idiopathic and symptomatic forms, and this clearly influences management as well as prognosis. The act of playing a wind instrument or of singing may trigger the attack. Medications, such as carbamazepine, phenytoin, or baclofen, may control the episodes. A variety of surgical procedures may be highly effective as well. The following unusual case is an example of a less favorable outcome.

A 35-year-old symphony orchestra clarinetist developed severe lancinating facial pain that was triggered almost exclusively by playing his instrument. No structural cause could be identified on imaging studies. Medications are poorly tolerated and the patient is unwilling to consider surgical intervention. He has changed careers because of the illness.

DISORDERS PARTICULARLY COMMON IN PERFORMING ARTISTS

The final category of disorders to be discussed are those that appear to be most common in performing artists seen by neurologists and perhaps are more common in performing artists than in other groups. As was mentioned previously, statistical confirmation of this is lacking. Among these disorders, we first discuss the regional pain syndromes, typically involving the neck, upper trunk, and upper extremity of the instrumentalist. Lower back problems are also quite common in instrumentalists as well as in dancers. The other types of disorders in this category include the focal neuropathies, mostly compression or entrapment neuropathies, and the occupational cramps or focal dystonias. These are discussed in some detail as they account for the large majority of neurologic ailments and, with the regional pain syndromes, make up the bulk of diagnoses in reported series from performing arts medicine clinics.[28,29]

Muscle Pain in Performing Artists: Overuse Syndrome

Definition.　Pain is the most frequent complaint among instrumentalists and dancers seen in performing arts medicine clinics. The bulk of these represent what has been called *overuse*, although this term admittedly is nonspecific and suggests a mechanism that has yet to be proved.[40] (For general discussion of overuse syndromes, see Chapter 9.) A number of other synonyms have been and continue to be used in various countries, including regional musculoskeletal pain syndrome, occupational cervicobrachial disorder, cumulative trauma disorder, repetition strain injury, repetitive motion disorder, tendinitis or tenosynovitis, and myofascial pain syndrome. Each of these has its proponents and critics. The term *overuse syndrome* is used in this discussion and is defined here as the symptoms and signs of presumed injury to tissues subjected to stresses that exceed their biological limits. Although any tissue may be so stressed, most disorders that affect instrumental musicians seem to involve the soft tissues of the musculoskeletal system, including muscle, tendon, ligament, and bursa.[41,42] Multiple tissues may be simultaneously or sequentially affected, and differentiation of involvement of one tissue from another may be difficult, such as separating bursitis from tendinitis at the shoulder. Most disorders appear to involve the muscle-tendon unit and this has become the common usage for the term *overuse syndrome*. Actual signs of inflammation, such as heat, swelling, and redness, are uncommon in this setting, and therefore the term *tendinitis*, although often used by patients and health care practitioners, is usually unwarranted.[43]

Symptoms and Signs.　The primary symptom of overuse, as implied above, is pain, although a variety of complaints are often voiced, including tightness, stiffness, cramping, fatigue, swelling, numbness, and impairment of control. Pain is sometimes aching and sometimes sharp and shooting although, again, numerous descriptions may be applied. Tenderness to palpation is the rule. Both the pain and tenderness may be unifocal or, more often, multifocal. The tender points often are at the muscle-tendon junction or over the belly of the muscle and less commonly along the length of the tendon itself or at its insertion.[43] As noted above, swelling is rarely identified despite the frequency of this as a complaint. An acute form of tendinitis can occur, with swelling and actual crepitation,[44] but this appears to be uncommon among performing artists. Pain is often elicited by activating the involved muscle-tendon unit against resistance or by stretching. This may lead to the impression on the part of both the patient and the examining physician that there is weakness, but in general no actual impairment of strength can be demonstrated in the overuse syndrome. As such, the neurologic examination is generally normal.

The largest group of instrumentalists who seek medical attention have developed pain in the hand, forearm, and wrist,[45] although shoulder and upper arm as well as neck and upper trunk are also commonly affected. Surveys of large numbers of musicians[17] also emphasize the involvement of lower and mid-back, although these seem to be tolerated by most performers much more readily than the pain syndromes that affect the upper extremity.

A number of observations have been made about the pain syndromes that appear to hold true for other occupational disorders of musicians, including the nerve entrapment syndromes and even the occupational cramps. In all but the latter, women outnumber men in virtually every series. Certain patterns of involvement are characteristic for specific instrument groups. For instance, violinists and violists have a preponderance of involvement of the left arm, whereas the right arm and hand are more frequently affected in keyboard instrumentalists.[9,13] The weight-bearing right thumb and associated muscle tendon units in oboists and clarinetists are more commonly affected than the opposite limb.[46] There appears to be a lesser tendency for asymmetry in more proximal locations, including shoulder, periscapular muscles, and neck. This impression is corroborated by data obtained in the ICSOM survey.[18]

Pathogenesis and Pathology. As discussed above, a number of predisposing factors and conditions may be identified in those who present with an overuse syndrome. These are outlined in Table 12.1 and are separated into intrinsic and extrinsic factors, terminology borrowed from sports medicine. One or several of these may be identified in most patients.

It should be stated at this point that the overuse syndromes seen in instrumentalists and other performers have many similarities to the muscle pain syndromes, variously labeled as noted previously, in other groups. Much of the controversy about these disorders relates to industrial injury and compensation issues.[47-49] This controversy, of course, is fueled by the frequency of muscle pain syndromes among industrial workers, particularly in those who perform repetitive and often monotonous tasks, by the lack of objective signs of injury clinically or pathologically, and by the financial implications, which lead to adversarial positions. While these issues are not inconsequential in the instrumental musician population, our experience suggests that there is a financial gain with continuing disability in only a minority of these cases and much more frequently a financial loss or even threat to a career. Thus, at least among the instrumental musicians, these overuse syndromes do not appear to represent forms of compensation neurosis.

Pathologic studies of muscle-tendon overuse have been few. Commonly quoted studies include that of Howard,[44] who reported tissue

TABLE 12.1
Factors Predisposing to Overuse in Instrumental Musicians

Intrinsic	*Extrinsic*
Body size, configuration (neck, arm, hand, finger length)	Faulty technique
Range of motion (hyperlaxity, restricted mobility of joints)	Change in technique, "excessive" playing (time, intensity)
Conditioning (muscle strength, flexibility, endurance)	Change in instrument
Degenerative musculoskeletal disorders	Faulty posture
Scoliosis	Stress (economic, psychosocial)
Metabolic, other systemic illness	Trauma (accidental, recreational, other work)

biopsy results in three manual workers with peritendinitis crepitans. Pathologic changes in the biopsies included edema, small vein thrombosis, and scattered inflammatory cells more commonly in the muscle or at the muscle tendon junction. Howard[44] assumed that the primary problem was in muscle itself. Thompson and associates[50] reported biopsy results in four cases out of a clinical study of 544 industrial workers with acute pain syndromes. Again histologic changes were quite variable and included edema and hypervascularization. Dennett and Fry[51] more recently reported muscle biopsy findings from the first dorsal interosseus of workers with apparent overuse syndrome. Changes identified included an increase in the proportion of type I fibers with type II fiber hypertrophy, increased frequency of central nucleation, and some mitochondrial abnormalities. These findings have been criticized for lack of specificity and inadequate control.[52] Further pathologic studies may clarify the issues, although other techniques of assessing muscle, such as magnetic resonance spectroscopy, may ultimately prove both more practical and more helpful. In this regard, the relevance of a number of studies on muscle fatigue is uncertain. Clearly, experimentally induced muscle fatigue does lead to tissue injury,[53] but whether the results of these acute experiments are applicable to the more chronic overuse syndromes remains to be determined.

Focal Peripheral Neuropathies

Localized or regional pain is often a presenting symptom of the focal neuropathies, including particularly the common nerve compression syndromes. Thus, the differential diagnosis of overuse syndrome often includes entrapment neuropathy. The frequency with which one identifies focal neuropathies in this setting often depends on the vigor with which the diagnostic evaluation is pursued. At the same time, one must be extremely cautious in interpreting modest evidence of nerve entrapment—

TABLE 12.2
Focal Peripheral Neuropathies in Instrumental Musicians*

Focal Peripheral Neuropathy	No. of Patients
Thoracic outlet syndrome	48
Carpal tunnel syndrome	42
Ulnar neuropathy, elbow	31
Cervical radiculopathy	20
Digital neuropathy	7
Median, other	7
Ulnar, other	5
Radial neuropathy	2
Other	22

*Seen at the Cleveland Clinic Medical Center for Performing Artists.

for instance, minimal slowing of ulnar nerve conduction at the elbow—as the mechanism for disabling pain in the instrumentalist. Careful weighing of all the factors and clinical judgment remain of critical importance in this situation as in all others involving patient care.

There are no peripheral nerve disorders unique to performing artists. Indeed, there is no epidemiologic evidence that peripheral nerve disorders, either generalized or focal, are more common in performing artists than in other segments of the population or that any individual group of performers, including instrumental musicians, are particularly prone to development of any of the compression mononeuropathies. What can be stated, however, is that in large groups of performers who seek medical consultation, particularly from the centers that provide specialized care for these groups, focal neuropathies account for a substantial proportion of the diagnoses.[9,29] Furthermore, the occurrence of certain mononeuropathies in specific instrumental groups and the fact that they tend to affect one side of the body more than the other suggest that some element of increased susceptibility may be present.

Since the peripheral nerve disorders are well known to neurologists, the specific syndromes seen in performers are only briefly reviewed, emphasizing the aspects that appear to be particularly relevant in this setting.

In our clinic, peripheral nerve disorders are identified in 25–30% of instrumental musicians seen. Among the 743 instrumentalists evaluated through December 1993, 184 (25%) were found to have a focal peripheral neuropathy. These are outlined in Table 12.2. The multiple selection factors that contribute to referral of patients to our center require that any conclusions regarding the distribution of these disorders among performers in general be made with extreme caution. Before discussing each of these specific disorders, a few general comments seem appropriate. The diagnoses are based on standard clinical and electrodiagnostic criteria, although not every patient underwent EMG or other ancillary study. A number of additional patients had symptoms that suggested one or another mononeuropathy, but clinical and electrical criteria were considered insufficient for specific diagnosis. The upper extremity involved showed the same lateralization as seen in the musculoskeletal syndromes. Thus, the left arm of string instrumentalists, particularly violinists and violists, was affected more frequently than the right, and the opposite held true for keyboard players. Among woodwind and brass instrumentalists, no definite lateralization was apparent, although there was a trend among flutists for the left arm to be preferentially involved.

Thoracic Outlet Syndrome.   The most common peripheral nerve disorder in our series, thoracic outlet syndrome, is also the most controversial. The difficulties with this diagnosis and the areas of disagreement about its existence, its frequency, the methods of diagnosis, and the treatment modalities are well known to most neurologists. A number of detailed reviews are available and should be consulted by those who want more discussion.[54–57]

The patients with thoracic outlet syndrome have unilateral or, occasionally, asymmetric bilateral arm pain and paresthesias. These are position related, often triggered by playing the instrument. Pain is most often in the forearm but may spread proximally to the upper arm and periscapular region as well as distally to the hand. Paresthesias include numbness and tingling as well as burning and sometimes a swollen sensation, generally following a C8-T1/lower brachial plexus distribution. Less frequently, the radial forearm and hand may be preferentially involved. These symptoms may be provoked by placing the patient's limb in specific positions during examination, including hyperabduction of the arm, the Adson maneuver, or the costoclavicular maneuver. I have found downward traction on the affected arm combined with internal rotation at the shoulder to be a particularly effective method of reproducing symptoms. Obliteration of the pulse does not seem to be a helpful sign, which further indicates that the contribution of arterial compression to the symptoms of this disorder is infrequent.[56] The neurologic examination is normal, although it may be difficult to exclude some muscle weakness because of the rapid fatigability these patients show in the provocative positions, and subjective sensory changes are common. However, using such methods as two-point discrimination and quantitative sensory testing, findings of actual impairment of sensation are infrequent and reflex changes are not seen. Despite considerable literature to the contrary, electrodiagnostic studies have been normal in our experience, and indeed abnormalities in EMG or somatosensory evoked potentials suggest an alternate diagnosis. About half our patients with thoracic outlet syndrome show the droopy shoulder configuration (Fig. 12.1). Women outnumber men by about 3 to 1 in this group, and the affected patients tend to be younger than the average instrumentalist referred to our center (mean age 25 years compared to 32 years for the entire group).

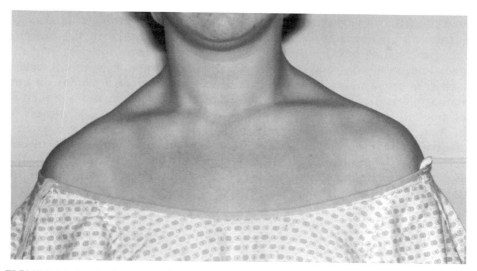

FIGURE 12.1   A pianist with typical upper trunk configuration and symptoms in the right arm suggestive of droopy shoulder syndrome. (From RT Sataloff et al. Textbook of Performing Arts Medicine. New York: Raven, 1991.)

Median Neuropathies.   Carpal tunnel syndrome (CTS) is also a common focal neuropathy among instrumental performers. The clinical configuration in these patients is no different from that of the general population. Pain in the affected extremity, both distal and proximal, paresthesias largely restricted to median nerve distribution, and impairment of dexterity or other manifestations of motor dysfunction are the most common complaints. Nocturnal symptoms are frequent; patients are often awakened by pain and paresthesias. The majority of our patients describe some interference with instrumental playing, as might be expected since this is what generally brings the performer to clinical attention. Examination reveals some sensory loss in about half; a particularly effective technique is to compare the sharpness of a pin on the radial and ulnar sides of the ring finger. Weakness and atrophy are seen much less commonly. Phalen's maneuver is positive in the majority, as is Tinel's sign. These are neither specific nor required for diagnosis but certainly can be helpful in some patients. All of our patients had abnormal nerve conduction studies, although most clinicians would agree that the diagnosis can occasionally, if cautiously, be made in the face of normal median nerve conduction across the carpal tunnel. As in the general population, CTS occurred more frequently in female than in male musicians, with 26 of the 42 being women. These patients were significantly older than the average age of the entire group of performers (mean age at diagnosis = 44 years).

Proximal median compression syndromes are seen much less frequently. Pain and paresthesias in median distribution may be seen in the pronator syndrome.[58] Nocturnal symptoms are less commonly reported than in CTS. There may be localized tenderness and a positive Tinel's sign in the proximal forearm. Weakness involves not only the thenar muscles but also the long flexor of the thumb and in some cases the flexors of the index and middle fingers. Our one patient with pronator syndrome developed this presumably as the result of repeated forceful pronation and supination required in tuning the harp. The anterior interosseous branch of the median nerve may occasionally be affected in isolation. Weakness of the long flexors of the thumb, index, and sometimes middle finger occurs, along with involvement of the pronator quadratus. One patient in our series had mild anterior interosseous neuropathy clinically and electrically. Five other patients had median neuropathies from trauma at various points proximal and distal to the carpal tunnel.

Ulnar Neuropathies.   Ulnar neuropathy also appears to be a particularly frequent neuropathy among musicians.[59] Compression at the elbow is most common, being identified in 31 of our patients. Some would separate those with compression at the intercondylar groove from others more distal ("cubital tunnel"), but this can be difficult both clinically and electrically.[60] Symptoms are similar, with pain, paresthesias in ulnar distribution on the hand, little and ring fingers, and motor impairment involving the interossei and lumbricals particularly. These muscles are especially critical in instrumental playing. Subtle deficits in motor function may be demonstrable on examination or, at times, in watching the performer play. Electrodiagnostic studies are often helpful but are less commonly abnormal than in CTS. Greater technical difficulties are involved in ulnar nerve conduction studies, including inherent problems with accurate distance measurement.[60] Mild degrees of apparent conduction slowing are frequently found in the elbow segment of asymptomatic individuals, rendering interpretation more uncertain.

Two patients in our series had ulnar neuropathies that could not be localized but were clearly proximal. One of these is a pianist with either a pure motor ulnar neuropathy or neuronopathy that has remained clinically and electrically stable for 7 years. Cause remains unknown.

The ulnar nerve may also be compressed distally. This will generally spare the dorsal ulnar sensory branch. Sensory loss on the palmar surface of the hand and little and ring fingers will be found if the entrapment is at the wrist, but a lesion further distally in the palm generally leaves sensation unimpaired and may spare the hypothenar muscles as well. One violinist in our series had ulnar neuropathy at Guyon's canal at the wrist, and another had a traumatic ulnar (and median) neuropathy after surgical fixation for a distal forearm fracture. A pianist appears to have ulnar nerve compression in the distal forearm, suggested by focal conduction block. He has to date declined surgical exploration.

Other Focal Neuropathies.   Cervical radiculopathy secondary to spondylosis or disk herniation is a common problem in the general population and has been seen among our performing artist patients. Symptoms again are well known to neurologists, including pain originating in the neck and radiating into the involved extremity, aggravated by neck movement or by Valsalva maneuver. Sensory and motor disturbances in appropriate distribution are commonly found. Reflex changes are frequent in these patients and help differentiate cervical radiculopathy from more distal nerve compression syndromes. These patients tend to be older, and in most series men are affected more frequently than women. One might hypothesize that the neck position required in playing violin and viola particularly could predispose to cervical radiculopathy over many years of the performer's career. While this may be the case, no such trend has been seen in our series; the numbers are obviously small, however, and no conclusion should be drawn.

Digital mononeuropathies are generally associated with external compression. The radial digital branch of the left index finger may be compressed against the neck of the violin or viola, or against the flute.[61] This represents a technical flaw since tight grip is neither necessary nor desirable. One of our patients developed a digital compression from gripping marimba mallets while repetitively practicing a piece that required the four-mallet technique (Fig. 12.2). Pain and sensory loss in digital branch distribution are commonly found. Electrodiagnostic studies are often normal in view of the distal site of compression.

Before leaving the upper extremity, radial entrapment should be briefly discussed. The most common site of radial nerve compression in the general population would be at the spiral groove. I have not seen this in an instrumental performer. Two patients with apparent radial compression in the "radial tunnel" have been included in this series.[62] One patient was seen following surgery at another institution. Another was a percussionist who had suggestive symptoms and signs. This diagnosis has some similarity to thoracic outlet syndrome, in that the clinical picture may be very difficult to define and neurologic signs are more difficult to verify. Tenderness is found in the proximal forearm distal to the lateral epicondyle, and pain may be provoked by resistive supination of the forearm or extension of the middle finger with the arm outstretched.[62] Weakness in the extensors of the digits or wrist may be found but is again difficult to interpret because of associated pain. Electrodiagnostic studies are technically difficult but may be extremely helpful.

Cranial mononeuropathies may be seen in performers. The only one that might be considered occupational in the usual sense would be that associated with compression of trigeminal branches subserving sensory function on the lips. These may be compressed against the mouthpiece of the brass instrument or between the flute and the lower dental arch. Patients describe localized numbness that clearly can be related to playing of the instrument. Sensory loss, if persistent, corresponds to the compressed branches.

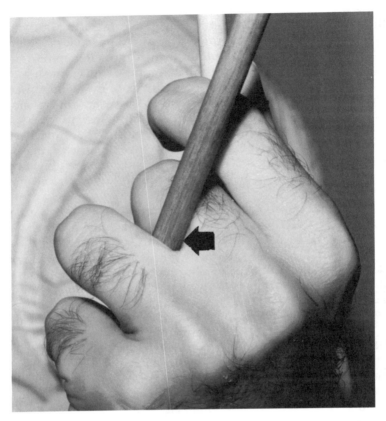

FIGURE 12.2   Marimba player demonstrating four-mallet grip, predisposing to digital compression neuropathy of the left middle finger. (From J Blum. Medical Problems of Musicians. Stuttgart: George Thieme, 1995.)

Two other common cranial mononeuropathies seen in the general population include idiopathic facial (Bell's) palsy and trigeminal neuralgia. Two examples of each of these are present in our series.

Lower-limb entrapment syndromes certainly might occur in instrumentalists. Lumbosacral radiculopathy may be an occupational hazard in the dancer, particularly the male ballet performer whose activities include frequent lifts. There are no specific features unique to performing artists, although one aspect of physical examination might be noted. Straight leg–raising may be unimpressive in the dancer despite L5-S1 root irritation because of the unusual flexibility these performers often have. Sensory, motor, and reflex changes would be similar to those seen in other groups. Saphenous[63,64] and peroneal mononeuropathies[65] have been described in association with playing the viola da gamba and guitar, respectively. These single case reports suggest that this is not a common occurrence.

Occupational Cramp (Focal Dystonia)

Historical Perspectives. Credit for the initial clinical description of writer's cramp, the prototype for occupational cramp, is generally given to Sir Charles Bell (1830),[66] although Ramazzini[67] was probably describing the same entity in his section on diseases of notaries and scribes. The first case in a musician may be that of Stromeyer, involving the right thumb of a pianist, as quoted in Romberg's textbook.[68] Poore[69] reported a series of 21 pianists with occupational cramp or, as he called it, hand failure. Most of these were women, with the left hand specifically involved. Subsequent to Poore's review, little interest was shown in the occupational cramp of musicians until the reports of Critchley,[70] Hochberg and his colleagues,[71–73] and others[74,75] in recent years. The clinical picture of occupational cramp was clearly delineated by Gowers[66] and Poore[69] in the late nineteenth century and little has been added since then. The concept of occupational cramp as a focal dystonia evolved much more recently. Marsden,[76,77] in a series of persuasive reports, has been the primary spokesperson for this conception of occupational cramp, which now appears to be generally agreed on by most neurologists.

The prevalence of occupational cramp among musicians is unknown. Estimates of its frequency among other groups in the population vary widely. A survey of telegraphers in Australia reported a prevalence of 14% in that selected group.[78] A larger survey among office workers in India found a prevalence of writer's cramp of 0.5%.[79] A population survey in Rochester, Minnesota, found a prevalence of 0.03% for all forms of focal dystonia, which would include torticollis and blepharospasm as well as writer's and other occupational cramp.[80] It was suggested that this was likely to be an underestimate.

Clinical Features. The characteristic history is of insidious development of difficulty with muscle control, speed, or dexterity involving the fingers or hands or, less commonly, the more proximal upper extremity. Wind players may describe similar symptoms involving the muscles of embouchure, particularly the lips. Additional complaints may include stiffness, tightness, cramping, or fatigue. A few patients describe pain, although this has not been prominent in our group[74] or in those reported by Newmark and Hochberg.[72] Involuntary movements may be noted by the patient, including undesired flexion or extension of the fingers or wrist, uncontrolled jerking, or tremor. Initially, these symptoms occur after prolonged playing, but as the disorder progresses, the cramping, fatigue, and involuntary movements may appear immediately after the afflicted patient begins to play.

A common, though not invariable feature, of the occupational dystonias is their task specificity. The same hand that may be contorted and twisted while an individual attempts to write or play an instrument may remain perfectly flexible and dextrous in other tasks that apparently involve the same groups of muscles. Another feature is that the patient often is able to identify specific maneuvers that at least partially ameliorate the dystonia. These may include a slight change in position of the limb or may involve touching the affected limb with the other hand, presumably providing a sensory stimulus. These sensory or proprioceptive "tricks" are well recognized in other forms of dystonia including torticollis.

We have identified 55 instrumentalists with focal dystonias. These include 13 violinists or violists, six guitarists, nine pianists, four percussionists, one harpist, 16 woodwind players, and six brass players. In eight of the wind instrumentalists, lip and other bulbar muscles were affected. One of the six guitarists, with focal dystonia involving the left hand, also had torticollis and multiple tics. The majority of these patients are in their fourth or fifth decade of life. Unlike virtually all other disorders among musicians, men in this series outnumber women by almost 3 to 1. This has been the experience of others as well.[72,75]

In occupational cramp, perhaps more than any other disorder among musicians, the part of the body affected is generally that which is particularly stressed by repetitive fine movement. Among the violinists and violists in our series, 10 of 13 involved the fingering hand and only three involved the bow arm. One violinist developed focal dystonia in the left (fingering) hand and successfully changed to playing left-handed (i.e., fingering with the right hand), only to develop the same problem in the right hand within a few years. He has now found that playing "normally," or right-handed, again is better, although he still has some difficulty with control of the left fingers. Among nine pianists, eight developed focal dystonia in the right hand and only two had left hand involvement (one bilateral). The right is the hand that generally carries the melody line and has the most repetitive work to do. Wind players have the susceptibility both in the hands and in the lips.[74] Newmark and Hochberg[72] have emphasized the frequency of certain patterns of involuntary movement, such as the curling of the fourth and fifth fingers of the right hand in pianists and involuntary flexion of the right middle finger in guitarists, but this has not been universally observed.[59,74,81]

Pathogenesis. The pathogenesis of focal dystonia remains uncertain. Gowers[66] suggested that this was a nervous system disorder (hence, his use of the term *neurosis*) but clearly recognized the possibility that peripheral factors contribute. Poore[69] emphasized the need for integrity of the entire sensorimotor system, both peripheral and central, in normal function. Current views on dystonia focus on the basal ganglia,[82] but much recent speculation centers on peripheral mechanisms as well. In several series of focal dystonias,[72,74,83] onset frequently seems to have followed some peripheral trauma or injury. Analogy has been made to reflex sympathetic dystrophy following trauma,[84] and some cases of coexistence of these two disorders have been described.[85] It may be that alteration of sensory input by peripheral injury disrupts the motor output centrally, either at the spinal level or more rostrally. Physiologic analysis of patients with focal dystonia typically shows poorly modulated muscular activity with simultaneous contraction of agonists and antagonists in long bursts.[81,86] A disruption of normal reciprocal inhibition has been suggested as one of the physiologic abnormalities underlying the disorder.[87] The contribution of psychological factors cannot be ignored, but most neurologists would not support the long-held view that these are largely psychogenic.

Disorders of the Senses

Vision and hearing are two of the most precious and vital commodities of the performing artist, particularly the musician. Occupational visual loss is infrequent in the performing artist and unlikely to have a neurologic basis. Musicians are sensitive to faulty lighting, particularly in orchestra pits and in other performance situations.[88] Aging and the problems of accommodation add to the burden. The need of the orchestra musician to be able to see the conductor, the music on the stand, and the fingers on the instrument may stress the usual refractive aids. Modern technology including enlarging copiers have been of considerable help in solving some of these problems. Vision is of less vital concern to the jazz or popular musician since improvisation is the norm rather than strict adherence to a score. There are, of course, a number of highly successful blind artists in these fields.

Occupational hearing loss is of great concern to the musician, who relies on this sense for ongoing feedback. Music itself can be damaging to the hearing apparatus and has become a subject of interest to symphony orchestra musicians who may be exposed to sound pressures that approach or are clearly within the toxic range.[89–91] Rock and some popular music forms that rely heavily on sound amplification pose exceptional risk to the performers, who often stand close to speakers, and even to members of the audience at some distance from the speakers.[92]

A number of symphony orchestras have become sufficiently concerned about hearing loss in some sections, particularly brass and those who sit immediately in front of these instrumentalists, to experiment with various protective devices. These include baffles and other deflectors as well as earplugs or attenuators; technology is imperfect but improving.[93]

Profound loss of hearing would severely impair if not prohibit active musical performance although other performing art forms are possible. A number of composers have progressively lost hearing, the most well known, of course, being Beethoven. His struggle against the ravages of deafness and his ability to compose sublime music despite profound hearing impairment suggest that once the necessary skills are acquired, the process of composition may continue successfully. Other composers who have suffered from disabling hearing impairment include Faure, Smetana, and Vaughan Williams.

Treatment and Prevention Strategies for Occupational Disorders of Performers

In dealing with the injured or impaired performer, the overriding consideration of the physician must be the health of the individual. Analogy is often made between sports medicine and performing arts medicine. While certain similarities clearly exist, in the area of treatment the approach to the injured individual may be very different. Most of us have witnessed an injury on the football field or other sports arena after which the injured athlete is quickly patched up at the sidelines or is given a local injection of anesthetic or steroid to allow completion of the game or even the season. This approach may be justifiable in view of the relatively short duration of the athlete's active career but in the performing arts it can hardly be condoned. At times management, in the case of a star performer, or even the performer him- or herself, may request a temporizing measure to get through a particular performance, audition, or jury. The long-term hazards must be considered in view of the length of some performance careers, which extend over many decades. At the same time, one cannot ignore the importance of that concert or audition, for which the performer has been preparing over many months, at times indeed precipitating the injury for which he or she is being seen. The physician's prescription of total rest or abstinence from playing may not be followed by the performer if alternative approaches are at all possible. Similarly, advice to stop playing or to take prolonged periods of rest is also difficult for performers and students to accept because of the potentially devastating effect of weeks or months of abstinence on performance skills and on the performer's psychological well-being.

In dealing with musicians, however, and particularly student musicians, it is sometimes important to emphasize how much may be accomplished away from the instrument. Many teachers stress this as well, but the fact remains that for most students long hours of practicing and repetition are necessary for acquiring technical skills and learning the repertoire.

Musculotendinous Overuse

The precise therapeutic approach to the common muscle-tendon overuse syndromes depends both on severity and an analysis of the factors that contribute.[41,94] While rest is the cornerstone of treatment, this may be accomplished by relative reduction in the total amount of playing as well as by interrupting playing sessions with breaks for brief rest, stretching, or relaxation exercise. If the basic problem underlying muscle-tendon overuse is the stressing of the tissues beyond biological limits, then reduction of the workload combined with increasing the tolerance of the tissues for such stresses is the most sensible approach. For the more severe overuse syndromes, brief abstinence from playing and other stressful activities may be required, along with analgesics or nonsteroidal antiinflammatory drugs, icing, other pain-reducing modalities, and occasionally local injection of anesthetic or steroids, or both. The rehabilitative phase, the principles of which are also applicable to prevention, should include a thorough assessment of technique, generally in conjunction with a teacher or colleague, to reduce inappropriate muscle tension or contraction, eradicate technical flaws that produce inefficient muscular activity, and correct improper posture. Alteration or repositioning of the chin rest or shoulder pad on a violin or viola, moving the thumb rest on a clarinet or oboe, modifying the keys on a flute, raising the fingerboard on a cello, and raising or lowering the piano bench, all again done with the advice of an expert teacher or instrument technologist, may be remarkably effective. Physical therapy, occupational therapy, and a variety of alternative techniques for body awareness and conditioning may be extremely useful. Recognition of sources of psychological stress, which may be manifest as muscular tension, must be addressed and similarly reduced. Through all of this, of course, the performer must assume primary responsibility for his or her own treatment program.

The rehabilitative phase must seek to improve the body's ability to withstand the stresses of performance. Gradual improvement of both general and local muscle conditioning must be a therapeutic goal.

Successful rehabilitation may require many months and occasionally one or more years. It has been our observation that the therapeutic response is often punctuated by periods of exacerbation. Sometimes these are triggered by even single sessions of prolonged or intensive playing and sometimes by nonmusical activities such as outside jobs, sports, or minor trauma. Depression may accompany these exacerbations and can be a serious problem in those required to undergo prolonged periods of rest or abstinence from playing. Counseling, psychotherapy, and sometimes antidepressant medications may be useful.

With these approaches, our follow-up data suggest that some 75–80% of performers are successfully rehabilitated, with either no pain or mild and readily tolerated pain that is related primarily to prolonged or unusual amounts of playing. Some of those who do not respond favorably clearly have not followed the prescribed programs, but others who have complied simply do not improve. These performers must either reduce their playing, alter their career goals, or tolerate the symptoms. Some will seek alternate modes of therapy.

COMPRESSION NEUROPATHIES

The principles of treatment for the various focal neuropathies are often quite similar to those reviewed above for musculoskeletal overuse. Brief periods of rest or reduction in playing, modification of technique or instrument, pain-relieving measures, and reconditioning are all useful in the compression neuropathies. Some therapeutic measures are specific for the individual compression syndromes. Thoracic outlet syndrome exercises are designed to improve posture and to strengthen the shoulder elevators.[95] Some have advocated specific braces for the droopy shoulder syndrome,[96] but we have found these impractical and only occasionally helpful. The controversies regarding surgery are well known but remain unsolved. We have carried out first rib resection in two such patients with excellent results and have recommended surgery in several others whose condition has so far declined.

Nocturnal splinting of the wrist for patients with CTS is well recognized as effective in relieving symptoms and may improve daytime symptoms as well. Some patients will respond to local steroid injection. The definitive treatment is surgical release; this is effective in about 90% of cases. Postoperative rehabilitation in the instrumentalist is particularly important and should be under the supervision of a skilled hand therapist. Instrumentalists are often reluctant to consider any type of surgery on their hands and at the same time are rightfully fearful of permanent nerve injury if they delay. This ambivalence must be met with frank discussion of pros and cons, careful explanation of the risks and benefits of surgery, and continuing support. In our experience, armed with this understanding, most performers opt for earlier rather than later surgical intervention, and our results with this approach have been extremely gratifying.

Therapeutic approach to the ulnar neuropathies is more of a problem. The diagnosis is often less certain and the confidence with which one approaches surgery is generally lower. Our initial approach is to encourage avoidance of external pressure on the ulnar nerves and to reduce elbow flexion as much as possible during playing and other activities including sleep. When these measures fail, surgical treatment is usually effective. There is some controversy regarding surgical approaches, ranging from simple decompression to extensive neurolysis with anterior transposition of the nerve or epicondylectomy. Charness[59] has reported a large series of musicians treated successfully with ulnar decompression and has advocated early surgical intervention, at times before any electrodiagnostic abnormalities can be identified. This approach requires a high level of confidence in the clinical diagnosis as well as in the surgeon and may be difficult for some neurologists to accept.

Treatment of cervical radiculopathy in the performer is not substantially different from that of other segments of the population. In general, a conservative approach is advocated unless progressive neurologic impairment occurs, in which case appropriate surgery should be done as early as possible to avoid irreversible injury. Digital neuropathies generally respond to alteration of playing position or technique in conjunction with orthotics as required. In our series, excluding those patients who failed to follow recommended therapy and those for whom no therapy was available (e.g., those with chronic traumatic nerve injuries), results of these various approaches have been successful in about 80% of instrumental musicians.

OCCUPATIONAL CRAMP

The treatment of occupational cramp remains largely unsuccessful. Although many patients continue to play by avoiding certain pieces or passages, playing at a slower tempo, and making technical adjustments such as refingering, few have actual improvement despite attempts with multiple modalities. Body awareness and relaxation techniques, along with other behavioral modification approaches, may be helpful for some.[97] A variety of drugs, including anticholinergics and dopaminergics, have been used for occupational cramp as well as for other forms of dystonia[98] with limited success. We have seen partial improvement with trihexyphenidyl, ethopropazine, and bromocriptine. One percussionist is able to get through a "gig" by taking 10–20 mg trihexyphenidyl before playing, but by the end of the evening he has great difficulty in controlling his right hand and feels some discomfort. The local injection of botulinum toxin has been used for various forms of focal dystonia including the occupational hand cramp of musicians.[99,100] Several of our patients have been so treated, with varying success. One clarinetist with hand cramp had 90% improvement after 6 months, although subsequent lessening of effectiveness was seen. In others, the results have been less gratifying and some have had little or no functional improvement.

Both Gowers[66] and Poore[69] advocated rest or abstinence from the offending activity as the cornerstone of treatment. For musician's cramp, Fry[94] particularly has advocated prolonged rest and has reported success with this approach. Our results have been less favorable. One patient with focal dystonia involving the lip has abstained from any significant playing for more than 13 years, but each time he picks up the instrument, even after 2–3 years without touching it, the problem immediately reappears. Some musicians and teachers, most notably Dorothy Taubman,[101] have argued that these problems are all related to improper technique and that they are reversible by correcting the technical faults. While most physicians, the author included, are not capable of providing such technical advice, many other teachers have questioned this approach, arguing that there is not just one way or even several "correct" ways to play any particular instrument. While the author has no reason to doubt that some performers may well benefit from this approach, these claims remain to be verified.

Future Goals

Many challenges remain both diagnostically and therapeutically for performing arts medicine. The recognition that performers have special needs and special problems is an important first step. Close collaboration among physicians, other health care professionals, educators, and performers has been initiated but needs to be expanded and improved. The language barriers among these groups must be broken down by mutual education and gradual increase in mutual trust. Much remains to be learned about basic mechanisms of the various disorders and the most appropriate ways to approach them therapeutically. Preventive strategies need to be developed based on assessment of various risk factors, which need to be enumerated and clarified. The ultimate goal, of course, is the preservation of one of society's most cherished resources, the performing artist.

Summary

Neurologic and musculoskeletal disorders appear to be common among performing artists, as indicated by surveys of groups of performers and by reports from performing arts medicine clinics. Evaluation of the performing artist requires some attention to the occupational factors that may contribute to the development of these symptoms. This chapter reviews the clinical approach to the performing artist with occupationally related disorders. Some of the most common neurologic diseases may, on occasion, affect the performing artist more profoundly than others in the patient population, largely because of the exquisite sensorimotor requirements of the performing arts. Pain is the most frequent complaint of the performing artist; the most common cause of this is musculotendinous overuse, which generally affects the upper extremity, neck, and upper trunk of musicians and the lower extremity of the dancer. Among neurologic disorders, entrapment neuropathies and occupational cramp or focal dystonia are most frequently seen. Clinical characteristics of these disorders in the performing artist, methods of evaluation, and treatment strategies are reviewed.

References

1. Lederman RJ. Performing arts medicine. N Engl J Med 1989;320:246–248
2. Singer K. Diseases of the Musical Profession: A Systematic Presentation of Their Causes, Symptoms and Methods of Treatment. New York: Greenberg, 1932.
3. Miller E, Schneider H, Bronson J et al. A new consideration in athletic injuries: the classical ballet dancer. Clin Orthop 1975;111:181–191.
4. Washington EL. Musculoskeletal injuries in theatrical dancers: site, frequency, and severity. Am J Sports Med 1978;6:75–98.
5. Brodnitz F. Hormones and the human voice. Bull N Y Acad Med 1971;47:183–191.
6. Punt NA. Applied laryngology—singers and actors. Proc Royal Soc Med 1968;61:1152–1156.
7. Sataloff RT. Professional singers: The science and art of clinical care. Am J Otolaryngol 1981;2:251–266.
8. Critchley M, Henson RA (eds). Music and the Brain: Studies in the Neurology of Music. London: William Heinemann, 1977.

9. Hochberg FH, Leffert RD, Heller MD et al. Hand difficulties among musicians. JAMA 1983;249:1869–1872.

10. Blau JN, Henson RA. Neurological Disorders in Performing Musicians. In M Critchley, RA Henson (eds), Music and the Brain: Studies in the Neurology of Music. London: William-Heinemann, 1977;301–322.

11. Lederman RJ. Neurological Problems of Performing Artists. In RT Sataloff, AG Brandfonbrener, RJ Lederman (eds), Textbook of Performing Arts Medicine. New York: Raven, 1991;171–204.

12. Lockwood AH. Medical problems of musicians. N Engl J Med 1989; 320:221–227.

13. Knishkowy B, Lederman RJ. Instrumental musicians with upper extremity disorders: a follow-up study. Med Probl Perform Art 1986;1:85–89.

14. Stanish WD. Overuse injuries in athletes: a perspective. Med Sci Sports Exerc 1984;16:1–7.

15. Caldron PH, Calabrese LH, Clough JD et al. A survey of musculoskeletal problems encountered in high-level musicians. Med Probl Perform Art 1986;1:136–139.

16. Fry HJH. Incidence of overuse syndrome in the symphony orchestra. Med Probl Perform Art 1986;1:51–55.

17. Fishbein M, Middlestadt SE, Ottati V et al. Medical problems among ICSOM musicians: overview of a national survey. Med Probl Perform Art 1988;3:1–8.

18. Middlestadt SE, Fishbein M. The prevalence of severe musculoskeletal problems among male and female symphony orchestra string players. Med Probl Perform Art 1989;4:41–48.

19. Cunningham LS, Kelsey JL. Epidemiology of musculoskeletal impairments and associated disability. Am J Public Health 1984;74:574–579.

20. Fry HJH. Prevalence of overuse (injury) syndrome in Australian music schools. Br J Ind Med 1987;44:35–40.

21. Revak JM. Incidence of upper extremity discomfort among piano students. Am J Occup Ther 1989;43:149–154.

22. Lockwood AH. Medical problems in secondary school-aged musicians. Med Probl Perform Art 1988;129–132.

23. Manchester RA. The incidence of hand problems in music students. Med Probl Perform Art 1988;3:15–18.

24. Newmark J, Lederman RJ. Practice doesn't necessarily make perfect: incidence of overuse syndromes in amateur instrumentalists. Med Probl Perform Art 1987;2:142–144.

25. Simons H. Health and the choral conductor. Med Probl Perform Art 1986; 1:56–57.

26. Chmelar RD, Fitt SS, Schulz BB et al. A survey of health, training, and injuries in different levels and styles of dancers. Med Probl Perform Art 1987;2:61–66.

27. Mutoh Y, Sawai S, Takanishi Y et al. Aerobic dance injuries among instructors and students. Phys Sports Med 1988;16:80–86.

28. Hochberg FH, Lederman RJ. The Upper Extremity Difficulties of Musicians. In JM Hunter et al. (eds), Rehabilitation of the Hand: Surgery and Therapy (3rd ed). St. Louis: Mosby, 1990;1197–1209.

29. Lederman RJ. Peripheral nerve disorders in instrumentalists. Ann Neurol 1989;26:640–646.

30. Dawson WJ. Hand and upper extremity problems in musicians: epidemiology and diagnosis. Med Probl Perform Art 1988;3:19–22.
31. Critchley M. Musicogenic Epilepsy. In M Critchley, RA Henson (eds), Music and the Brain: Studies in the Neurology of Music. London: William Heinemann, 1977;344–353.
32. Forster FM, Klove H, Peterson WG et al. Modification of musicogenic epilepsy by extinction technique. Trans Am Neurol Assoc 1965;90:179–182.
33. Daly DD, Barry MJ. Musicogenic epilepsy: report of three cases. Psychosomatic Med 1977;19:399–408.
34. Benton AL. The Amusias. In M Critchley, RA Henson (eds), Music and the Brain: Studies in the Neurology of Music. London: William Heinemann, 1977;378–397.
35. Brust JCM. Music and language: musical alexia and agraphia. Brain 1980;103:367–392.
36. Calabrese LH. AIDS in the performing arts. Med Probl Perform Art 1987;2:113–116.
37. Dalakas M, Wichman A, Sever J. AIDS and the nervous system. JAMA 1989;261:2396–2399.
38. Nubé J. Beta-blockers: effects on performing musicians. Med Probl Perform Art 1991;6:61–68.
39. Brandfonbrener AG, MacLean IC, Johnsen JA. Myasthenia gravis in wind players: two case studies. Med Probl Perform Art 1988;3:155–157.
40. Lambert CM. Hand and upper limb problems of instrumental musicians. Br J Rheumatol 1992;31:265–271.
41. Lederman RJ, Calabrese LH. Overuse syndromes in instrumentalists. Med Probl Perform Art 1986;1:7–11.
42. Hoppmann RA, Patrone NA. Musculoskeletal Problems in Instrumental Musicians. In RT Sataloff, AG Brandfonbrener, RJ Lederman (eds), Textbook of Performing Arts Medicine. New York: Raven, 1991;71–109.
43. Fry HJH. Physical signs in the hand and wrist seen in the overuse injury syndrome of the upper limb. Aust N Z J Surg 1986;56:47–49.
44. Howard NJ. Peritendinitis crepitans: a muscle-effort syndrome. J Bone Joint Surg 1937;19:447–459.
45. Newmark J, Hochberg FH. "Doctor, it hurts when I play": painful disorders among instrumental musicians. Med Probl Perform Art 1987;2:93–97.
46. Fry HJH. Patterns of overuse seen in 658 affected instrumental musicians. Int Music 1988;11:3–16.
47. Armstrong TJ, Silverstein BA. Upper Extremity Pain in the Workplace—Role of Usage in Causality. In NM Hadler (ed), Clinical Concepts in Regional Musculoskeletal Illness. New York: Grune & Stratton, 1987;333–354.
48. Hadler, NM. Is Carpal Tunnel Syndrome an Injury That Qualifies for Workers' Compensation Insurance? In NM Hadler (ed), Clinical Concepts in Regional Musculoskeletal Illness. New York: Grune & Stratton, 1987;355–360.
49. McDermott FT. Repetition strain injury: a review of current understanding. Med J Aust 1986;144:196–200.
50. Thompson AR, Plewes LW, Shaw EG. Peritendinitis crepitans and simple tenosynovitis: a clinical study of 544 cases in industry. Br J Ind Med 1951;8:150–160.

51. Dennett X, Fry HJH. Overuse syndrome: a muscle biopsy study. Lancet 1988;1:905–908.
52. Semple JC, Behan PO, Behan WM. Overuse syndrome. Lancet 1988;1:1464–1465.
53. Friden J, Sjostrom M, Ekblom B. Myofibrillar damage following intense eccentric exercise in man. Int J Sports Med 1983;4:170–176.
54. Gilliatt RW. Thoracic Outlet Syndromes. In PJ Dyck, PK Thomas, EH Lambert (eds), Peripheral Neuropathy (2nd ed). Philadelphia: Saunders, 1984;1409–1424.
55. Lederman RJ. Thoracic outlet syndrome: review of the controversies and a report of 17 instrumental musicians. Med Probl Perform Art 1987;2:87–91.
56. Roos DB. Thoracic outlet syndromes: symptoms, diagnosis, anatomy and surgical treatment. Med Probl Perform Art 1986;1:90–93.
57. Wilbourn AJ, Porter JM. Thoracic outlet syndromes. Spine: State Art Rev 1988;2:597–626.
58. Kopell HP, Thompson WAL. Pronator syndrome: a confirmed case and its diagnosis. N Engl J Med 1958; 259:713–715.
59. Charness ME. Unique Upper Extremity Disorders of Musicians. In LH Millender, DS Louis, BP Simmons (eds), Occupational Disorders of the Upper Extremity. New York: Churchill Livingstone, 1992;227–251.
60. Kincaid JC. The electrodiagnosis of ulnar neuropathy at the elbow. Muscle Nerve 1988;11:1005–1015.
61. Cynamon, KB. Flutist's neuropathy. N Engl J Med 1981;305:961.
62. Lister GD, Belsole RB, Kleinert HE. The radial tunnel syndrome. J Hand Surg 1979;4:52–59.
63. Howard, PL. Gamba leg. N Engl J Med 1982;306:115.
64. Schwartz E, Hodson A. A viol paresthesia. Lancet 1980;2:156.
65. Mladinish EK, DeWitt J. A newly recognized occupation palsy. JAMA 1974;228:695.
66. Gowers WR. A Manual of Diseases of the Nervous System (2nd ed). Vol. II. 1893. Reprinted by Hafner Publishing Company, Darien CT, 1970;710–730.
67. Ramazzini B: Diseases of workers (1713). Revised and translated by WC Wright. Chicago: University of Chicago, 1940;420–425.
68. Romberg MH. A Manual of the Nervous Diseases of Man. Translated by EH Sieveking, Vol. 1. London: Sydenham Society, 1853;320–324.
69. Poore GV. Clinical lecture on certain conditions of the hand and arm which interfere with the performances of professional acts, especially piano-playing. Br Med J 1887;1:441–444.
70. Critchley M. Occupational Palsies in Musical Performers. In M Critchley, RA Henson (eds), Music and the Brain: Studies in the Neurology of Music. London: William Heinemann, 1977;365–377.
71. Merriman L, Newmark H, Hochberg FH et al. A focal movement disorder of the hand in six pianists. Med Probl Perform Art 1986;1:17–19.
72. Newmark J, Hochberg FH. Isolated painless manual incoordination in 57 musicians. J Neurol Neurosurg Psychiatry 1987;50:291–295.
73. Hochberg FH, Harris SV, Blattert TR. Occupational hand cramps: professional disorders of motor control. Hand Clin 1990;6(3):417–428.
74. Lederman RJ. Focal dystonias in instrumentalists: clinical features. Med Probl Perform Art 1991;6:132–136.

75. Jankovic J, Shale H. Dystonia in musicians. Semin Neurol 1989;9(2):131–135.
76. Marsden CD. The problem of adult-onset idiopathic torsion dystonia and other isolated dyskinesias in adult life (including blepharospasm, oromandibular dystonia, dystonic writer's cramp, and torticollis, or axial dystonia). Adv Neurol 1976; 14:259–276.
77. Sheehy MP, Marsden CD. Writers' cramp—a focal dystonia. Brain 1982;105:461–480.
78. Ferguson D. An Australian study of telegraphists' cramp. Br J Ind Med 1971;28:280–285.
79. Sarkari NBS, Mahendru RK, Singh SS. An epidemiological and neuropsychiatric study of writers cramp. J Assoc Physicians India 1976;24:587–591.
80. Nutt JG, Muenter MD, Melton LJ et. al. Epidemiology of dystonia in Rochester, Minnesota. Adv Neurol 1988;50:361–365.
81. Cohen LG, Hallett M. Hand cramps: clinical features and electromyographic patterns in a focal dystonia. Neurology 1988;38:1005–1012.
82. Fross RD, Martin WRW, Li D et al. Lesions of the putamen: their relevance to dystonia. Neurology 1987;37:1125–1129.
83. Scherokman B, Husain F, Cuetter A et al. Peripheral dystonia. Arch Neurol 1986;43:830–832.
84. Schott GD. Induction of involuntary movements by peripheral trauma: an analogy with causalgia. Lancet 1986;2:712–715.
85. Schwartzman RJ, Kerrigan J. The movement disorder of reflex sympathetic dystrophy. Neurology 1990;40:57–61.
86. Marsden CD, Rothwell JC. The physiology of idiopathic dystonia. Can J Neurol Sci 1987;14:521–527.
87. Panizza ME, Hallett M, Nilsson J. Reciprocal inhibition in patients with hand cramps. Neurology 1989;39:85–89.
88. Marmor MF. Vision and the musician. Med Probl Perform Art 1986;1:117–121.
89. Westmore GA, Eversden ID. Noise-induced hearing loss and orchestral musicians. Arch Otolaryngol 1981;107:761–764.
90. Johnson DW, Sherman RE, Aldridge J et al. Effects of instrument type and orchestral position on hearing sensitivity for 0.25 to 20 kHz in the orchestral musician. Scand Audiol 1985;14:215–221.
91. Hart CW, Geltman CL, Schupbach J et al. The musician and occupational sound hazards. Med Probl Perform Art 1987;2:22–25.
92. Dey FL. Auditory fatigue and predicted permanent hearing defects from rock-and-roll music. N Engl J Med 1970;282:467–470.
93. Chasin M, Chong J. A clinically efficient hearing protection program for musicians. Med Probl Perform Art 1992;7:40–43.
94. Fry HJH. The treatment of overuse syndrome in musicians: results in 175 patients. J Royal Soc Med 1988;81:572–575.
95. Peet RM, Henriksen MD, Anderson TP. Thoracic outlet syndrome: evaluation of a therapeutic exercise program. Mayo Clin Proc 1956;31:281–287.
96. Swift TR, Nichols FT. The droopy shoulder syndrome. Neurology 1984;34:212–215.
97. LeVine WR. Behavioral and biofeedback therapy for a functionally impaired musician: a case report. Biofeedback Self Reg 1983;8:101–107.
98. James I, Cook P. Bromocriptine for horn players' palsy. Lancet 1983;1:1450.

99. Cohen LG, Hallett M, Geller BD et al. Treatment of focal dystonias of the hand with botulinum toxin injections. J Neurol Neurosurg Psychiatry 1989;52:355–363.
100. Cole RA, Cohen LG, Hallett M. Treatment of musician's cramp with botulinium toxin. Med Probl Perform Art 1991;6:137–143.
101. Wolff K. Dorothy Taubman: the pianist's medicine woman. Piano Quart 1986;133:25–32.

CHAPTER 13

Occupational and Environmental Exposures and the Risk of Developing "Naturally Occurring" Neurologic Disorders

Neil L. Rosenberg, M.D.

Earlier chapters discussed in detail the role that various occupational and environmental exposures play in the development of different neurologic disorders. These disorders have primarily been nonspecific syndromes such as peripheral neuropathy, encephalopathy, and myelopathy, among others. There has been a great deal of interest in recent years in looking at various environmental factors and trying to define their roles in specific neurodegenerative disorders.[1] This has been particularly true in Parkinson's disease, amyotrophic lateral sclerosis, and senile dementia of the Alzheimer's type. Most of these have been either clinical-pathologic studies in humans or experimental studies in animals and have yielded important information that has led to the development of hypotheses to be developed regarding environmental exposures and these conditions.

Like other disorders, neurologic disease does not occur randomly in populations. Disease susceptibility may be influenced by a wide variety of factors, including those beyond individual control such as age, sex, and genetic makeup of the individual. Factors related to an individual's environment are also important and include lifestyle, diet, and home and work environments. Epidemiology involves the study of disease occurrence in populations with the aim of relating disease occurrence to these aspects of individuals and their environment. Unlike clinical-pathologic and experimental studies, epidemiology uses populations, rather than individuals, as the unit of analysis.

Epidemiologic studies have been valuable in analyzing the occurrence of potential occupational hazards. Occupational epidemiologic studies either try to investigate determinants of disease or attempt to monitor disease rates over time so that potential health problems may be recognized early.

Epidemiologic studies related to important occupational neurologic disorders are discussed in other chapters. In this chapter the occupational epidemiology of certain naturally occurring neurologic disorders, including brain tumors, multiple sclerosis, amyotrophic lateral sclerosis, and Alzheimer's disease, is discussed.

Brain Tumors

Most scientists accept the fact that factors regulating the growth and differentiation of brain tumors are based on the paradigm that oncogenesis is a multistep process. In this model a carcinogenic substance is thought to act on a target cell and to induce biochemical change in the deoxyribonucleic acid (DNA) of the host cell. It is hypothesized that to firmly establish an inheritable change in the altered host genome, the cell must undergo a round of cellular proliferation. Once "initiated," the cell evolves through a series of changes aided by certain "promoting" agents that eventually lead to the malignant phenotype. Complete discussion of the present knowledge of the process of central nervous system oncogenesis and the roles that chemicals and other factors may play in the process is beyond the scope of this text. A more thorough review of possible occupational risks and exposures is the purpose of this review.

Studies of occupational risks for the development of brain tumors consist predominately of epidemiologic studies in four major areas: general epidemiologic studies,[2-16] general occupational epidemiologic studies,[17-27] specific occupational or industrial studies,[28-59] and studies of childhood brain tumors and parental occupation.[60-67]

GENERAL EPIDEMIOLOGIC STUDIES

General epidemiologic studies consist of epidemiologic surveys of brain tumors and attempts at associating various risk factors. Although most studies in this category do not mention any association with occupational risks or exposures,[3,6-11] at least four specifically address the issues of occupational risk.[2,4,5,12] In one such study performed in Southeast Wales, United Kingdom, comment was made on the presence of the possible etiologic significance of the association of brain tumors with the chemical industries within Southeast Wales. Specific epidemiologic data were not gathered in this regard; however, data did not show clustering around the chemical plants. If anything, therefore, this study did not show an association of brain tumors with living near or working in chemical plants. Another study performed in Los Angeles County[4] revealed an excess of gliomas among workers in the aircraft industry. Workers in the petroleum industry and the rubber and plastics industry were found to have an excess of meningiomas in this study. In addition, specific occupational groups at increased risk include dentists, who were shown to have an increased risk of all types of brain tumors, and electricians, whose excess risk is limited to gliomas. In another study performed in Los Angeles County, where risk factors for gliomas and meningiomas in males was evaluated,[5] it was found that employment in occupations likely to involve high exposure to electric and magnetic fields (EMF) increased the risk for development of gliomas but not for meningiomas. This study defined those occupations at risk from EMF exposure to include electrical engineers, radio operators, telegraph operators, electricians, electrician apprentices, data processing machine repairmen, household appliance and accessory installers and mechanics, office machine mechanics and repairmen, radio and television repairmen, and telephone linemen and splicers. More glioma cases were found in individuals who worked in the rubber industry and in "hot" processes using plastics. More meningioma cases were found in individuals who had jobs that involved exposure to metal dust and fumes. Another study[12] found that occupation in the rubber industry was associated with a significant relative risk although no other occupational risks were seen.

Recent studies have looked at both meningiomas[13–16] and gliomas[14–16] and at possible environmental risk factors. Increased risk factors for meningioma include ionizing radiation and head trauma,[13] dental x-rays (in men),[14] and occupations where cooling, cutting, or lubricating oils are used on a daily basis.[16] Increased risk of gliomas has been reported in women working with cathode ray tubes[15] and in individuals who work in the rubber industry,[16] which may be related to exposure to *N*-nitroso compounds (NOC). In this latter study, there were no other occupations involving NOC exposure, other than the rubber industry, in which workers were found to be at increased risk for the development of gliomas.

Many other risk factors have been identified separate from occupational risks in these studies. In general, it is found that all of these tumors increase with age and there are certain sex differences. Meningiomas have been clearly shown in almost all studies to be increased in women over men and gliomas increased in men over women. Numerous other factors include birthplace, religion, social class, rural living, infection by *Toxoplasma gondii*, familial tumors (particularly neurofibromatosis), and physical trauma (head injury), to name a few. In addition, it is difficult to compare these studies because both the definition of brain tumor and how it was diagnosed vary among the studies, and no information on specific exposure data in the various occupations are noted.

GENERAL OCCUPATIONAL EPIDEMIOLOGIC STUDIES

General occupational epidemiologic studies are generally designed to look at the specific occupational risks associated with the development of brain tumors. The findings in these studies are variable and difficult to interpret regarding occupational exposure and risk of the development of brain tumors.

In one study performed in east Texas[17] the risk of developing brain cancer was found to be increased in male workers employed in the transportation, communication, and utilities industries. After further analysis it was believed that these workers were specifically at risk because their occupations were associated with electricity or electromagnetic fields. Although no exposure data were available, it was believed that there was a linear relationship between the probability of exposure to electromagnetic fields and brain cancer. This same study showed a significantly elevated risk for brain cancer in men working in the trucking industry who were clearly not exposed to electricity or electromagnetic fields to any excess degree.

A case control epidemiologic study performed in Italy revealed a statistically significant risk increase for the development of brain tumors in farmers.[18] This risk increase was attributable to those farmers who reported the use of chemicals such as insecticides or fungicides, herbicides, and fertilizers. In another case control study from New Zealand,[27] an increased risk for the development of brain tumors was seen in the category of agriculture/forestry/fishing, which was entirely due to an excess of brain tumors in farmers, with the highest risk found for livestock farmers.

In a study performed in Sweden,[21] statistically significant increases in the frequency of intracranial gliomas were observed among a wide variety of individuals in professional and white-collar occupations as well as in blue-collar workers. It was somehow believed that white-collar workers had an increase in incidents of diagnosis of gliomas in part because of the higher level of diagnosis and reporting of the particular neoplasm. Why this is not believed to be so in blue-collar workers is not clear; however, among white-collar workers significantly elevated rates of brain tumors were noted among a variety of professionals, including male dentists, agricultural research workers, and public prosecutors. Increases in brain tumors were seen among female physicians and other employees in the health care industry. Among blue-collar workers, significant increases in the numbers of brain tumors were noted among welders and metal cutters; glass, porcelain, or ceramic workers; cellulose plant employees; brick and tile workers; and women employed in the wool industry. In a similar study, in which cases were identified through the Missouri Cancer Registry,[26] elevated risks for the development of brain tumors were seen both in occupations with no obvious exposure to carcinogens (e.g., engineering and the social science profession) and in those occupations with potential exposure to carcinogens (e.g., agricultural crop production, printing and publishing, and brick masonry and tile setting). These different occupational groups have no obvious similar risk factors and similarities of any particular exposures between these groups have not been found.

In a case control study performed in Sweden looking at occupational factors associated with astrocytomas, several answers to an extensive questionnaire seemed to be associated with an extreme risk of astrocytoma: "Working at an airfield," "living near a petrochemical plant," "living near a municipal sewage treatment plant," and "living in a neighborhood of a paper mill or a sawmill" all gave increased relative risks for the development of astrocytomas. Once again, what common bond exists among those answering positively to any one of these questions is not clear. Inquiries concerning individual chemicals or category of chemical in this particular study did not reveal a significantly increased risk for the development of astrocytoma.[20]

In a case reference study,[22] links between development of astrocytic brain tumors and occupational chemical exposures were assessed. It was found that no statistically significant increased risk was associated with employment in the chemical industry; however, the risk of astrocytic tumors was increased among individuals with production or maintenance jobs in the petroleum refining industry. Of particular interest is the fact that this risk decreased with increasing length of time employed. Numerous insignificant increases of astrocytic brain tumors were seen in men exposed to other chemicals including cutting fluids and organic solvents. In another study using a case referent death certificate analysis,[23] small insignificant increases of brain tumors were seen among persons whose usual employment was in the petroleum refining, electrical equipment manufacturing, health services and educational services industries. Compared with other white-collar professionals, health diagnosticians, teachers, and artist/designers had a significantly elevated risk of brain tumor. Among blue-collar workers, the only group with a significantly elevated brain tumor risk were precision metal workers who are exposed to metal dust and fumes and who use substances such as coolants, lubricants, and degreasers. Again, in this latter study no apparent link is seen among the different white- and blue-collar jobs described and increased risks; therefore, the reason for the slightly increased risk of development of brain tumors is not clear.

A descriptive study of 100 patients with established diagnoses of glioblastoma multiforme (GBM) was concerned specifically with exposure to herbicides.[24] The study focused on place of residence and occupation during the year before the diagnosis of GBM. More than one-third of cases came from just three counties in which rice, cotton, or wood products were produced. In addition, these industries were reported as the occupations of almost one-third of cases for whom occupations involved a risk of herbicide exposure.

A population-based case control study from Germany found no significant effects for most occupations.[25] Some categories showed slightly elevated risks, but the only significant occupational risk for the development of brain tumors was seen in women employed in "electrical occupations."

SPECIFIC OCCUPATIONAL EXPOSURE STUDIES

Specific occupational studies are conducted variably on specific industries or general occupational studies that have pointed to specific industry risks and use a variety of methodologies. The findings of all of these studies are mixed with many contradictory findings.

Many studies have examined the association between brain tumors and working in the petrochemical industry.[28–34] Some have found an excessive risk for the development of brain cancer in the petrochemical industry.[28,29] Other studies have found no association between working in the petrochemical industry and an increased risk of brain tumors.[30–34]

Several additional isolated studies have suggested an increased risk for brain tumors in veterinarians,[36] chemists,[38] asbestos insulation workers,[42] farmers,[37,54] embalmers,[41] rubber workers, nuclear facility workers,[47,48,55] and those exposed to numerous other chemical agents.[49,56]

A study showing that dentists and dental nurses had an increased risk for the development of brain tumors suggested that some common occupational factors such as amalgam, chloroform, or radiography are the associated risk factors in the development of brain tumors in these individuals.[45]

Another study revealed an increased risk of gliomas in woodworkers.[46] In this study it was believed that exposure to wood preservatives in solvents occurred more often than not in woodworkers who develop brain tumors. However, in the same study an increased risk was seen in teachers who had no exposure to wood preservatives or solvents.

In two studies performed at nuclear facilities in Oakridge, Tennessee, there appeared to be no association between deaths from brain tumors and exposure to ionizing radiation.[47] In these studies there are a small number of monitor subjects, and the author could not rule out a modest association. However, in a second study performed at the same facility, a strong association was found between the development of brain tumors and a history of epilepsy.[48] This is in keeping with prior epidemiologic studies that have suggested that individuals with a history of epilepsy or head injury have a higher incidence of brain tumors, and therefore no apparent occupational risk factors at these nuclear facilities could be strongly suggested. Overall, it has been estimated that United States nuclear workers have a 15% increased risk of brain cancer.[55]

An increased incidence of brain tumors was reported in laboratory workers at the Pasteur Institute in Paris.[56] Three cases of primary brain tumors were also reported in three laboratory workers from one laboratory in a district general hospital, which may have been due to geographic clustering or merely to coincidence. Nevertheless, laboratory workers may be at increased risk for the development of brain tumors because of the multiple chemicals to which they are exposed.

A review[49] on the epidemiology of brain tumors and the relationships with exposure to chemical agents emphasizes the difficulty of interpreting such studies that show some correlation to some sort of chemical exposure or occupational exposure in the development of brain tumors. Because of the relatively low incidence of brain tumors in humans, cohort studies need to be large in order to accrue sufficient numbers of cases for meaningful interpretation. The evidence for any chemical causation of brain cancer in humans was inconclusive based on this review.

Other studies have suggested an association between exposure to electromagnetic fields and brain tumors.[50–53,57–59] The results of these studies have likewise been variable, with some showing an association of occupational exposure to electromagnetic fields and increased risk of brain tumors[51–53,57–59] and others showing no increased risk of brain tumors in those occupations exposed to high electromagnetic fields.[52] A Swedish study found no increased risk of brain tumors for "all electrical occupations"; however, increases were seen in certain areas: increase in brain tumors and GBM in assemblers and repair workers in the radio and television industries, increase in brain tumors in all welders, and increase in brain tumors in all welders in the iron and steel works industries.[57] In this same study, no major changes in relative risk estimates were noted after the exclusion of persons who were over the age of 65 at the time of diagnosis. Other studies that have shown some association with some "electrical occupations" and the development of brain tumors have also failed to confirm some previously reported associations.[58,59]

In an editorial, no strong evidence for an association between exposure to electromagnetic fields and brain tumors was believed to exist; however, that same editorial ends with this quote: "Thus, with all the reservations one may have toward the ultimate validity of this new information, EM energy, which is with us to stay, must be considered an environmental hazard and must be dealt with accordingly, until proven otherwise."[59A] The association between occupational exposure to electromagnetic fields and the development of brain tumors needs further study.

CHILDHOOD BRAIN TUMORS AND PARENTAL OCCUPATION

Epidemiologic studies have suggested there may be associations between the environmental exposures of residential electromagnetic fields[60] and home pesticide use[61] and the development of brain tumors in childhood. In addition to possible direct environmental influences, other studies have examined the occupations of parents of children in whom brain tumors developed.

Of the six studies published that looked at parental occupation and development of brain tumors in their children,[62–67] one revealed that fathers of children in whom brain tumors developed were more likely than control fathers to have been employed in agriculture, metal-related jobs, structural work jobs in the construction industry, electrical assembling, installing, and repairing occupations in the machinery industry.[63] This was a mortality-based, case-controlled study and therefore the results must be interpreted with caution.

Another case control study of environmental factors and childhood brain tumor risk revealed several associations between that risk and parental occupation:[66] Increased risk was seen for several parental occupations (agriculture, benchwork, transportation) and parental employment in several industries (agriculture, construction, metal, food/tobacco). This study also attempted to assess risk for the development of a brain tumor and timing of exposure. The greatest excess risks were associated with parental exposure during the preconception period. Fathers of children with brain tumors were more likely to have had jobs linked to exposure to aromatic amino and aromatic nitro compounds; however, in this situation, exposure was more likely to occur in the postnatal period. Few associations were found between maternal exposures and the development of brain tumors; however, the numbers of mothers employed outside the home was small in this study.

A study of childhood brain tumors in children with fathers in the aerospace industry[64] is difficult to interpret. An apparent increased risk for the development of brain tumors varies with the age at diagnosis. This study must be interpreted with caution because of small numbers of inconsistent associations.

A case control interview study of environmental factors and childhood brain tumors revealed an interesting space-time cluster in rural Ohio.[65] Six genetically unrelated children were diagnosed with primary brain tumors in a 2.4-year period, and each child had one parent employed by the same company (an electronics firm). This company used over 100 chemicals in a manufacturing process, so the possible link was believed to be through one or multiple chemicals. This study is obviously limited by the small number of affected individuals but is compelling nevertheless.

The most carefully performed studies in this group are epidemiologic case control studies examining parental (not just paternal) occupational exposures in children with brain tumors.[62,67] One study[62] failed to show any consistent association between childhood brain tumor risk and paternal exposures to hydrocarbons, electromagnetic fields, employment in the aerospace industry, or pulp and paper manufacturing.

Only one study focused on a particular type of brain tumor.[67] In this case-control study, parental occupation was investigated as a possible risk factor for the development of childhood astrocytoma. Over a 6-year period from eight hospitals in three states, 163 cases were identified. No strong associations were seen, although significantly more fathers of these patients were electrical or electronic repairmen. An excess of cases in children below the age of 5 years was seen in mothers employed as nurses. Elevated, but not significantly increased, odds ratios were seen in the following categories: some white-collar and professional occupations, paternal exposure to paint (for the period after the child's birth), employment in the paper and pulp mill industry (for period after child's birth), and maternal occupation as a hairdresser.

Several studies have shown associations between parental occupational exposures and the development of childhood brain tumors; however, there appears to be no consistent or strong association.

CONCLUSIONS OF OCCUPATIONAL EPIDEMIOLOGIC BRAIN TUMOR STUDIES

Numerous epidemiologic studies have been performed that address occupational risks and the development of brain tumors. No consistent pattern of occupational risk appears from these studies. Numerous white-collar and professional occupations, as well as blue-collar jobs, have been associated in these studies with an increased risk of the development of brain tumors. A wide variety of agents, including chemicals, electromagnetic fields, ionizing radiation, and others, have been variably linked to the development of brain tumors.

It appears that nonoccupational risks, such as age, head trauma, and epilepsy, are greater potential risk factors for the development of astrocytic brain tumors (including GBM), and that sex (i.e., hormonal factors) is probably the greatest risk factor for the development of meningiomas.

Multiple Sclerosis

Gowers suggested in 1888[68] that a possible etiology of multiple sclerosis (MS) was "overwork." However, a possible connection between occupational exposures and the development of MS did not appear in the literature until 1947, when four of seven researchers studying swayback in lambs were reported as having developed this disease.[69]

The possibilities for such an outbreak were considered and included a number of different workplace factors, but none could be substantiated. A later study of these same individuals revealed that among the original seven research workers, a fifth later developed MS.[70] Although the odds of four or more of a random group of eight men developing MS were calculated to be about 1 in 109, this disease has not occurred in other research workers studying swayback, which has subsequently been found to be related to a nutritional disorder.[71]

OCCUPATIONS ASSOCIATED WITH INCREASED RISK OF MULTIPLE SCLEROSIS

Neuroepidemiologic studies have provided important clues about the cause and pathogenesis of MS. These studies have not dealt with occupational or environmental toxic exposures, with few exceptions. Reports of possible occupational risks for the development of MS have been few,[72-82] but primarily associated with solvents,[72-74] zinc,[75] lead,[74] methanol,[76] or combinations of organic solvents and welding.[79]

Evaluation of the occupational pattern of MS patients compared to the general population or control groups reveals inconsistent results. Individuals in the few occupations or industries that have been associated with an increased risk of MS include shoe and leather workers,[72] workers in paper manufacturing,[77] hairdressers,[83] and those who had professional contact with pathology specimens,[84] but these associations are weak at best, however.

ORGANIC SOLVENTS AND MULTIPLE SCLEROSIS

A study from Norway failed to show an association between exposure to organic solvents and multiple sclerosis.[78] This was a case-control study in western Norway and included 93% of the patients who had clinical onset of MS in a western county of Norway during the years 1976–1986 (N = 155) and 200 age-, sex- and residence-matched controls. No statistically significant difference was found between MS patients and controls with regard to exposure to organic solvents or exposure to combinations of either organic solvents/welding or organic solvents/other chemicals. This study contradicts a prior observation, which demonstrated that solvents, especially in combination with welding, appeared to be associated with an increased risk for MS in men.[79]

MERCURY AND MULTIPLE SCLEROSIS

Reports in the lay press as well as the scientific literature have tried to make a link between mercury liberated from dental fillings and MS.[85,86] Because of this association, one study looked at the mercury content from the frontal lobes of eight MS autopsy brains and eight controls.[85] Mercury content was assayed by neutron activation. While no differences were seen between the two groups and total mercury content, the lipid-soluble mercury was significantly decreased in the MS brain tissue. This study not only fails to support a toxic effect of mercury in MS but actually contradicts this as a viable hypothesis.

CONTAMINATED WATER AND MULTIPLE SCLEROSIS

Two recent cluster analysis studies have tried to link toxic contaminants in water and focal geographic locations with an increased incidence of MS compared to normative incidence data.[87,88] One study suggests that where the incidence of MS was higher, the water contained an excess of heavy metal wastes, especially cadmium and chromium.[87] There was virtually no evidence to support this assertion as well as that of the other study from

Henribourg, Saskatchewan,[88] which suggests that both certain deficiencies in the water (e.g., selenium and sulfate) and excesses (e.g., barium, calcium, chloride, chromium, magnesium, molybdenum, nitrate plus nitrite, strontium, zinc) are associated with increased risk of developing MS.

CONCLUSIONS

Several studies have been published and there has been much speculation in the lay press regarding occupational or environmental toxic exposures and an increased incidence of MS. To date, the strongest environmental links to MS are nontoxic in nature.

Alzheimer's Disease

Chronic occupational exposures to a variety of industrial chemicals are linked to several cognitive disorders (see Chapter 5). In particular, organic solvents have been associated with abnormalities of several aspects of central nervous system function (see Chapter 4). Numerous epidemiologic studies have suggested a possible link between chronic occupational organic solvent exposure and neurobehavioral abnormalities and dementia. A case-control study in Massachusetts evaluated 98 patients with Alzheimer's disease and 162 matched control subjects for occupational risk factors.[89] This study failed to find an association between Alzheimer's disease and occupational exposure to organic solvents or lead. While this exposure can certainly cause central nervous system dysfunction, it is not associated with Alzheimer's disease or other neurodegenerative disorders.

Several factors have been identified that are associated with an increased risk for the development of Alzheimer's disease. These include advanced age (which shows the strongest association with increased risk), family history of dementia, female sex, Down's syndrome, and depression.[90] Other nonoccupational factors occur less frequently as associated risks in various studies, including head trauma. Some recent studies have noted an association between occupational factors and the development of Alzheimer's disease.[91,92]

Since decline in memory performance is a strong predictor of dementia in the elderly, investigators in the Bordeaux area of France conducted an epidemiologic study on brain aging.[91] They studied the relationship between lifetime occupation and memory performance in visual recognition. Independent of educational level, the risk of poor memory performance was two to three times greater than that of professionals/managers in farmers, domestic service employees, and blue-collar workers. In another study, manual labor was correlated as a risk factor for the development of Alzheimer's disease[92]. This same study also found alcohol abuse and family history among the risk factors.

Epidemiologic studies have only recently identified occupation as a relatively minor risk factor for the development of Alzheimer's disease, which may be linked primarily to education or declining complexity of work tasks with aging.[90]

Amyotrophic Lateral Sclerosis

There has been a great deal of interest in recent years in the hypothesis that amyotrophic lateral sclerosis (ALS) can be caused by environmental or occupational exposures. The data come from three sources: studies of ALS being related to occupational exposures,[93-100] heavy metals and trace elements,[101-112] and organochlorine insecticides,[113] and also from studies of the western Pacific parkinsonism-dementia-ALS complex.[114-122]

OCCUPATIONAL EXPOSURES AND AMYOTROPHIC LATERAL SCLEROSIS

There is very little evidence that occupational exposures are associated with ALS. Studies have suggested a slightly increased risk in individuals who have contact with carcasses and hides or those who are exposed to organic solvents while working in the leather industry.[94,95]

After an initial observation that identified 16 cases of ALS in leather industry workers based on unpublished tables of the Decennial Supplement on Occupational Mortality,[94] a more in-depth search for ALS cases in leather industry workers was undertaken.[95] Thirty-three cases of ALS in leather industry workers were compared to 131 controls randomly selected from deaths of all causes in the same period. Although no statistically significant difference was seen between the two groups in regard to various occupational subdivisions, there may have been a deficit of ALS cases among tanners. This would suggest that the apparent excess of ALS cases in the leather industry was not related to individuals involved in the tanning process.

Individuals with ALS were found to have worked more frequently (though this was not statistically significant) in blue-collar jobs and at welding and soldering in one study.[96] In recent epidemiologic studies, other possible occupational risk factors have been identified. Farmers were found in three separate studies to have an increased risk of ALS.[97-99] One of these studies[97] also found an increase in individuals exposed to chemical products. In a case control study from Sweden,[99] an increased risk was seen in women employed as medical service workers and in men employed as office workers and farm workers. In another study, an increased risk for the development of ALS was seen in individuals employed in hard labor and in individuals who had exposure to heavy metals.[100]

HEAVY METALS AND TRACE ELEMENTS

Numerous metals and trace elements have been evaluated in serum, muscle, and spinal cord tissue samples of patients with ALS. The possible role that these substances may or may not play in the pathogenesis of ALS has been recently reviewed.[101] Although no epidemiologic study has addressed metals and trace elements specifically, certain ones are discussed here because of their past links to ALS and the workers who are exposed to them.

Occupational and other exposure to lead has been said to produce a clinical picture that closely resembles ALS.[102–106] In those individuals in whom this "ALS-like" picture occurs, removal of the patient from the exposure or chelation therapy, or both, will improve the patient's condition. However, individuals with typical ALS and no history of exposure do not improve with these measures. Therefore, while the clinician needs to be aware of occupational lead exposure in individuals who present with a clinical picture of ALS, the likelihood that lead plays a role in the pathogenesis of naturally occurring (i.e., without history of significant lead exposure) ALS is remote.

The same conclusion can be drawn with exposure to mercury, where an ALS-like clinical picture may occur with occupational exposure,[107–109] and may respond to chelation therapy, but where the naturally occurring disorder does not respond to treatment with these agents.[110,111] In a study from Japan,[112] extensive evaluation was performed on 83 ex–mercury workers who had been poisoned or exposed to mercury vapor 18 years previously at a large mercury mine, to look for possible links between mercury and ALS. Neurologic examinations and measurements of mercury in blood, urine, and hair failed to disclose these links. Causes of death in an additional 65 deceased workers were analyzed in this study. Of the 148 cases reviewed, no cases of ALS were found. Although this study does not eliminate the possibility of mercury being associated pathogenetically with ALS, it seems unlikely to be a common mechanism given the lack of cases in this study, in which individuals had very high levels of exposure to mercury (see discussion of dose-response relationship in Chapter 2).

Trace elements of possible importance to ALS with regard to occupational exposures include aluminum, selenium, manganese, chromium, and copper.[101] The evidence linking exposure of these elements to ALS is even weaker than that for lead and mercury. However, since the cause of ALS remains unknown, further studies evaluating exposures to these and other occupational and environmental elements need to be considered.

ORGANOCHLORINE INSECTICIDES AND
AMYOTROPHIC LATERAL SCLEROSIS

One study reports the association between organochlorine pesticides in two patients with chronic motor neuron disease.[113] What was intriguing about these two individuals is that they worked together (employer and employee) spraying crops with organochlorine insecticides (prepared by mixing with their bare hands) during agricultural seasons and they did not use protective equipment. One of these individuals had been hospitalized with acute insecticide poisoning. Both had elevated levels of pesticides, including aldrin, lindane, and heptachlor, in the peripheral blood. Both developed typical features of ALS and progressed and died despite lack of continued exposure. These cases were reported from Brazil, where, like other Third World countries, adequate protective equipment is usually not worn by workers. Intriguing as these two cases may be, other links between organochlorine insecticides and ALS have not been reported.

EXCITATORY DIETARY AMINO ACID AND WESTERN PACIFIC AMYOTROPHIC LATERAL SCLEROSIS

There has been a great deal of interest recently in the role of excitotoxic amino acids (EAAs) in causing the cell damage in stroke, epilepsy, and several degenerative neurologic disorders, including ALS.[114–122] The relationship of EAAs to possible occupational or environmental exposures and ALS is controversial, but an awareness of this area is important for clinicians in evaluating this active area of research.

The western Pacific ALS and parkinsonism-dementia complex is a neurodegenerative disorder seen in Guam, and certain areas of New Guinea and Japan (see Chapter 7).[114–116] Environmental factors, nonviral in nature, peculiar to these regions seem to play an important etiologic role. In particular, individuals in these regions who developed ALS have been found to consume large amounts of raw or incompletely detoxified seed (in the form of a flour made from the seed) of certain cycad plants that contain BMAA, an excitotoxic amino acid. Macaques fed BMAA developed clinical and pathologic features of both motor neuron degeneration, like ALS, and parkinsonism-dementia.[115] However, a study of levels of BMAA in cycad flour found that only very low levels of this amino acid survive the usual processing procedure, suggesting that BMAA may not be the cause of this syndrome in humans.[116]

One study of this syndrome focused on mineral composition of soil and drinking water.[122] This environmental study revealed identical mineral composition in soils and drinking water: low calcium and magnesium, and high aluminum and manganese. Trace element analysis of central nervous system tissues from patients with ALS has revealed high contents of aluminum and calcium, with significant positive correlations between aluminum and calcium and/or between calcium and manganese, which suggests the possibility that prolonged exposure to these trace elements may cause abnormal mineral metabolism in neurons. It was also found that aluminum seemed to preferentially bind to nucleic acids, which may lead to progressive inhibition of protein synthesis of ribosomal ribonucleic acid (rRNA) leading to neuronal degeneration.

Additional studies of glutamate, a naturally occurring EAA in the brain, have also yielded conflicting results.[119,120] Finally, a recent epidemiologic analysis of this disorder revealed that purely environmental, Mendelian dominant, and Mendelian recessive hypotheses could be rejected.[121] However, a two-allele additive major locus hypothesis could not be rejected, suggesting that a genetic component could by itself explain the occurrence of this disorder.

In conclusion, environmental and genetic factors alone or in combination may explain the occurrence of the ALS and parkinsonism-dementia complex of the western Pacific. Further studies of this disorder may lead to increased understanding of how environmental exposures may be linked to the pathogenesis of ALS and other neurodegenerative diseases.

References

1. Henneberry R, Spatz L. The role of environmental factors in neurodegenerative disorders. Neurobiol Aging 1991;12:75–79.
2. Cole GC, Wilkins PR, West RR. An epidemiological survey of primary tumors of the brain and spinal cord in southeast Wales. Br J Neurosurg 1989;3(4):487–493.
3. Mills PK, Preston-Martin S, Annegers JF, Beeson WL, Phillips RL, Fraser GE. Risk factors for tumors of the brain and cranial meninges in Seventh-Day Adventists. Neuroepidemiology 1989;8:266–275.
4. Preston-Martin S. Descriptive epidemiology of primary tumors of the brain, cranial nerves and cranial meninges in Los Angeles County. Neuroepidemiology 1989;8:283–295.
5. Preston-Martin S, Mack W, Henderson BE. Risk factors for gliomas and meningiomas in males in Los Angeles County. Cancer Res 1989;49:6137–6143.
6. Helseth A, Mork SJ, Johansen A, Tretli S. Neoplasms of the central nervous system in Norway. IV. A population-based epidemiological study of meningiomas. APMIS 1989;97:646–654.
7. Helseth A, Mork SJ. Neoplasms of the central nervous system in Norway. III. Epidemiological characteristics of intracranial gliomas according to histology. APMIS 1989;97:547–555.
8. Helseth A, Langmark F, Mork SJ. Neoplasms of the central nervous system in Norway. I. Quality control of the registration in the Norwegian Cancer Registry. APMIS 1988;96:1002–1008.
9. Lona C, Tabiadon G, Curro Dossi B, Mohsenipour I. Incidence of primary intracranial tumors in the provence of Bolzano 1980–84. Ital J Neurol Sci 1988;9:237–241.
10. Abu-Salih HS, Abdul-Rahman AM. Tumors of the brain in the Sudan. Surg Neurol 1988;29:194–196.
11. Kallio M. The incidence of intracranial gliomas in southern Finland. Acta Neurol Scand 1988;78:480–483.
12. Burch JD, Craib KJP, Choi BCK, Miller AB, Risch HA, Howe GR. An exploratory case-control study of brain tumors in adults. JNCI 1987;78:601–609.
13. Longstreth WT Jr, Dennis LK, McGuire VM, Drangsholt MT, Koepsell TD. Epidemiology of intracranial meningioma. Cancer 1993;72(3):639–648.

14. Ryan P, Lee MW, North B, McMichael AJ. Amalgam fillings, diagnostic dental x-rays and tumours of the brain and meninges. Part B. Oral Oncology. Eur J Cancer. 1992;28B(2):91–95.

15. Ryan P, Lee MW, North B, McMichael AJ. Risk factors for tumors of the brain and meninges: results from the Adelaide Adult Brain Tumor Study. Int J Cancer 1992;51(1):20–27.

16. Preston-Martin S, Mack W. Gliomas and meningiomas in men in Los Angeles County: investigation of exposures to *N*-nitroso compounds. IARC Sci Pub 1991;105:197–203.

17. Speers MA, Dobbins JG, Miller VS. Occupational exposures and brain cancer mortality: a preliminary study of east Texas residents. Am J Ind Med 1988;13:629–638.

18. Musicco M, Sant M, Molinari S, Filippini G, Gatta G, Berrino F. A case-control study of brain gliomas and occupational exposure to chemical carcinogens: the risk to farmers. Am J Epidemiol 1988;128:778–785.

19. Kessler E, Brandt-Rauf PW. Occupational cancer of the brain. Occup Med 1987;2:155–163.

20. Olin RG, Ahlbom A, Lindberg-Navier I, Norell SE, Spannare B. Occupational factors associated with astrocytomas: a case-control study. Am J Ind Med 1987;11:615–625.

21. McLaughlin JK, Malker HSR, Blot WJ, Malker BK, Stone BJ, Weiner JA, Ericsson JLE, Fraumeni JF Jr. Occupational risks for intracranial gliomas in Sweden. JNCI 1987;78:253–257.

22. Thomas TL, Stewart PA, Stemhagen A, Correa P, Norman SA, Bleecker ML, Hoover RN. Risk of astrocytic brain tumors associated with occupational chemical exposures. Scand J Work Environ Health 1987;13:417–423.

23. Thomas TL, Fontham ETH, Norman SA, Stemhagen A, Hoover RN. Occupational risk factors for brain tumors: a case-referent death-certificate analysis. Scand J Work Environ Health 1986;12:121–127.

24. Smith-Rooker JL, Garrett A, Hodges LC, Shue V. Prevalence of glioblastoma multiforme subjects with prior herbicide exposure. J Neuroscience Nursing 1992;24(5):260–264.

25. Schlehofer B, Kunze S, Sachsenheimer W, Blettner M, Niehoff D, Wahrendorf J. Occupational risk factors for brain tumors: results from a population-based case-control study in Germany. Cancer Causes Control 1990:1(3):209–215.

26. Brownson RC, Reif JS, Chang JC, Davis JR. An analysis of occupational risks for brain cancer. Am J Public Health 1990;80(2):169–172.

27. Reif JS, Pearce N, Fraser J. Occupational risks for brain cancer: a New Zealand Cancer Registry-based study. J Occup Med 1989;31(10):863–867.

28. Waxweiler RJ, Alexander V, Leffingwell SS, Haring M, Lloyd JW. Mortality from brain tumor and other causes in a cohort of petro chemical workers. JNCI 1983;70:75–81.

29. Thomas TL, Waxweiler RJ, Crandall MS, Moure-Eraso R, Itaya S, Fraumeni JF. Brain cancer among OCAW members in three Texas oil refineries. Ann N Y Acad Sci 1982;381:120–129.

30. Austin SG, Schnatter AR. A case-control study of chemical exposures and brain tumors in petrochemical workers. J Occup Med 1983;25:313–320.

31. Austin SC, Schnatter AR. A cohort mortality study of petrochemical workers. J Occup Med 1983;25:304–312.

32. Divine BJ, Barron V, Kaplan SD. Texas mortality study I. Mortality among refinery, petrochemical, and research workers. J Occup Med 1985;27:445–447.
33. Hanis NM, Holmes TM, Shallenberger LG, Jones KE. Epidemiologic study of refinery and chemical plant workers. J Occup Med 1982;24:203–212.
34. Hanis NM, Shallenberger LG, Donaleski DL, Sales EA. A retrospective mortality study of workers in three major U.S. refineries and chemical plants. J Occup Med 1985;27:283–292.
35. Alexander V, Leffingwell SS, Lloyd JW, Waxweiller RJ, Miller RL. Investigations of an apparent increased prevalence of brain tumors in a U.S. petrochemical plant. Ann N Y Acad Sci 1982;381:97–107.
36. Blair A, Hayes HM Jr. Mortality among U.S. veterinarians, 1947–1977: an expanded study. Int J Epidemiol 1982;11:391–397.
37. Musicco M, Filippini G, Bordo BM, Melotto A, Morello G, Berrino F. Gliomas and occupational exposure to carcinogens: case-control study. Am J Epidemiol 1982;116:782–790.
38. Olin GR, Ahlbom A. Cancer mortality among three Swedish male academic cohorts: chemists, architects, and mining engineers/metallurgists. Ann N Y Acad Sci 1982;381:197–201.
39. Reeve GR, Bond GG, Lloyd JW, Cook RR, Waxweiler RJ, Fishbeck WA. An investigation of brain tumors among chemical plant employees using sample-based cohort method. J Occup Med 1983;25:387–393.
40. Savitz DA, Moure R. Cancer risk among oil refinery workers. J Occup Med 1984;26:662–670.
41. Walrath J, Fraumeni JF Jr. Mortality patterns among embalmers. Int J Cancer 1983;31:407–411.
42. Seidman H, Selikoff IJ, Hammond EC. Mortality of brain tumors among asbestos insulation workers in the United States and Canada. Ann NY Acad Sci 1982;381:160–171.
43. Theriault G, Goulet L. A mortality study of oil refinery workers. J Occup Med 1979;21:367–370.
44. Thomas TL, Waxweiler RJ, Moure-Eraso R, Itaya S, Fraumeni JF. Mortality patterns among workers in three Texas oil refineries. J Occup Med 1982;24:135–141.
45. Ahlbom A, Norell S, Rodvall Y. Dentists, dental nurses, and brain tumors. Br Med J 1986;292:662.
46. Cordier S, Poisson M, Gerin M, Varin J, Conso F, Hemon D. Gliomas and exposure to wood preservatives. Br J Ind Med 1988;45:705–709.
47. Carpenter AV, Flanders WD, Frome EL, Crawford-Brown DJ, Fry SA. CNS cancers and radiation exposure: a case-control study among workers at two nuclear facilities. J Occup Med 1987;29:601–604.
48. Carpenter AV, Flanders WD, Frome EL, Cole P, Fry SA. Brain cancer and nonoccupational risk factors: a case-control study among workers at two nuclear facilities. Am J Public Health 1987;77:1180–1182.
49. Jones RD. Epidemiology of brain tumors in man and their relationship with chemical agents. Fd Chem Toxic 1986;24:99–103.
50. Modan B. Exposure to electromagnetic fields and brain malignancy: a newly discovered menace? Am J Ind Med 1988;13:625–627.
51. Lin RS, Dischinger PC, Farrell KP. Brain Tumors in Electrical Workers. In SK Dutta, RM Millis (eds), Biological Effects of Electropollution: Brain Tumors and Experimental Models. Philadelphia: Information Ventures, 1986;21–32.

52. Tornquist S, Norell S, Ahlbom A, Knave B. Cancer in the electric power industry. Br J Ind Med 1986;43:212–213.
53. Lin RS, Dischinger PC, Conde J, Farrell KP. Occupational exposure to electromagnetic fields and the occurrence of brain tumors: an analysis of possible associations. J Occup Med 1985;27:413–419.
54. Morrison HI, Semenciw RM, Morison D, Magwood S, Mao Y. Brain cancer and farming in western Canada. Neuroepidemiol 1992;11(4–6):267–276.
55. Alexander V. Brain tumor risk among United States nuclear workers. Occup Med 1991;6(4):695–714.
56. Rutty GN, Honavar M, Doshi B. Malignant glioma in laboratory workers. J Clin Pathol 1991;44(10):868–869.
57. Tornqvist S, Knave B, Ahlbom A, Persson T. Incidence of leukaemia and brain tumors in some "electrical occupations". Br J Indust Med 1991;48(9):597–603.
58. Mack W, Preston-Martin S, Peters JM. Astrocytoma risk related to job exposure to electric and magnetic fields. Bioelectromagnetics 1991;12(1):57–66.
59. Juutilainen J, Laara E, Pukkala E. Incidence of leukaemia and brain tumours in Finnish workers exposed to ELF magnetic fields. Int Arch Occup Environ Health 1990;62(4):289–293.
60. Savitz DA, Kaune WT. Childhood cancer in relation to a modified residential wire code. Environ Health Perspectives 1993;101(1):76–80.
61. Davis JR, Brownson RC, Garcia R, Bentz BJ, Turner A. Family pesticide use and childhood brain cancer. Arch Environ Contamination Toxicol 1993;24(1):87–92.
62. Nasca PC, Baptiste MS, MacCubbin PA, Metzger BB, Carlton K, Greenwald P, Armbrustmacher VW, Earle KM, Waldman, J. An epidemiologic case-control study of central nervous system tumors in children and parental occupational exposures. Am J Epidemiol 1988;128:1256–1265.
63. Wilkins JR, Koutras RA. Paternal occupation and brain cancer in offspring: a mortality-based case-control study. Am J Ind Med 1988;14:299–318.
64. Olshan AF, Breslow NE, Daling JR, Weiss NS, Leviton A. Childhood brain tumors and paternal occupation in the aerospace industry. JNCI 1986;77:17–19.
65. Wilkins JR 3d, McLaughlin JA, Sinks TH, Kosnik EJ. Parental occupation and intracranial neoplasms of childhood: anecdotal evidence from a unique occupational cancer cluster. Am J Indust Med 1991;19(5):643–653.
66. Wilkins JR 3d, Sinks T. Parental occupation and intracranial neoplasms of childhood: results of a case-control interview study. Am J Epidemiol 1990;132(2):275–292.
67. Kuijten RR, Bunin GR, Nass CC, Meadows AT. Parental occupation and childhood astrocytoma: results of a case-control study. Cancer Research 1992;52:782–786.
68. Gowers WR. Diseases of the Nervous System. Philadelphia: Blakiston, 1888;919.
69. Campbell AMG, Daniel P, Porter RJ, Russell WR, Smith HV, Innes JRM. Disease of the nervous system occurring among research workers on swayback in lambs. Brain 1947;70:50–58.
70. Dean G, McDougall EI., Elian M. Multiple sclerosis in research workers studying swayback in lambs: an updated report. J Neurol Neurosurg Psychiatry 1985;48:859–865.

71. Fell BF, Mills CF, Boyne R. Cytochrome oxidase deficiency in the motor neurones of copper deficient lambs: a histochemical study. Res Vet Sci 1965;6:170–171.

72. Amaducci L, Arfaioli C, Inzitari D, Marchi M. Multiple sclerosis among shoe and leather workers: an epidemiological survey in Florence. Acta Neurol Scandinav 1982;65:94–103.

73. Noseworthy JH, Rice GPA. Trichlorethylene poisoning mimicking multiple sclerosis. Can J Neurol Sci 1988;15:87–88.

74. Juntunen J, Kinnunen E, Antti-Poika M, Koskenvuo M. Multiple sclerosis and occupational exposure to chemicals: a co-twin control study of a nationwide series of twins. Br J Ind Med 1989;46:417–419.

75. Stein EC, Schiffer RB, Hall WJ, Young N. Multiple sclerosis and the workplace: report of an industry-based cluster. Neurology 1987;37:1672–1677.

76. Henzi H. Chronic methanol poisoning with the clinical and pathologic-anatomical features of multiple sclerosis. Med Hypothesis 1984;13:63–75.

77. Lauer K. Risk of multiple sclerosis in relation to industrial activities: an ecological study in four European countries. Neuroepidemiology 1989;8:38–42.

78. Gronning M, Albrektsen G, Kvale G, Moen B, Aarli JA, Nyland H. Organic solvents and multiple sclerosis: a case-control study. Acta Neurol Scand 1993;88:247–250.

79. Flodin U, Soderfeldt B, Noorlind-Bruge H, Fredriksson M, Axelson O. Multiple sclerosis, solvents and pets. Arch Neurol 1988;45:620–623.

80. Lauer K, Firnhaber W. Epidemiological investigations into multiple sclerosis in southern Hesse. III.The possible influence of occupation on the risk of disease. Acta Neurol Scand 1985;72:397–402.

81. Sourbielle BE, Martin-Mondiere C, O'Brien ME, Carydakis C, Cesao P, Degos JD. A case-control epidemiological study of MS in the Paris area with particular reference to past disease history and profession. Acta Neurol Scand 1990;82:303–310.

82. Swank RL, Lerstad O, Strom A, Backer J. Multiple sclerosis in rural Norway. Its geographic and occupational incidence in relation to nutrition. N Engl J Med 1952;246:721–728.

83. Souberbielle BE, Martin-Mondierre C, O'Brien ME, Carydakis C, Cesaro P, Degos JD. A case-control epidemiological study of MS in the Paris area with particular reference to past disease history and profession. Acta Neurol Scand 1990;82(5):303–310.

84. Clausen J. Mercury and multiple sclerosis. Acta Neurol Scand 1993;87:461–464.

85. Ingalls TH. Epidemiology, etiology and prevention of multiple sclerosis. Am J Forensic Med Pathol 1983;4:55–61.

86. Ingalls TH. Endemic clustering of multiple sclerosis in time and place. Am J Forensic Med Pathol 1986;7:3–8.

87. Ingalls TH. Clustering of multiple sclerosis in Galion, Ohio, 1982–1985. Am J Forensic Med Pathol 1989;10(3):213–215.

88. Irvine DG, Schiefer HB, Hader WJ. Geotoxicology of multiple sclerosis: the Henribourg, Saskatchewan, cluster focus. I. The water. Sci Total Environ 1989;84:45–59.

89. Shalat SL, Seltzer B, Baker EL Jr. Occupational risk factors and Alzheimer's disease: a case-control study. J Occup Med 1988;30:934–936.

90. Friedland RP. Epidemiology, education, and the ecology of Alzheimer's disease. Neurology 1993;43:246–249.
91. Dartigues JF, Gagnon M, Mazaux JM, Barberger-Gateau P, Commenges D, Letenneur L, Orgogozo JM. Occupation during life and memory performance in non-demented French elderly community residents. Neurology 1992;42:1697–1701.
92. Fratiglioni L, Ahlbom A, Viitanen M, Winblad B. Risk factors for late-onset Alzheimer's disease: a population-based case-control study. Ann Neurol 1993;33:258–266.
93. Hannisch R, Dworsky RL, Henderson BE. A search for clues to the cause of amyotrophic lateral sclerosis. Arch Neurol 1976;33:456–457.
94. Hawkes CH, Fox AJ. Motor neurone disease in leather workers. Lancet 1981;1:507.
95. Hawkes CH, Cavanaugh JB, Fox AJ. Motoneuron disease: a disorder secondary to solvent exposure? Lancet 1989;1:73–76.
96. Armon C, Kurland LT, Daube JR, O'Brien PC. Epidemiologic correlates of sporadic amyotrophic lateral sclerosis. Neurology 1991;41(7):1077–1084.
97. Chio A, Meineri P, Tribolo A, Schiffer D. Risk factors in motor neuron disease: a case-control study. Neuroepidemiology 1991;10(4):174–184.
98. Kalfakis N, Vassilopoulos D, Voumvourakis C, Ndjeveleka M, Papageorgiou C. Amyotrophic lateral sclerosis in southern Greece: an epidemiologic study. Neuroepidemiology 1991;10(4):170–173.
99. Gunnarsson LG, Lindberg G, Soderfeldt B, Axelson O. Amyotrophic lateral sclerosis in Sweden in relation to occupation. Acta Neurol Scand 1991;83(6):394–398.
100. Provinciali L, Giovagnoli AR. Antecedent events in amyotrophic lateral sclerosis: do they influence clinical onset and progression? Neuroepidemiology 1990;9(5):255–262.
101. Mitchell, JD. Heavy metals and trace elements in amyotrophic lateral sclerosis. Neurol Clinics 1987;5:43–60.
102. Campbell AMG. Calcium versenate in motor neurone disease. Lancet 1955;2:376–377.
103. Campbell AMG, Williams ER, Barltrop D. Motor neurone disease and exposure to lead. J Neurol Neurosurg Psychiatry 1970;33:877–885.
104. Currier RD, Haerer AF. Amyotrophic lateral sclerosis and metallic toxins. Arch Environ Health 1968;17:712–719.
105. Livesley B, Sissons SE. Chronic lead intoxication mimicking motor neurone disease. BMJ 1968;4:387–388.
106. Simpson JA, Seaton JA, Adams JF. Response to treatment with chelating agents of anaemia, chronic encephalopathy and myelopathy due to lead poisoning. J Neurol Neurosurg Psychiatry 1964;27:536–541.
107. Adams CR, Ziegler DK, Lin JT. Mercury intoxication simulating amyotrophic lateral sclerosis. JAMA 1983;250:642–643.
108. Barber TE. Inorganic mercury intoxication reminiscent of amyotrophic lateral sclerosis. J Occup Med 1978;20:667–669.
109. Brown IA. Chronic mercurialism: a cause of the clinical syndrome of amyotrophic lateral sclerosis. Arch Neurol Psychiatry 1954;72:674–681.
110. Conradi S, Ronnevi LO, Nise G et al. Long-time penicillamine treatment in amyotrophic lateral sclerosis with parallel determinations of lead in blood, plasma andurine. Acta Neurol Scand 1982;65:203–211.

111. House AO, Abbot RJ, Davidson DLW et al. Response to penicillamine of lead concentrations in CSF and blood of patients with motor neurone disease. BMJ 1978;2:1684.

112. Moriwaka F, Tashiro K, Doi R, Satoh H, Fukuchi Y. A clinical evaluation of the inorganic mercurialism—its pathogenic relation to amyotrophic lateral sclerosis. Rinsho Shinkeigaku-Clinical Neurology 1991;31(8):885–887.

113. Fonseca RG, Resende LAL, Silva MD, Camargo A. Chronic motor neuron disease possibly related to intoxication with organochlorine insecticides. Acta Neurol Scand 1993;88:56–58.

114. Spencer PS, Kisby GE, Ludolph AC. Slow toxins, biological markers, and long-latency neurodegenerative disease in the western Pacific region. Neurology 1991;41(Suppl 2):62–68.

115. Spencer PS, Nunn PB, Hugon J, Ludolph AC, Ross S., Roy DN, Robertson RC. Guam amyotrophic lateral sclerosis-parkinsonism-dementia linked to a plant excitant neurotoxin. Science 1987;237:517–522.

116. Duncan MW, Steele JC, Kopin IJ, Markey SP. 2-amino-3-(methylamino)-propanoic acid (BMAA) in cycad flour: an unlikely cause of amyotrophic lateral sclerosis and parkinsonism-dementia of Guam. Neurology 1990;40:767–772.

117. Plaitakis A. Glutamate dysfunction and selective motor neuron degeneration in amyotrophic lateral sclerosis: a hypothesis. Ann Neurol 1990;28:3–8.

118. Perry TL, Krieger C, Hansen S, Eisen A. Amyotrophic lateral sclerosis: amino acid levels in plasma and cerebrospinal fluid. Ann Neurol 1990;28:12–17.

119. Rothstein JD, Tsai GC, Kuncl RW, Clawson L, Cornblath DR, Drachman DB, Pestronk A, Stauch BL,Coyle JT. Abnormal excitatory amino acid metabolism in amyotrophic lateral sclerosis. Ann Neurol 1990;28:18–25.

120. Young AB. What's all the excitement about excitatory amino acids in amyotrophic lateral sclerosis? Ann Neurol 1990;28:9–11.

121. Bailey-Wilson JE, Plato CC, Elston RC, Garruto RM. Potential role of an additive genetic component in the cause of amyotrophic lateral sclerosis and parkinsonism-dementia in the western Pacific. Am J Med Genet 1993;45(1):68–76.

122. Yoshida S. Environmental factors in western Pacific foci of ALS and a possible pathogenetic role of aluminum (Al) in motor neuron degeneration. Rinsho Shinkeigaku-Clinical Neurology 1991;31(12):1310–1312.

Index